CW01521215

Rethinking
General Practice

Rethinking General Practice

DILEMMAS IN
PRIMARY MEDICAL CARE

Margot Jefferys
and Hessie Sachs

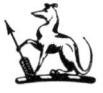

TAVISTOCK PUBLICATIONS
London and New York

First published in 1983 by
Tavistock Publications Ltd
11 New Fetter Lane, London EC4P 4EE
Published in the USA by
Tavistock Publications
in association with Methuen, Inc.
733 Third Avenue, New York, NY 10017
© 1983 Margot Jefferys and Hessie Sachs
Printed in Great Britain by
J. W. Arrowsmith Ltd, Bristol

All rights reserved. No part of this book may be reprinted or
reproduced or utilized in any form or by any electronic, mechanical or
other means, now known or hereafter invented, including photocopying
and recording, or in any information storage or retrieval system,
without permission in writing from the publishers.

British Library Cataloguing in Publication Data

Jefferys, Margot
    Rethinking general practice.
    1. Family medicine – Great Britain – Social
    aspects
    I. Title   II. Sachs, Hessie
    362.1'72'0941   R729.5.G4

    ISBN 0-422-78630-6

Library of Congress Cataloging in Publication Data

Jefferys, Margot.
    Rethinking general practice

    (Social science paperbacks)
    Bibliography: p.
    Includes index.
    1. Family medicine – Practice – Great Britain –
Addresses, essays, lectures.   2. Physicians (General
practice – Great Britain – Addresses, essays, lectures.
I. Sachs, Hessie. II. Title. III. Series. [DNLM:
1. Family practice. 2. Primary health care. WB 110
J45r]
R729.5.G4J43   1983   610.69'52   83-4962
ISBN 0-422-78630-6 (pbk.)

Contents

vi Contents

In order to save costs we have not provided a full
account of our methodology in this book. Readers who wish to know more about the methods
used, including the questions asked, or who wish
to examine and further exploit the quantitative
data sets from the patient interviews and taped
consultations should consult the Social Science
Survey Archive where these are lodged. The
address is:

> Social Science Survey Archive
> University of Essex
> Wivenhoe Park
> Colchester
> Essex CO4 35Q
> England.

Acknowledgements

The project on which this monograph is based began in May 1970 and ended in September 1982. Throughout those twelve and a half years the Department of Health and Social Security provided the financial support for it. We believe that its willingness to continue to fund the project owes much to the sympathetic support of some of its members who saw us through some difficult moments.

Mr J. B. Cornish, our link with the Department, was the first of its 'human faces' for those of us who worked on the project. He was followed by Mr Arthur Forsdick. More recently Dr Doreen Rothman was our liaison officer. In the course of so long a study it was inevitable that changes should take place in the study's design, its scope, and, even, its objectives. All three of them sought to understand our reasons for wanting to make a change, and helped us to make them.

The material we have used in this monograph is the product of the creative and investigative efforts of a considerable number of people who worked on the project for varying lengths of time. The names of those who were members of the team at some time during the project are given on page ix. It is not possible to give details of the contributions made by each member but there are some we feel we must mention individually. Peter Mansfield was the medical research officer on the project from 1970 to 1974. His vision, enthusiasm, and commitment to the project sparked off an answering enthusiasm and commitment in those who worked with him. Hilda Forman, a senior member of the team, was the person mainly responsible for liaison with the personnel in the units we were studying. The good relations between researchers and re-searched over so long a time can, to a very great extent, be attributed to her good sense, humour, sensitivity and insight. Clive

Russell, mathematician and statistician, joined the study in 1975, virtually at the end of the data collection period. He cannot, therefore, be held responsible for weaknesses in the data. We are indebted to him, however, for the systematic, rigorous, and imaginative ways in which our data were processed and examined. Jacqueline Kelly joined the team as a research officer in 1975 bringing with her a keenness to try out current social theories. She infused the team with fresh excitement. Lilian Angell was the project's administrator throughout the study and our main liaison with the Department of Health and Social Security. Janette Costello was project secretary from 1976 and, among her other duties, typed and retyped the many drafts as well as the final manuscript for this book.

In the course of the long years of the study there were times when we felt we had lost our way, were sinking in a morass of data, or, simply, could not see the wood for the trees. On two occasions when our floundering appeared to be reaching crisis proportions, we appealed to Yette Glass. She helped us to prepare the interim report which we presented in 1973 and again, in 1981–82, to select and organize the material for this book.

We want also to thank the colleagues and friends who patiently read the manuscript in draft and commented helpfully on it. Mike Bury, Ann Cartwright, Wilfrid Harding, John Horder, Doreen Rothman, and members of the staff of one of the practices we studied all performed this useful function and we are most grateful to them.

Finally, we want to thank those who allowed us to study them, the staff and patients of the practices and Family Health Clinics in our sample. But for their forbearance with our ubiquitous and sometimes, we fear, intrusive presence, there would have been no study. We hope they will derive some benefit from it.

MARGOT JEFFERYS
HESSIE SACHS

January 1983
Bedford College

Those who worked on the study at some time between 1970 and 1982

Project Director	:	Margot Jefferys
Research officers and assistants	:	Susan Barham, Lynn Bennett, Jean Betteridge, Margaret Ellwood, Hilda Forman, Anita Heller, Jacqueline Kelly, Michael Larkin, Peter Mansfield, Anne Mast, Elizabeth Mindline, Stephanie Munn, Jenny Naidoo, Clive Russell, Hessie Sachs, Betsy Thom.
Administrative and secretarial staff	:	Lilian Angell, Janette Costello, Ann Goddard, Jane Hooper, Karen Keane, Rani Saund, Deborah Vowles, Elizabeth Young.
Interviewers and coders	:	Angela Brewer, Linda Candy, Lillian Carson, Martin Coles, Barbara Cuff, Elizabeth de Keller, Mary Furness, Lilian Griffiths, Alison Halse, Ann Hickey, Brenda Laker, Oliver Merrington, Andrew Munro, Nairne Plouviez, Alison Probert, Edward Rooney, Marjorie Sachs, Donald Sassoon, Katherine Schneider, Nora Spowart, Adele Tansey, Jenny Trad, Elizabeth Verber, Elizabeth Webb, Jacqueline Wirth.
Students	:	Jean Harris, Madelon Lubin, Linda Lowe, Janice Moore, Jacqueline Rugless, Hilary Smith, Pamela Wagstaff.
Consultants	:	Yette Glass, Ray Meddis, John Reynolds, Richard Stephens.

The Cast

This is not a play. In the pages of this book we describe the opinions and activities of real people as they were given to us. However, we do not want to reveal their identities, and so we have given them fictitious names.

We have listed these fictitious names here to help the reader keep track, if necessary, of the status and location of the various *dramatis personae* mentioned in the text. The list does not include all the personnel of each unit, only those named in the text.

THE GENERAL PRACTITIONERS

The Avesbury Practice : Doctors Adams (senior partner); Adair; Alexander; Amery; Attenborough; Ashton (trainee, then, after Dr Adams retired, a partner)

The Barr Practice : Doctors Bourne (senior partner); Balfour; Barrett; Bennett; Bowen; Bridges; Binet (trainee)

The Charlton and Cox Practice : Doctors Charlton (retired in 1974); Cox

The Erickson Practice : Doctors Erickson; Edmunds (joined in 1973)

The Osmond Practice : Doctor Osmond (included in the study in 1974)

THE CONSULTANTS

Dr Stevens (psychiatrist) at the Avesbury
Dr Smythe (psychiatrist) at the Barr

Mr Stimson (obstetrician and gynaecologist) } at both practices
Dr Jones (paediatrician)

THE EMPLOYED SURGERY NURSES

Ms Anstey } at the Avesbury
Ms Abbott

Ms Bond } at the Barr
Ms Denton

THE ATTACHED DISTRICT NURSE

Ms Bligh   at the Barr

THE ATTACHED HEALTH VISITORS

Ms Almont } at the Avesbury
Ms Auden

Ms Blane
Ms Boston } at the Barr
Ms Brodie

THE ATTACHED GERIATRIC VISITOR

Ms Bulmer   at the Barr

THE ATTACHED SOCIAL WORKERS

Ms Atkin } at the Avesbury
Ms Audrey

Ms Bancroft   at the Barr

Ms Dalby   at both practices

THE EMPLOYED ADMINISTRATIVE STAFF

Ms Armstrong (practice manager) } at the Avesbury
Ms Aldiss   (secretary)

Ms Bryce   (secretary)   at the Barr

PART I

Setting the Scene

1 Introducing the Study

The concern shown by the Department of Health and Social Security (DHSS) and shared by many medical practitioners and others with the state of general practice during the late 1960s and early 1970s forms the backcloth to the research reported in this book. To those responsible for the National Health Service the continued viability of general practice was seen as essential yet precarious; essential because a strong community-based medical service seemed to offer the only hope of containing mounting health care costs which, given an Exchequer-funded service, could only be met by increasing taxation in some way; precarious because young doctors appeared to be turning away from general practice and seeking careers within hospital-based specialties to the extent that total numbers of general practitioners were declining, as, given an increase in the population, was the ratio of general practitioners to patients (DHSS 1969a: 6).

As the 1960s advanced, both the DHSS and the bodies representing general practitioners, jealous of the reputation of their members, realized, although perhaps for different reasons, that what was seen as an imbalance between hospital and general practice medicine was not likely to right itself. Purposive strategies designed to revivify a general practice sector diagnosed as ailing began to take shape (Ministry of Health 1963; Medical Practitioners' Union 1963). They were posited on the assumption that if general practice was not merely to survive but to take an increasing share of the care of those requiring medical care and attention, it was at least necessary to make it financially and professionally an attractive career choice for young doctors (*BMJ* 1960a: 487).

Naturally enough there was no unanimity about what was wrong

with general practice nor about what was required to restore it to
health, still less about what its function should be in a world where
the pattern of disease and need for medical care was demonstrably
changing (McWhinney 1964; McKeown 1965: 177; Draper 1967).
Nevertheless a kind of consensus appeared to be developing
between the DHSS on the one hand and the leaders of the general
practitioners on the other to the effect that low morale in this
health service sector and reluctance on the part of newly qualified
doctors to enter it could be attributed to a combination of
economic disincentives and professional dissatisfactions.

The economic disincentives were of two kinds. First, while those
who entered general practice early had an initial advantage over
junior hospital doctors aspiring to become consultants, the latter
could be expected to earn considerably more over a life-time if
they were successful (Royal Commission on Doctors' and Dentists' Remuneration 1960: 9). If they were not, on the other hand,
they might have to be reluctant recruits to general practice having
made the initial sacrifice in vain. Hardly a state of affairs to endear
them to a career in general practice. Second, under the pool
system of remuneration negotiated for general practitioners in the
early years of the National Health Service, they were financially
penalized for any steps they might take to improve the quality of
their premises, increase their equipment, or employ ancillary
professional or administrative support staff, in that the additional
expenditure had to come out of their own earnings, not from the
'pool' which met only *per capita* payments for registered patients
and some minimal practice allowances (*BMJ* 1963a: 134).

The professional dissatisfactions were attributed to a number of
causes. There was first the separation of general practice from the
hospital service in a world which increasingly paid tribute to the
specialist and denigrated the generalist (Moran 1960). Allied to
this was the image of general practice work as essentially trivial,
unexciting and unrewarding as compared to the work of the
specialties (Scott 1963). On top of this was the unrelieved time
commitment of the general practitioner's contract which was felt
to enslave him to his patients, especially if he was in single-handed
practice, isolated from or suspicious of nearby peers with whom he
could make satisfactory arrangements to allow him some leisure
for relaxation and opportunities for professional renewal (Eimerl
1956; Hewitt 1963).

The strategy which emerged gradually was multi-faceted. A variety of measures were taken to encourage general practitioners to work together in groups from common premises, to employ support staff, to provide facilities for local health authority health visitors, midwives, and district nurses to work from the same premises with the same patients, to use hospital-based diagnostic services directly instead of through specialists, and to refresh their professional expertise by attendance at suitable courses.

The main instrument of this strategy was the Family Doctor's Charter – a negotiated settlement reached in 1966 between the Government and the General Medical Services Committee of the British Medical Association representing the general practitioners (BMA 1965). The Charter encouraged the formation of groups of general practitioners by giving additional allowances to those who could show that they shared central premises with at least two other principals. There were secondary gains from this provision, those of ending the isolation of the doctor from his professional peers and making easier mutually advantageous arrangements for after hours and weekend coverage. The Charter gave a positive economic incentive to employ ancillary staff by enabling doctors to claim reimbursement for 70 per cent of the salary bill for such workers. It was also intended to foster continuing education by linking a scheme of seniority payments to attendance at approved courses. In the next year, following the annual review of doctors' and dentists' incomes, the general practitioners obtained a substantial increase in the initial practice allowance and in *per capita* payments, including a higher rate for registered patients over statutory retirement age (Review Body on Doctors' and Dentists' Remuneration 1966). These increases had the effect of making general practice a relatively more attractive career financially than hospital-based medicine.

The Family Doctor's Charter was not the only action taken to enhance the attraction of general practice for the potential recruit. Government reactivated the idea of the local authority Health Centre, embedded in the National Health Service Act 1946 (section 21) as a proper milieu for general practice. Local authorities were encouraged to build Health Centres in which general practitioners would be provided with good facilities at reasonable rents and in close proximity to a range of preventive and domiciliary support services (Ministry of Health 1965). Local authorities were also encouraged, where possible, to attach their health visitors, district nurses, and midwives to work with patients on the list of a general practitioner rather than with those in a specific locality (Health Services and Public Health Act 1968, sections 10 and 11). It was hoped that schemes of this kind would create an integrated health team. Within such a team there would be benefits for doctors, attached workers, and patients. The closer work associations between general practitioners and attached workers would result in a greater appreciation of their respective roles. This, in turn, it was hoped would improve the morale and job satisfaction of the staff. It also appeared to promise less likelihood of neglect of patients who could fall between the gaps of specific provisions as well as less unnecessary duplication of services with patients playing off one professional worker against another. Further, the attached workers would be able to assist the general practitioners to take a broader view of health problems, especially those of the very old and the very young, by informing them of social circumstances involved in the aetiology or the course of their condition (Jefferys 1965: 87).

During the same period the Royal College of General Practitioners had identified training as crucial in improving the self-esteem of general practitioners and the quality of their service. The College argued that so long as it was possible for any qualified medical practitioner to become a principal in general practice without further training he must necessarily appear less skilled than the specialist in other branches of medicine. To right this situation it campaigned for the establishment of regular training posts in general practice and for a qualifying examination for all new entrants. (College of General Practitioners 1956). The Report of the Royal Commission on Medical Education (1968: 118) lent support to these proposals. The Commission both emphasized the necessity for a strong general practice sector and recommended that entry into it as a principal should be comparable to entry into any other specialty as a consultant, namely by showing that a recruit had had the relevant post-qualification training experience.

RESEARCH ISSUES

While there was a general shared presumption on the part of the DHSS and the leaders of the general practitioners that, taken together, these measures would strengthen general practice, they had still to be put to the test and a number of questions answered. Would young doctors choose positively to enter general practice in sufficient numbers? Would they welcome and make use of the services of attached local authority staff? Would they employ more ancillary staff? What tasks would doctors delegate to other health workers? How would doctors react, if, for example, the nurses employed in or attached to their practices were to demand a greater share in decision-making relating to patient care and perhaps even some autonomy in their clinical work within the general practice unit? Would doctors, who had a long tradition of being independent single-handed practitioners, take to working in groups with other doctors? Indeed, would the expected professional benefits of group practice necessarily be realized? Further would such practices reduce the pressure on specialist out-patient clinics and on hospital beds? Could the relationship with hospital consultants on the one hand and the social services departments of local authorities on the other be predicted?

The list of uncertainties did not end there. What of the acceptability of the Health Centre idea to patients? Would they find it less easy to consult the doctor of their choice at a time of their own choosing? Would they resent nurses and others undertaking work once performed for them by doctors? What would their feelings be about the range and quality of the services provided in these larger and better-equipped premises? Would they bring less pressure to bear on their general practitioners to refer them to specialist out-patient clinics?

It was also not clear what effect changes in general practice structure might have on the character of the services provided. Would general practitioners become more interested in disease prevention and health promotion as a result of their closer contact with the local authority attached staff? Would they become more involved in the psycho-social aspects of their patients' problems as a way of differentiating their work from that of hospital specialists? In their turn, would patients consider these new directions as a legitimate extension of the doctor's role? Or, would general practitioners concentrate even more on the physiological aspects of disease leaving the psycho-social aspects to the health visitors, social workers, and others? And, if they did so, would they see themselves as substitutes – superior ones perhaps – for the hospital-based doctor? Would they become more self-critical, less complacent about the quality of the services they offered?

COMMISSIONING THE RESEARCH

It was the general concern with questions of this kind which presumably led the research management division of the DHSS to commission the research which is reported here. Since Health Centres built under section 21 of the National Health Service Act 1946 were to be one of the most crucial developments of the 1970s, the research division in 1969 felt that it would be useful to know what happened when two general practice units, which already had a reputation as innovators practising good-quality care, moved to a section 21 Health Centre due to be completed in the early 1970s. It was not suggested that the research should try to measure the effect of the shift to Health Centre practice on the health of the practices' patients. Apart from the problems of constructing and applying measures of physical and mental health which such an enterprise would have demanded, it was also appreciated that changes in such measures substantial enough to show up in general practice populations in the short run and which could be unequivocally attributed to changes in clinical procedures, practice location, or organizational policy were unlikely. It was, however, anticipated that there would be new initiatives made possible by the change of premises, new ways of working occasioned by larger more diverse units, and problems both envisaged and unforeseen to be overcome, and it was to these that the research was to address itself as well as to the task of assessing the response of patients and staff to the move and subsequent developments.

The local authority, whose enthusiastic medical officer of health had initiated the proposal for the planned health centre to house the two group practices and the authority's own family health clinic staff, agreed to a study as did the principals of the two group practices.

The objectives of the practices and the local authority coincided with those of the DHSS in wishing to know what the effect of the move to the Health Centre in 1972 would be on their patients and themselves. Both group practices had positive if not totally similar reasons for wanting to move. However, they also had fears for the future and they hoped that the research would alert them to changes which could be potentially dysfunctional. Both were jealous of their professional reputations and were anxious to know what criticisms patients had of various aspects of their practice arrangements. Each had concerns about the consequences of the move for some of their fundamental practice philosophies. One group, for example, feared that the move might further encourage a tendency on the part of their patients to be prepared to consult any doctor in the group rather than one in particular. The other group felt that the family atmosphere which they had experienced in their old and in most ways unsatisfactory premises might be lost when they had to share the public spaces of the Health Centre with the staff and patients of other units. So their requirements, and those of the family health clinic, included information both about the move and about their patients' more general perception of the service they rendered.

The Social Research Unit at Bedford College, which had undertaken a number of studies in the London borough in which the Health Centre was to be built, was asked to undertake the research with assistance from the Department of Medicine at University College Hospital with whom it had close working relations. (Rosenheim *et al.* 1968) and a team was recruited in 1970. Besides a willingness to try to meet the expectations of the DHSS and the units who had agreed to be studied, the research team wished to apply a sociological perspective in its analysis since there were then no previous sociological studies of general practice units or local authority family health clinics. We did not set out with any specific theory or model to apply to our observations, but our decisions on what and how to observe were loosely founded on the propositions suggested by previous studies in this country and in North America of the behaviour and attitudes of doctors, other health workers, and patients, and of people in small groups and formal organizations. We adopted from these studies those perspectives which offered us the most cogent explanations of the behaviours we observed or the attitudes we heard expressed.

The research brief which we had accepted demanded that we study the behaviour and attitudes of all those involved both before and after the Health Centre move in 1972. It seemed to us, however, to call for more than this. We felt, and our sponsors agreed, that our findings would be worth more to them and be more generalizable beyond the individual parties if these behaviours and attitudes were to be compared and contrasted over the same period with those of doctors, other health workers, and patients living and working in comparable surroundings but where no health centre move was planned. No true perfectly matched control practices, in the strict experimental sense of the word control, could be found. However, in a neighbouring, socially comparable district there were two practices, whose principals also had a reputation for good quality practice and forward thinking, which were not contemplating a Health Centre move and which were willing to allow us to study them and to give us access to their patients. One of the principals was single-handed: the other two were in partnership. The contrast in the size of these practices with those entering the Health Centre appeared to us to be of intrinsic interest and to compensate in some sense for the absence of a close match. Furthermore, a newly developed local authority family health clinic was situated close to the practices for comparison with the one destined to move to the Health Centre.

The value of studying the smaller practices was brought home to us when we examined the data obtained from patients at the end of the first phase of the enquiry. They showed distinct differences in the views of the patients registered with the single-handed practitioner and those registered elsewhere. As a consequence and with encouragement from one of the group practices we decided in the second phase of the enquiry to include another single-handed practitioner in our study. In this instance, of course, we do not have, as we do for the original four practices, data for both 1972 and 1975.

RESEARCH METHODS

The patients' perspectives

Our research objectives meant observing or questioning patients registered with the practices as well as the doctors in the practices, the other health and administrative staff employed by or attached to the practices, and those working in the Family Health Clinics.

Where patients were concerned we wished to ascertain their patterns of consultation, their expectations of the services, and their satisfaction with the ways in which these services were delivered. We were interested to discover whether differences over time or between practice units could be attributed to unit structures, procedures, or attitudes, to the type of patient commenting or, indeed, to the interaction of all these component factors. We obtained information about the patients from doctors' records, from interviews with samples of them in their own homes, and at the doctors' surgeries, and from taped recordings of their consultations with doctors.

For a number of reasons, most of them pragmatic, the sample of patients we studied in some depth was not representative of all registered patients. First, for example, we deliberately excluded children (i.e. those aged fifteen and less) on the grounds that questioning their adult guardians involved developing and testing a different set of questions. We considered our resources to be too limited to do this. Second, but only after finding that the time required to obtain good quality data from many of those aged seventy-five and over was too great, we imposed an upper age limit of seventy-four. Third, because our initial focus was intended to be on the Family Health Clinics as much as on the general practices, we chose to limit our enquiries to registered practice patients residing in the Family Health Clinics' catchment areas.

The sample of patients we eventually interviewed in their own homes was chosen in a three-stage process. In the first stage we sent a brief postal questionnaire through the practices to all their registered adult patients in the catchment areas. Their responses enabled us to categorize people rather crudely into, first, those suffering from long-term chronic conditions such as diabetes, chronic bronchitis, anxiety, or depression; second, those with disabling conditions affecting mobility such as osteo-arthritis; third, those whose health was vulnerable because they were heavy smokers, or those who were likely to use the services with some frequency for contraceptive advice or care in pregnancy and in early motherhood because they were young women in the fertile age group; and fourth, the rest.

Having done this we then drew a random sample from each category, not in proportion to the numbers in each of the categories but weighted to provide sufficient numbers in the first three categories. We monitored the use which this sample made of the services by regular inspection of the record cards held by the doctors in the four practices. In the third stage of selection we interviewed a sub-sample of this sample in their own homes before the group practices moved to the Health Centre in order to obtain their views of the services which they were then receiving. We re-interviewed all those in the sub-sample still registered with the practices and residing in the catchment areas a year after the group practices' move. These interviews were supplemented by interviews with members of the original sample not previously interviewed, that is, uncontaminated by the interview process, as well as by interviews with a sample of new arrivals, that is, patients joining the practices after the first sample was drawn. We used the same method to sample new arrivals as we had done for the original sample.

Besides their comments on the services provided by their practice and Family Health Clinic, the patients interviewed in their homes were asked to talk about their state of health as they perceived it, their belief in the efficacy of remedies, their willingness to self-treat, and about such personal details as their age, occupation, family and household composition, and proximity to kin and friends. In short, the interviews were to provide data on the patients themselves as well as on how they saw the health units.

Patients interviewed in their own homes had not necessarily been recent users of the services. We therefore supplemented our information on patients' views and experiences of the practices by interviewing a sample of current users. Patients visiting all practice surgeries during sampled sessions in the spring and autumn in the years before and after the group practices' move to the Health Centre were asked to complete a simple questionnaire. The questionnaire was in two parts: the first, put to patients before their consultation with their doctor, focused on their decision to consult and on their expectations of the consultation: the second, completed after seeing the doctor, asked what had happened during the consultation and what they felt about it.

The clinical records kept by the doctors on their patients were central to our sampling and monitoring procedures. We had therefore to ensure that all the doctors used the same conventional abbreviations and definitions on their patients' record cards. The steps we took included discussions with doctors on their current methods and experiments with new but still essentially simple forms of recording. Ultimately, agreement was reached by all the doctors concerned to use a new card for all their patients, at least for the duration of the study. Once the new card came into use we instituted spot checks to make sure that the agreed conventions were implemented. These checks were on the whole reassuring, although they revealed some under-recording, especially of home visits. We might have secured a higher level of recording if we had tagged the records of the sample of patients we had drawn. We felt, however, that this might have altered the doctors' normal clinical procedures with these patients. In the second phase of our enquiry our capacity to make checks on recording levels declined and in the end we were unable to make as much use of the records as we had intended.

The doctors' decisions to allow the research team privileged access to patients' records were not taken lightly. They and the DHSS insisted that every precaution should be taken to prevent the identification in any research results of any individual patient or the disclosure of any confidential material whether potentially damaging or not. All those engaged in abstracting from the records were made fully aware of the likely consequences of any breach of confidence and hence of the need not to comment, even casually, to anyone else on any patient data. None of the abstracted material contained names, and the identification codes which linked it back to the patients' records were separately filed under lock and key. As far as we are aware there was no breach of confidence throughout the study.

Interviewing doctors and other health workers

Information from doctors and other practice and Health Clinic staff was gained in a variety of ways including interviews, observations, short questionnaires on specific topics, and attendance at meetings. The longest and most detailed interviews were those held with the doctors. They were free-ranging and gave them an opportunity to talk not only about their work but also about themselves. The interviews with other practice and clinic staff and with consultants who conducted regular sessions in the Health Centre tended to be both more formal and shorter.

There are many ways of looking at relationships between individuals and in our lengthy interviews with doctors we asked them to examine the relationships they formed with their patients from a number of different perspectives. The perspectives themselves were those we considered likely to further our understanding of the ways in which general practitioners came to terms with their day-to-day work with their patients and with their working colleagues. We were particularly interested in how far they had been consciously influenced in their attitudes, beliefs, values, and practices by the various reports of the 1960s and 1970s from official or professional bodies which had attempted to define or lay down a blueprint for the general practitioner's role in patient care (Ministry of Health 1963; BMA 1970; DHSS 1971) or by the burgeoning social and psychological literature relating to the doctor-patient relationship (Parsons 1951; Freidson 1961; Balint 1964; Bloom 1965; Cartwright 1967; Balint *et al.* 1970; Freidson 1970). We also wanted to know whether they felt that patients' attitudes and behaviours had undergone recent changes and, if so, of what kind and from what causes. We were equally interested in how they saw their relationships with their fellow general practitioners and with the health and administrative staff with whom they were drawn into closer and closer contact.

The dialogue form of our interviews with the general practitioners, their leisurely pace, their conduct outside usual working hours and off working premises, and the use of an unobstrusive tape-recorder to make note-taking unnecessary were deliberately designed to encourage the doctors to be reflexive, to acknowledge and ruminate on difficulties or conflicts if they existed. We recognized, nevertheless, that our questions could be seen as challenging since they probed into the very core of the general practitioners' work, to their professional *raison d'être*, namely into the character of their work with those who consulted them or their relations with those who worked beside them. We often asked ourselves how many of us, in any walk of life, would be able or willing to expose our professional activities, warts and all, to the gaze of an outsider, however sympathetic and well-disposed.

For these reasons we expected some defensiveness, some anxiety on the part of the doctors to cover up self-perceived weaknesses or limitations, a tendency to present a somewhat idealized picture of their relationships with their patients or colleagues. In the event, we were more struck by their candour than by their reticence, by their self-criticisms than by their self-assertions. This perhaps should not have surprised us since those willing enough to become objects of social science research would in all probability be those most likely to seek opportunities for self-appraisal and to see research in this light rather than as a threat to self-esteem or established defences. We cannot, of course, assert that we have an uncontrived, un-doctored (*sic!*) account of their relationships with their patients or of the role they played in meeting their patients' needs. Nevertheless, we felt fairly confident that we had obtained a relatively undistorted picture of how the general practitioners viewed their work and relationships with patients and fellow workers. Our confidence was enhanced by the reception the doctors themselves gave to our draft report which they accepted as providing a reasonably accurate portrayal of their attitudes and behaviour.

Observing behaviour

Systematic direct observation was mainly undertaken at practice and clinic meetings. At least one member of the research unit was allowed to attend such meetings throughout the period of the study. The researchers took no active part in any of the proceedings but kept notes of the verbal exchanges. These records provided material on the issues discussed, on decision-making, and on inter-professional and inter-personal relationships. The reception, waiting, treatment, and patient record areas, together with the canteen and corridors of the Health Centre, made possible further direct observation. There were few such opportunities in the old premises of the group practices or in the old or new settings of the smaller general practice units which we had included for comparative purposes.

The main activity of general practice – whatever its setting – is not readily observable. The consultation between doctor and patient is a private, privileged occasion, although in recent years, because general practitioners have become involved in medical education and post-qualification training, patients may have been asked to permit the presence of a student or a trainee. In the early stages of the study we did not ask permission to observe consultations systematically, although a member of the research team who subsequently left did attend a few without the team as a whole gaining much from her experience. In the second phase of the study, however, we felt the need to make such systematic observations, and, with two exceptions, all the principals and trainees, with the consent of the patients, agreed to allow us to tape-record a sample of their consultations. This resulted in the recording of some eight hundred consultations of fifteen doctors and we selected a random tenth of them to construct a coding scheme. We then analysed the content of 215 consultations, 93 of them from the Avesbury group, 95 from the Barr group, and the remaining 28 from two of the smaller practices. We did not obtain a high inter-rater agreement on some of the more qualitative measures and the quantitative data were relatively limited. The systematic yield from this indirect observation of the core activity in general practice, therefore, was less than we had hoped for.

Nevertheless, listening to the tapes was a rewarding experience for the research team and one which helped us gain greater insight into the meaning of doctor-patient interaction. We learnt of the various ways patients present their problems to doctors and react to their suggestions, diagnoses, and directions. We were made aware of the different styles of consultative behaviour displayed by the doctors. We also heard how doctors initiated the delegation of tasks to nurses and others and how they typically took decisions to refer to hospital or to maintain responsibility for continuing care. These were valuable experiences which helped us understand the variety and complexity of the general practitioner's daily care tasks.

THE RESEARCHERS' PROBLEMS

Researchers know that any study can be even more difficult and frustrating than they had anticipated. The most carefully pre-tested designs and instruments are not immune to unpredictable factors. In longitudinal studies, the time dimension can compound the unpredictability. Our initial plans were over-ambitious. They provided for the collection of data which, in the event, through lack of resources, we were unable to obtain. Even more seriously, we had insufficient time to make full use of those data we did collect. The departure of most of the original members of the research team and their replacement by a succession of other research workers, some of them for short periods only, were also responsible for some of the difficulties which we found in carrying through our objectives and analysing our findings.

We encountered other problems – problems probably inherent in all kinds of social science research, but which had particular salience in this study. They can be characterized as issues of consent, objectivity, interference, and expectations, about which we think it fruitful to say something here.

Let us first take *consent*. Without it we could not have proceeded. In the opening phases of the study, we negotiated our access to the practices, clinics, their staff and patients with the general practitioner principals and the medical officer of health. In short, we were recognizing the authority structure of the units we were proposing to study. How far these authority figures consulted other members of the units at this stage was not clear to us. Once the project started we used unit meetings of all kinds as a means of communicating plans and securing consent for them from other members of the units. One or two complaints about lack of consultation were heard from late arrivals who had not been adequately briefed on the study. When conducting our systematic interviews we made it clear that there was no obligation on anyone to respond; but since the senior unit members had given their consent, others may have felt that they had little choice in the matter. Most displayed interest in and commitment to the study and welcomed the opportunity to express their opinions and make their assessments. There were even some who sought us out. None refused, but a few doctors and other health workers were less than enthusiastic in their participation, a reflection perhaps of our failure to overcome their initial scepticism of its utility.

Consent was also an ethical issue in the tape-recording of patients' consultations with their doctors. By custom, the medical consultation has been regarded as a privileged confidential occasion, so that doctors and researchers agreed that patient consent was required before switching on the recorder. Evidence on the tapes confirmed that this was generally obtained but that, on a few occasions, patients were either not asked, or were asked in such a way that they would have found it difficult to refuse. As far as we know only a few did not agree. Again the tacit authority of the doctor was probably responsible for there being only a small number of refusals. As researchers we were relying on it and hence confirming, if not reinforcing, that authority. Similarly, in consenting to be interviewed either at home or in the surgery – and there were few refusals, especially in the surgery – patients may have felt under some obligation to cooperate, despite our efforts to assure them that participation was entirely up to them.

These thoughts lead us logically to *objectivity* which posed particular problems in our long-term project. It is easier for researchers to maintain a degree of detachment from their subjects if they do not spend a great deal of time with them. The greater the time, the greater the likelihood that the observer will begin to see situations through the eyes of the participants with whom there is closest contact (Denzin 1970: 188). This process, in itself, is not a bad thing. The more exposure the researchers have to day-to-day experiences of their subjects the greater the opportunity for learning and understanding. The complications lie in unequal exposure to different participants and in appraising situations where there is some explicit or implicit conflict between them. Greater empathy with one party could influence both the observation and the interpretation of the facts observed.

The public generally and the medical profession in particular have an image of the sociologist as favouring the underdog, in the case of medicine, the 'powerless' patient as against the 'powerful' doctor (Backett 1976). Among some sociologists there is a contrary belief. Sociologists of medicine have been accused of seeing the consultation or the medical team through the eyes of the dominant profession under whose aegis their research has largely been carried out (Johnson 1975). In the present study we could perhaps be accused of such a bias given that we were constantly in contact with the health workers and, apart from our interviews with samples of patients, had restricted opportunities for eliciting patient opinions.

It is also true that during the course of our study some of us were more likely to discuss matters with doctors than with the other health workers in the practices and, in the course of time, to build up relationships with the former which extended beyond the limits of the research enterprise. These personal relationships could have acted as powerful inducements to explain the doctors' behaviour in their own terms. It goes without saying that doctors, like other professional workers, are apt to believe they act primarily in their clients' interests and not in their own, and a sociologist working with them may come to accept uncritically that this is so. There were others in the research team, however, who did not interact mainly, if at all, with doctors. Their links were with the other health workers. Indeed, one member of the research team, who was located first in one of the group practice premises and subsequently in the Health Centre itself, gained a reputation for neutrality and discretion and was used by many doctors and other health workers as a repository for confidences. In short, while our continued close association with the units put strains upon us which challenged our capacity to sustain our objectivity, we felt that the very variety of our relationships helped us to maintain a balance of perspective and our role as objective observers, analysts and interpreters of data.

We next turn to *interference*, to the impact of our continued presence on the people and situations we were studying. It is axiomatic in prospective behavioural research in real life situations – except in the case of 'action' research – that, as far as possible, the effects of the research enterprise itself should not be confused with the effects of the experimental innovation – in this situation the move to the Health Centre (Bulmer 1977). It followed that we did our best to be self-effacing, non-participant observers interfering as little as possible with the normal functioning of the units. We emphasize 'as little as possible' advisedly for there was no guarantee that our ubiquitous presence over a long time span, our attendance at most practice meetings during which we kept detailed notes, and our interviews with participants did not affect their behaviour.

Not surprisingly, given the length of time we were there, many changes took place in the group practices which might have been attributed, in part at least, to our presence (Mayo 1933). The doctors at the end of the study told us that our presence at meetings and our interviews with them had made them more self-conscious about their work and about their relationships with others. Furthermore, we had had in 1973 to prepare an interim report for the DHSS and did not feel, on ethical as well as on practical grounds, that we could withhold it from the practices who responded to it by examining some of their own procedures and relationships. Changes were, however, proceeding at the smaller practices where we did not have such an intense presence and we can only conclude that our research project was therefore probably only one among the many stimuli making for self-examination, re-appraisal, and change.

Organizational research also gives rise to *expectations* (Scott 1965: 261). Those who give of their time, their thoughts, and their trust want, at the very least, to know what the outcome of their efforts has been. In longitudinal research, objectives themselves may change and make fulfilment of some initial expectations impossible. In our study our own objectives were modified as time proceeded and we gained greater experience and as new members with fresh ideas joined our team. We therefore had to disappoint some of the perfectly legitimate expectations of members of the units which we were studying. Sometimes, too, expectations may not have been realistic. For example, after the appearance of our interim report some members of the group practices wanted to cast us in the role of management consultants as well as researchers, a role for which we did not have the necessary expertise. They had interpreted our findings as evidence of deficiencies in their practice arrangements and felt we should be able to recommend remedies. There was inevitably some disappointment, if not resentment, when we told them that we could not fulfil these expectations. However, some expectations we could fulfil, if not as expeditiously as the practices would have wished. For instance, we were able to give the practices some information as the research proceeded about their patient loads and the effects of modifying appointment systems.

There was, however, another more serious failure to meet the expectations which we had aroused in those we involved in the research. It became clear to us at the end of the first phase that our resources would not allow us to continue to study the developments taking place in the Family Health Clinics as well as those in the general practice units. We therefore restricted our enquiries after 1973 to the personnel and patients of the general practice units. This of course included the professional staff attached by the Area Health Authority to these units; but it was no longer possible to compare their work with that of those who had district-based assignments.

INTERPRETING THE FINDINGS: THE INFLUENCE OF
EXTRANEOUS FACTORS

Longitudinal research is more difficult than cross-sectional research, and presents more difficulties of interpretation and explanation. We have already mentioned the time dimension when referring to the move to the Health Centre and to the research design. We have to consider change, however, in an even more fundamental way.

Our research began in the early 1970s at a time marked by great social changes in Britain and in the rest of the world. It continued into a period when, if anything, the rate of change accelerated. Changes in the socio-cultural milieu inevitably affected our own perspectives and, as important, must have been major influences on the behaviour and attitudes of the doctors, other health workers, and patients we studied. In accounting for the changes we observed and in interpreting their meaning we have therefore had to bear in mind the generally shifting social, economic, and cultural climates of the 1970s, especially as they were likely to apply to those living and working in central London. Equally, we recognize that, writing in the early 1980s, what we now decide to highlight in this study of the 1970s will reflect present-day concerns and values as much as it does the concerns and values of the past decade.

This is not the place to make a detailed analysis of the social trends of the period covered by our research. It is however worth reminding readers of some of the major features of the 1970s, which must have affected the research effort itself and its subjects.

The social and economic climate of the late 1960s was still relatively buoyant and expansive. There was a manifest desire to understand social problems and a high degree of political commitment to extend public expenditure where there was evidence of social need. At the same time it was clear that the traditional social order was being questioned. The growing iconoclasm took many forms and involved many different groups. During the 1970s the demands of the young, of women, of lower status occupations, and of ethnic minorities for recognition became more strident and their criticisms of those they saw as responsible for their subordination became more outspoken (Miliband 1978). Expectations increased while economic expansion slackened and in the middle of the 1970s virtually came to a halt. All these developments cannot but have made an impact on general practice and health care in general.

Take first, for example, the question of the young. It was during the 1960s that we became aware of a social phenomenon – 'the generation gap' – manifested in a rejection by many young people of the traditional norms of deference to the authority of older people in the family and the wider society (Cohen 1973; Martin 1981). It was no longer possible for doctors to treat adolescents as though they were the property of their parents, nor could they use age as sufficient in itself to justify a demand for compliance. Younger people were also no longer so ready to accept conventional ideas about sexual relationships before, during, and after marriage. It also became more acceptable to reveal homosexual and bisexual propensities (Home Office 1967). Because doctors are inevitably involved in sexual aspects of behaviour, such changes in the behaviour and outlook of their patients could require them to reconcile their own, often more conforming, outlook with that of their less conventional patients, not necessarily an easy process.

The 1960s also saw the beginning of a new wave of feminist consciousness (Friedan 1963; Greer 1971; Mitchell 1971). An increasing number of women began not only to question their own roles but also the relationships derived from and shaped by them, including their relationships with their medical advisers. Many started to insist that they be treated with a greater degree of genuine respect as human beings and not subjected to subtle or not so subtle forms of demeaning stereotyping. Again these changes could have challenged the customary behaviours and attitudes of general practitioners, the majority of whose consulting patients were women.

A related trend which can be traced back to the 1960s has been in the relationship between people drawn from different social classes (Runciman 1966; Westergaard and Resler 1975). Working-class groups have increasingly and in many different forms challenged the legitimacy of the conventional assumption governing the conduct of their face-to-face encounters with members of other social classes. Younger workers, in particular, were often reported to be less willing to show the deference in interaction with professional people which the latter expected, especially in such situations as in the doctor's surgery.

This change in attitude among some members of one social class to those of another has also been accompanied by a rising tide of scepticism in society in general about the work of professional groups (Haug and Sussman 1971). The sapiential authority of the latter has been increasingly challenged, not least through the medium of newspapers, television, and a growing industry devoted to debunking inflated claims to superior knowledge. The tendency of some professional groups to retain their authority by mystifying rather than communicating elements of their expertise is more likely to be criticized now than formerly (Waitzkin 1979).

Another manifestation of the rejection of subordination was the growing trend amongst some health workers, who had previously accepted a lesser professional status, to review their situation and to make bids for greater recognition and autonomy at the expense of the long-established profession (Carpenter 1977).

During the late 1950s and the 1960s, too, we witnessed the arrival of immigrants from many Commonwealth countries (OPCS 1971). They brought with them their traditional cultural patterns and accustomed modes of interpersonal relationships. Their reception in the host society varied widely depending on their country of birth, their racial origin, their date of arrival, their educational, occupational, and financial position, the community they settled in, and their ability to meet the manpower needs of the country. Doctors thus encountered attitudes to and expectations of medicine which often lay outside their own experience (RCGP 1967). Opportunities for misunderstanding and for mutual non-comprehension abounded, especially with the first generation immigrants. Relationships with the children of immigrants could also be fraught with tensions; young members of black minority groups, in particular, often experienced discrimination and began to question the treatment accorded to them by the host society (Rex and Tomlinson 1979). Their relationship with doctors might be predicated on the assumption that no white doctor could fully understand illness in a black person. In the London borough in which this study was done, immigration was not new. It was an area which had received successive waves of immigrants from the middle of the last century and some of its doctors were themselves drawn from the longer established communities of migrants from Europe and Asia which still retained their identities.

Doctors are more vulnerable than most other professional people to changes of the kind we have outlined. Their vulnerability stems from the fact that they are more visible to a large number of people than most other professional people. A majority of the population visits a general practitioner at least once a year. Further because few people escape feelings of physical or even mental discomfort for any length of time, the medical profession is more likely to hold a salient position in the lives of the population than is, say the lawyer, architect, or accountant.

Our findings will therefore reflect these and other general changes in the times and in the people as well as changes in the specific activities of the units we studied. A fuller understanding of what we present will depend on a conscious awareness by the reader that these changes, as well as the relatively discrete change, the move of the group practices to the Health Centre, will have influenced what we discerned and described. To disentangle these effects as one would wish to do in a classical experimental situation is not possible.

FOCUSING THE REPORT

In the initial phases of the research, as we have stated, we had a broad, largely unfocused approach to the general field. Virtually any item of information was grist to our mill. We were not committed to a single approach or to narrow boundaries. As we proceeded, resources of time and personnel as well as the development of greater discrimination on our part limited the range of phenomena that we observed and recorded. We had to focus down and ignore aspects of the situations which we had originally intended to cover. In particular, as we have already indicated, we had had to make a decision at the end of the first phase of the study to concentrate on the general practice units at the expense of the Family Health Clinics.

Nevertheless, by the time we had called a halt to further data collection we were metaphorically drowning in the data we possessed. They presented us with a wide variety of possibilities for analysis and presentation from which we had to make a choice. What should we select? What sort of story should we tell? Who should be the prime audience to whom we should address ourselves? After much deliberation we decided, in this, our major report, to focus on the general practitioners and to tell the story with them as the centrepiece.

A first reaction may well be that to focus on general practitioners contradicts our opening non-partisan assertions, for are we not implying that the doctor's role is the one most worthy of consideration? We claim, however, that an understanding of other workers and of patients is not diminished by the choice of focus. Some focal reference point was necessary to contain the study and, within the general practice setting, the general practitioners themselves were the natural choice. Within general practice the centrality of the general practitioners cannot be denied. They are independent contractors, not employees: indeed they employ some members of the practice unit. It is on the premises which they own or rent that health service or local authority attached workers are accommodated. Only they have the right to accept or reject patients who elect to register with them for general medical services. While employed and attached nurses and health visitors are legally responsible for their own actions (Standing Medical Advisory Committee 1981: 33), the general practitioners have a continuing contractual responsibility to provide medical services to patients on their lists and have to satisfy themselves that those whom they ask to carry out any task are qualified to do so. Finally, most of those who use the service do so to consult a doctor and not the other health workers who may be associated with the general practitioner (see Chapter 16).

These indications of the general practitioners' centrality, although not the sole determinants of our decision to focus this book on them, and their place in the network of roles and relationships, were enough to reinforce our belief that our choice was the most likely to yield results of use to policy-makers and to all the participants in the primary health care services, whatever their occupational allegiances.

The contents and order of the rest of this book flow from this decision. We conclude Part I by a chapter which describes the practices as we found them at the outset of our study largely in terms of the philosophies espoused by their most prominent members. In Part II, comprising Chapters 3–11, we first examine in some detail the relationships of the general practitioners with the other occupational groups whose work intermeshed with theirs. We also look there at organizational forms and the expanding role of the general practitioner as teacher. In Part III, Chapters 12–16, we examine the information we obtained from both doctors and patients on the primary functions of the general practitioner's role.

In both Parts II and III we concentrate essentially on the views of doctors, other health workers, and patients as they gave them to us. In these chapters, although we have not always been able to resist the temptation to comment on the data from our own sociological perspective, we have deliberately tried to refrain from giving our own interpretation of the meanings which we felt could properly be attached to the views expressed by the participants. At the end of each chapter, to be sure, we do essay a brief capitulation which inevitably embodies our view of the significance which should be attached to the views and experiences of our informants. However, it is in Part IV, which contains our final chapter, that we draw the threads together and ask what can legitimately be inferred from the study, what light it throws upon the developments in general practice and primary care in the recent past, and what lessons may be learned for its future.

2 The Practices: their Structures and Philosophies

THE AREA AND THE PRACTICE PATIENTS

In order to safeguard the anonymity of the practices and their members we have given them fictitious names. The names of those associated with a particular practice start with the same letter. The cast list is given on page x. The words in quotation marks in this and subsequent chapters are taken verbatim from tape-recorded interviews or from records of meetings.

The Avesbury practice, one of the groups which moved into the Health Centre in 1973, took its name from the road in which it was initially located, in a converted house. The other group to move to the Health Centre was still known by the name of the doctor, Thomas Barr, who had founded it some eighty-five years earlier. It was located in converted commercial premises at a busy street intersection. Of the three smaller practices studied one was a partnership between Drs Charlton and Cox; but Dr Charlton retired in 1975 leaving Dr Cox single-handed. A second practice presented a change in the opposite direction. Dr Erickson was in practice on his own at the start of the study but towards the end of 1972 joined forces with Dr Edmunds to form a two-man partnership. Dr Osmond, whose practice was only studied from 1974 onwards, was at that time and remained throughout the period of our study a single-handed practitioner. In 1975 these three small practices, all located in small converted houses or shops, moved into a single house, partly rebuilt and specifically adapted for general practice purposes. While maintaining their separate practice identities, they thereby acquired group practice status with its financial advantages (DHSS 1966).

All five practices were situated fairly close to each other in a densely populated area of London. A main shopping street traversed the area from north to south. The Avesbury and Barr practices were located to the east of it, as was the Health Centre into which they subsequently moved. The smaller practices were a quarter mile to the west, both before and after their move.

The district had undergone a series of changes, resulting in a very heterogeneous population at the time of our study. Until the mid-1960s it had been a predominantly working-class area, populated by considerable numbers of public utility workers as well as by successive waves of Commonwealth immigrants, some of whom were self-employed, but many of whom worked in the garment and catering trades. During the 1960s there was a steady infiltration of predominantly young middle-class people, working in commerce or in government and other public sector agencies. As the market for private rented dwellings declined, they bought houses for owner-occupation and adapted and improved them, the process thus 'gentrifying' the area. (Glass 1964: xviii; Hannett and Williams 1979: 1). Many of them as well as of the overseas migrants were essentially transients in the area, with the result that there was a large annual turnover of patients registered with the practices. At the same time, the local authority began a long-term urban renewal programme, and during the 1970s their new blocks of flats began to replace many of the terraced and semi-detached Victorian houses which had previously characterized the area. This process developed furthest in the immediate vicinity of the smaller practices in the west of the district. Almost the whole ward in which they were situated was scheduled for redevelopment and in 1971 over half the households were local authority tenants. Gentrification and the settlement of immigrant populations, on the other hand, occurred more commonly in the east of the district in the vicinity of the group practices. In the ward surrounding those practices 28 per cent of the heads of household were born overseas compared to 19 per cent in the ward which included the smaller practices. There was about the same percentage difference in the social class composition of the household heads in the two wards, those in the group practice area being the more middle-class.

The smaller practices drew the great majority of their patients from the immediate vicinity of their practices; the two group practices had a wider geographical spread. A not inconsiderable proportion of the Avesbury group's patients came from a socially mixed area to the north: the Barr group up to 1972 had another surgery to the south-west of the area in a relatively well-to-do district. They closed it shortly after they moved to the Health Centre, and most of the patients who had used it chose to stay on their list. They, like the more distant patients of the Avesbury group, were more likely than those in close proximity to the practice to be middle-class.

Since we did not obtain a random sample of the entire registered population of each practice (see Chapter 1, p. 11), we are not able to say with certainty how far they differed from one another on many demographic criteria. Only the age and sex distribution of the registered population as a whole was available to us from age/sex registers which we helped the practices to erect and maintain. However, the samples we selected for interview and longitudinal study were chosen on the same principles for each practice; hence we believe that the similarities and differences we found among these practice samples in respect of their demographic characteristics reflect real similarities and differences in the composition of at least that part of each practice's population living within its immediate vicinity. Similarly, we obtained some limited information about the demographic characteristics of a sample of those who consulted their general practitioners in each practice in 1972; these also permit us to draw some conclusions about their similarities and differences.

Using all these data, we concluded that there were some marginal differences in the demographic composition of each practice's patient population. For example, one of the smaller practices (Drs Cox and Charlton) had rather more men registered in 1971 than did the other three. By 1974 the sex difference between this practice and the others had diminished, but the practice we only began to study in 1975 (Dr Osmond's) had an even greater proportion of males on its list. The Cox-Charlton practice had also a substantially larger proportion of patients aged sixty-five and over of both sexes than did the others, and this was reflected in the age compositions of the sample of attenders and of home interviewees. The sex composition of the home interview sample and the proportion of over sixty-five year-olds in that sample are shown in *Table 1*.

The original two smaller practices, reflecting the composition of

Table 1   *Some demographic characteristics of the four study practice samples in 1972. (Home interview sample)*

characteristic	practice			
	Avesbury	Barr	Cox	Erickson
	%	%	%	%
males	41	42	45	39
over 65s	23	24	28	21
local authority tenants	50	30	56	48
owner-occupiers	20	23	10	7
privately rented	30	47	34	45
non-manual (social class I, II and III non-manual)	50	40	23	24
leaving full-time education at 16 or less	79	75	96	94
native-born Londoners	53	46	61	68
born elsewhere in UK and Ireland	36	36	36	26
born overseas	11	18	3	6
N = 100%	(151)	(132)	(101)	(117)

the ward in which they were situated, also had more patients living in local authority property than had the Barr practice, but not the Avesbury; more in manual occupations (Office of Population Censuses and Surveys 1970); and more native-born Londoners than did both the two larger practices. They had fewer patients who had continued full-time education beyond the minimum school-leaving age. The size of the practice differences in each of these respects is shown in *Table 1*. The table also draws attention to some interesting differences in the social composition of the two group practice samples. Although each had similar proportions of social class I and II patients, the Avesbury had more individuals in routine non-manual occupations (social class III non-manual) than the Barr; the latter had fewer council housing dwellers and more individuals born outside the British Isles.

We cannot say with certainty why there were differences in the social composition of the group practices. Although situated within 200 yards of one another they probably each tapped the population of particular streets with rather different social mixes.

It is also possible that patients with particular kinds of demographic and/or personality characteristics may have been drawn to one practice rather than another.

To us, as observers, however, it was soon clear that there were certain unique features of each of the practices we studied, and it is with these that we now deal. In depicting each of the practices at the time when we first began to study them, we start with the single-handed practice and finish with the more complex structures of the two group practices. In the case of the latter we have done so largely through the eyes and the biographies of the 'old men' of the practices, to use an anthropological term, that is the senior partners. We have done so both to avoid repetition and because it was they who gave us the fullest accounts of their practices' histories and philosophies.

THE ERICKSON PRACTICE

The first solo practice in our sample was acquired by Dr Erickson in 1959. It had been in existence for at least fifty years, but by 1959 the practice list had dwindled to some 900 patients, many of them very elderly. On taking over Dr Erickson had started a maternity and baby clinic which very quickly attracted younger patients. Within three years his list had grown to 3,000. In 1970 he took a partner; but the partnership was not a success and a year later was dissolved. So, at the outset of our study Dr Erickson, then forty-six years of age, was on his own.

Dr Erickson was born and received his early education in an eastern European country, leaving it during the war, after which he started his medical education in France, completing it in the UK in 1953. He wanted to specialize but resented having to be under someone for a long period of time; so, after working in hospitals for two years and subsequently in a series of general practice assistantships, he sought and found his London practice.

Dr Erickson had always supported a nationalized health service and was not then opposed to the idea of a salaried service, although he was an articulate critic of what he called 'the bureaucratic tendencies in the National Health Service'. He attributed his resistance to such tendencies, not only in the National Health Service but in all spheres, to his own early life experiences. These had turned him against bureaucracy and radicalism, whether in politics or in life more generally, and towards a belief in liberal democracy. This, he thought, accounted in part for his desire to work autonomously and to manage and control his environment.

Despite the failure of his first partnership, Dr Erickson in 1972 was again looking for a partner because, as he said, the advantages of working alone were outweighed on balance by its disadvantages. He still maintained that, as a vocation, doctoring was intrinsically most satisfying when working alone, because it was only in solo practice that particular types of doctor-patient relationships developed. Moreover, he felt that he was not a good team man. Yet there were times when he found working alone well-nigh intolerable:

> 'In all these years that I have been in single-handed practice, I have been practically on the verge of giving up every year. While in some ways it is very satisfactory, perhaps more satisfactory than working in a partnership, it is so much more exhausting. The only way to get a second opinion is by referring a patient to a consultant at the hospital or asking a consultant for a domiciliary visit.'

Besides the secretary-receptionist whom he employed, Dr Erickson had accepted the local authority's offer of the services of a health visitor, seconded on a part-time attachment to his practice; but there was no room in his surgery premises for her to see patients there or to use it as her office.

In 1972, he was contemplating life in a group practice building as a solution to his difficulties in obtaining adequate surgery premises. Besides being cramped and inadequate in other ways, his own premises were scheduled for local authority redevelopment. That authority had asked whether he would like to practise in a Health Centre building but he had not accepted the offer. He believed that Health Centre practice would diminish his control over his practice premises and affect his relationship with his patients. He was currently negotiating with the local authority for group practice accommodation in premises to be solely leased to general practitioners with no strings attached.

Dr Erickson's early history left him a second legacy, a proficiency in a number of languages. As a result, his most important spare-time activity was translating papers from foreign language medical journals into English, which also served to keep him abreast of developments in medicine.

THE CHARLTON-COX PRACTICE

The two-man practice of Drs Charlton and Cox could trace its origin to a single-handed practice started in 1890. In 1925 it became a partnership which Dr Charlton joined in 1948. He was then fifty years old and had been in general practice in the provinces; he moved to London mainly because his wife wanted to live there. In 1952, he became the senior member and took over the house, the ground floor of which accommodated the practice's surgeries, an arrangement he described as one of necessity, not of choice. The vacancy left by the retiring partner was filled by Dr Cox, who had qualified five years earlier having served for a year in hospital posts and in a number of other 'small jobs'. Thus at the start of the study, Drs Charlton and Cox had been in partnership for twenty years; the former was in his seventies and the latter about to turn fifty.

The doctors shared the expenses and income of the practice on a fifty-fifty basis with each virtually retaining his own list. Except when one was absent or if there was an emergency, each doctor was, in the main, consulted only by the patients on his list. The main advantage of their partnership was the opportunity it gave each for some off-duty time and informal professional consultation, although they consulted each other about patients only infrequently. Basically their relationship was an uncomplicated one. They knew each other's habits and practices and were comfortable with each other, although Dr Cox instanced some small differences in approach.

The partnership shared the services of the health visitor working with Dr Erickson; but like him the partners did not think of themselves as members of a team. Dr Charlton was not opposed to Health Centre practice: he felt that 'life in ordinary practice in London was becoming impossible' and that organizational changes were long overdue. Had he been younger he would have welcomed salaried service in a local authority Health Centre. Although their present premises were inadequate, his retirement was imminent and the future location and structure of the practice was no longer his concern.

Dr Cox, on the other hand, did not think a Health Centre was the best solution to his accommodation needs. Since the building in which their practice premises was situated was scheduled for redevelopment, the partnership had been offered local authority

Health Centre accommodation. While attracted to such advantages of a local authority Health Centre as relief from the responsibility for the upkeep of surgery premises and the maintaining of domestic supplies, he did not accept the offer. He feared the consequences of loss of control over his own premises and anticipated restriction of doctor and patient rights to 'free choice'. He was not, however, as unequivocal in his opposition to Health Centre practice as was Dr Erickson. It is possible that had it not been for the latter's emphatic rejection of the proposal for a Health Centre put to both their practices – and to a third one in the redevelopment area, the Osmond practice – the partnership might have found itself in such a Health Centre. If this had happened, it would have reflected lack of strong opposition to the idea of a Health Centre rather than positive support of it. As it was, he was well pleased that his move was to be to a group practice building and not a Health Centre: it would, he felt, suit him better and be a vast improvement on the practice's present premises.

THE OSMOND PRACTICE

Dr Osmond, a single-handed practitioner, was asked to join the study in 1974 shortly after the move of the group practices to the Health Centre and the issue of the research team's interim report (see Chapter 1, p. 10). His practice premises housed only himself and a receptionist. It had a small waiting room and surgery and was in a rented converted corner shop which was also due to be demolished in the local authority's redevelopment plan.

Dr Osmond, then in his early fifties, had been in general practice for twenty-seven years. Looking back on this experience he was not sure he would choose to undergo it again. He was somewhat uncertain and ambivalent about nearly all forms of practice structure. He thought of single-handed practice, in which he had spent most of his professional life, as 'impoverished – not good from the professional point of view' and on the decline. He saw the trend as moving towards group practice and teams and commented 'as far as I'm concerned, that's OK'. Yet his one short-lived experience of a partnership had not been a success. The difficulties in dissolving it and unravelling the finances when it ultimately broke down had deterred him from entering formal partnership again.

Unlike all the other doctors in the study, with the exception of Dr Edmunds who joined Dr Erickson after the study began, Dr Osmond was not totally convinced of the value of the National Health Service. He held that it was good for politicians but not necessarily for patients or doctors since patient access to the general practitioner was now so easy that the doctor's services had been devalued. He was also apprehensive of being pressured by the Area Health Authority into accepting health workers into his practice at too fast a rate, thereby being forced to expand his practice into a team when he might not want to do so. In the meantime, he had made reciprocal arrangements with Dr Cox to cover each other's patients at night, weekends, and during holidays, and he participated with the other small practices in the local authority's health visitor and geriatric visitor attachment scheme. He had also agreed to join the small practices in renting a converted building from the local authority for group practice purposes.

THE GROUP PRACTICES

The Barr practice

The Barr practice was founded in 1887. Dr Thomas Barr began and remained in single-handed practice until 1929 when his son, Peter, joined him as an assistant. Six years later Thomas retired and Peter Barr took over. Dr James Bourne joined the practice in 1949, first as an assistant in training: in 1951 he became a partner, and in 1968, when Dr Barr retired from full-time practice, the senior partner.

Dr Bourne was born in the early 1920s and studied classics until he was called up in World War II. After the war, in which he served in the armed forces, he decided to study medicine with the intention of becoming a psychiatrist, but his experience in a psychiatric hospital convinced him that full-time psychiatric practice was not for him. Nevertheless, he retained his interest in mental illness and for a number of years was a member of one of the early Balint groups, the first of which had been established by the psychoanalyst Michael Balint (1964) to encourage and train general practitioners in 'whole person' medicine. As a consequence Dr Bourne's work was psychologically oriented at a time when such an orientation was unusual.

At the beginning of the study Dr Bourne was already convinced of the value of working in a group of general practitioners. It was the only kind of practice structure in which he had worked as a principal, for when Dr Barr had offered him a partnership, he had offered one to a doctor who had also been his assistant at the same time. By 1972, the number of partners had increased to six. For Dr Bourne group practice meant the mutual support of colleagues and, not least, the opportunity to pursue professional interests outside the practice. These last were directed to improving the professional standing of British general practice as a whole and the quality of the care it delivered.

While the practice moved purposively to group practice, its development into a primary care team composed of health workers other than general practitioners was, to some extent, haphazard. In the late 1960s the group had accepted the local authority's offer of attachment to the practice of, in turn, a midwife, a home nurse, a health visitor, and a geriatric visitor. Before their move to the Health Centre they had no practice nurse and did not really feel the need for one. In 1972, the local authority social services department, under pressure from the Avesbury group to second a social worker to work with them, agreed to place one such worker with both practices since they were shortly to share common premises. The Barr practice accepted the offer, which they had not initiated.

In short, at that time, the attitude of Dr Bourne and his partners to other health workers was that they were not essential in the general practice setting but that, if they were available, they might be able to help the doctors manage their patients' problems. Nevertheless, they did recognize that, with technical advances in medicine and the advent of the National Health Service, the comprehensive service which had come to be expected from the general practitioner could not be provided by any one person. In an interesting aside to us, Dr Bourne referred to the contrast between the work of the practice in the late 1960s and its work at the turn of the century, to which his former colleague, Dr Barr, had drawn his attention. The founder of the practice, working on his own, assisted only by his wife as receptionist, had covered an area almost identical to that covered by the group's six partners, two trainees, four receptionists and the various local authority attached workers. Yet he lived a relaxed life, mainly because at that time medicine was directed towards alleviating suffering rather than to saving life: 'People in Queen Victoria's day', he reported Dr Peter Barr, the founder's son, as saying, 'did not really believe that medical men had much more control over disease than meteorologists of our age have over the weather.'

Thus at the outset of the study the Barr practice was both a group practice and at least in embryo a primary care team. The partners, however, subscribed to relatively traditional ideas about the ordering of the practice and the team. They held that in clinical matters, that is in relation to patients, each doctor in the group was autonomous. However, in regard to administrative and organizational matters, that is to matters affecting the group as a whole, responsibility for their regulation needed to be vested in one person, the senior partner. Finally they held that because what happened to patients in general practice was always the responsibility of the doctor, the doctor was *de facto* as well as *de jure* in authority over non-medically qualified members of the practice.

Besides internal growth and development the practice had, by 1972, established many external connections. They had and made direct use of the pathology laboratories and X-ray facilities of local hospitals. Dr Bourne, and later a second practice doctor, participated in seminars on psychiatry in general practice at an independent psychiatric institute, and a member of that institute in turn attended the practice as a visiting psychiatric consultant on a weekly basis. This connection, Dr Bourne felt, was of great help to the practice members in improving their interpersonal skills and in understanding patients' needs. The practice was also a teaching outlet for the nearby Masters Hospital Medical School. In the early 1960s, Dr Barr had been appointed adviser in general practice to this school and looked after what little general practice training was given to its students. Dr Bourne subsequently took over the position, and was followed, as pressure of other work mounted, by another doctor in the Barr practice, Dr Bridges, who, in due course, became responsible for the co-ordination of the school's considerably expanded general practice teaching programme.

Perhaps most important for the standing of the practice as a whole, was Dr Bourne's connection with the Royal College of

General Practitioners, of which he was a foundation member. Through it he was involved in seeking to establish model standards of education for general practitioners and general practice as a specialty equivalent in status and regard to other medical specialties. He was also involved in the work of the World Health Organisation, representing the interests of general practitioners, and again, in particular, their training needs.

The decision of the Barr partners to move to a Health Centre was based almost entirely on their recognition of their need for better premises. They were still occupying those in which Thomas Barr had started practice eighty-six years earlier. The Health Centre would, they hoped, provide them with the setting and facilities to do better what they were already doing. They anticipated too that it would enable them more easily to accommodate the medical student teaching to which the group was committed. They did not have the fears of the effects of tenancy in a local authority building expressed by Drs Erickson and Cox, although they did have some anxieties about what the move might mean to their patients. In particular, they felt that the size of the new building and the scale of activity in it might be too reminiscent of institutionalized hospital-like settings and thus might alienate patients. There was also some concern among them about what it would be like to work alongside a practice as dynamic and forceful as they thought the Avesbury practice to be. Would they be swept up, perhaps even against their wills, in radical policies designed by that practice for the Centre as a whole?

The Avesbury practice

The Avesbury practice, established in 1953, was from its inception a radical departure from the then general pattern of general practice. It was in essence even then already a group practice and a rudimentary health care team, and it aspired to work in a comprehensive Health Centre.

When the practice began, its founding member, Dr Adams, was deeply involved in debates on the nature of post-war Britain and its health service. He saw himself as 'a political animal' committed to the radical left and his approach to medicine was a reflection of his political orientation. He came to medicine, he told us, believing it could be only part of the response to people's demands for a healthier and a better quality of life:

'Things like poverty, conditions of work, inadequate food, housing, all these things had taken me into the left-wing movement. To be concerned with politics was not contradictory to the practice of medicine. Rather for me, it was an inseparable part of it.'

Throughout his career he had remained politically active. Although a foundation member of the Royal College of General Practitioners and a long-standing member of the Royal Society of Medicine, his main medico-political allegiance was to the Medical Practitioners' Union, one of the few associations of professional workers affiliated to the Trades Union Congress.

Born just before the First World War, Dr Adams reached adulthood during the great depression. He began his working life as a social worker in the East End of London, and entered medical school in the mid-1930s, qualifying in 1943. After serving in the armed forces he returned to civilian life in 1947. He was in favour of a general practitioner salaried service, working from comprehensive Health Centres provided by funds from national or local government.

Although his major medical interest was in paediatrics he chose to become a general practitioner because he considered it to be the point at which health needs would be most readily met. He described general practice at the time as a 'cottage industry' (Brotherston 1967) comprised of small businesses, differing little from those of commercial tradesmen, and in open competition with one another. When general practitioners spoke about the opposition, he said they meant the practitioner in the next road. None of them spoke to each other. It seemed to him that they had a very bad life, working in miserable isolation, exploited and exploiting themselves for very little money, and unable to afford the basic equipment required to practise up-to-date medicine. In consequence they were not giving a good service to patients.

Despite this view of the profession the only way he could begin in general practice in the working-class area of his choice was to become a single-handed practitioner. This he did in 1948, at the same time calling on his local authority to build a Health Centre – as set out in the National Health Service Act of 1946 – in which he and others in the neighbourhood could practise. The idea of group practice as a viable alternative in the absence of a comprehensive

Health Centre was first suggested to him by a lecturer in social medicine. It appealed to him and so, as a first step, he persuaded a number of colleagues working close by to form a rota to provide off-duty coverage for their combined lists (*BMJ* 1954c: 34). Next he discussed with them the possibility of group practice. Group practice, as Dr Adams interpreted it, was significantly different from a partnership. It implied a state of mind and a commitment on the part of each doctor to act as a member of a collectivity serving all the patients on the combined lists of the doctors in the group. The essence of a group practice was that patients could expect help from *any* doctor in the group. He was aware that the corollary to such commitment by the doctors was the education and encouragement of patients to move away from what he labelled the 'bourgeois concept' of personal property embodied in the phrases 'my doctor' and 'my patient'. It was a view of a group of doctors as a corporate family doctor. Group practice for him was the antithesis of the highly individualistic practice which existed when medical services were primarily provided in the private sector of the economy.

Although, as he saw it, co-operation between general practitioners was both a desirable end in itself and a necessary prerequisite for good medical care, it was not sufficient to achieve the goals of a comprehensive community service and a satisfactory working life for its practitioners. Other forms of co-operation were needed, particularly with the hospital services and with workers in other health-related disciplines. Although group practices could afford facilities which single-handed practitioners could not, facilities such as X-ray and pathology laboratories could only be provided and economically justified at hospital level. On both practical grounds, and principle, Dr Adams wanted general practitioners to have unquestioned right of direct access to these facilities. For him, consultants' exclusive access to diagnostic equipment symbolized a hierarchical relationship which encouraged consultants to regard general practitioners as inferior doctors. Dr Adams believed too that relations between consultants and general practice would improve if consultants attended some general practice surgeries and saw how practitioners worked, but such developments were possible only in a large group practice or a Health Centre setting.

Perhaps as a result of his social work background, Dr Adams

also maintained that many patients' needs could be dealt with by someone other than a doctor, and hence he was an advocate of inter-disciplinary teamwork. He considered that doctors were brainwashed into believing that they had a special relationship with patients into which no one else might intrude, and that this attitude was an obstacle to providing good medico-social care. It was paradoxical too that many doctors who resented patients consulting them because, for instance, they were unhappy or could not find a flat, were yet reluctant to work with social workers who had some responsibility for helping with such problems. Moreover, many people needed, not the skills of a doctor or of a social worker, but the support and aid of health visitors to help them to understand how to look after their own health. If doctors worked closely with such other health workers then their élitism would go and they would pay proper respect to the skills and expertise of other workers. Nor was he convinced that a doctor was necessarily the best person to lead a primary care team. In fact, he argued that leadership should not be held by a single person. He recognized that someone had to take responsibility for ensuring continuity and consistency in the implementation of policy, but he defined this as a managerial function for which health workers had neither the training nor adequate time. It was a team secretary or manager that was required and a separation of professional and managerial functions in primary care. He felt that his view of the structure of primary health care teams, based on his egalitarian beliefs and now more generally accepted, had been regarded as revolutionary and 'shocking' in the 1950s.

Finally, Dr Adams throughout the 1950s and 1960s continued to campaign for Health Centres as places in which medical and social workers could best meet community needs. For him a Health Centre was: 'A jumping off place for involving health workers and others in the community, in the environment and for being active in changing that environment.' Dr Adams's account of the philosophies and principles which he held when he started practice as a general practitioner were given to us retrospectively in 1974 and may thus have reconstructed the reality to suggest consistency and continuity of purpose; but the early history of the practice did suggest that it had been innovative in many ways. For example, Dr Adams and two other doctors sufficiently in agreement with his views obtained surgery premises in the house of a doctor about to retire and entered into a formal partnership contract. Within a few weeks, a practice secretary/manager and a surgery nurse joined them to form a team. In the mid-1960s, two health visitors and a geriatric visitor were seconded to the practice, and in the late 1960s, as part of an experiment funded by a private trust, a social worker was attached to the group. On the termination of this funding the local authority agreed to the part-time attachment of a social worker. By 1972 the group practice had grown to number five principals with, at any one time, two trainees. Dr Adams felt that the collectivity – the organization which had grown and developed – had created the kinds of relationships he had intended. In his view, it was egalitarian and leaderless, arriving at decisions by democratic debate and consensus involving not only the doctors but all the non-medically qualified team members as well. Further, as the other members of the practice team confirmed, they experienced their relationships with one another as informal, warm, intimate, and supportive – as those of a 'family'. They had also succeeded within a year of establishing the practice in making arrangements for direct access to hospital diagnostic facilities, and in 1971 a hospital consultant psychiatrist had agreed to hold regular sessions in their practice premises.

It was not surprising, therefore, that Dr Adams and the other members of the practice believed that they had achieved many of their long-term organizational goals before their move to the Health Centre. There were at least two objectives, however, which they felt their limited accommodation had prevented them from realizing. One was their association on the scale desired with hospital consultants. They hoped that consultants in a range of other specialties would participate actively in the Health Centre once the practice had moved. The other unmet objective was 'the co-ordination and streamlining of methods of case-finding and surveillance of unmet needs'. However, they intended to have a moratorium on change for at least a year after the move. They wanted time to ease their organization into its new premises, which, they hoped, would enable them to maintain, but with greater ease, the relationship they had developed with their patients and among themselves. In fact, their major anxiety concerning the move was that sharing a canteen and communal spaces with members of other units might disrupt their highly valued close-knit 'family' type relationships.

THE SIMILARITIES AND THE DIFFERENCES

From these accounts of the practices at the start of the study certain points of similarity and contrast stand out. To take first those of similarity. All the doctors working in them enjoyed the reputation within the London area of concerned forward-looking practitioners rather than merely notional 'average' ones. They were all ready to allow a team of social scientists to scrutinize their practices. They all occupied premises which they recognized as inadequate for the type of medicine they wished to practise and had entered into negotiations to remedy the situation. They all supported the broad principles of the NHS and the place of the general practitioner in it, and they all rejected the negative self-image held by many general practitioners which inferred an inferior status for them *vis-à-vis* the hospital consultants. They subscribed to the view that general practice was a specialty in its own right.

One set of differences was that between the doctors in the group practices and those in the smaller units. While the doctors in the smaller units were not isolationists, in that they were willing to accept the proffered services of attached staff and to share accommodation, they were not prepared to become part of a large formal practice partnership, or to enter a local authority-owned Health Centre. By contrast, the group practices had come to the conclusion that their type of practice organization had considerable advantages and were willing to work from a purpose-built Health Centre. They did not appear to share the small practices' fear of the 'bureaucracy', the statutory bodies of central and local government. For the most part, they had more extensive medical interests outside their own practices and greater previous experience in the initiation of and participation in research.

There were also differences within the group and within the small practices, many of which emerged as the study progressed, but some of which we were apprised of from the start. For example, the Charlton-Cox practice was known to attract a significantly larger proportion of the local Irish-born patients than the other small practices: the Osmond practice, on the other hand, had proportionately more Cypriots. The Avesbury practice also had something of a reputation locally for radical politics, while the Barr practice had one for wishing to maintain a close, almost paternalistic relationship between doctors and patients.

In the chapters which follow we examine the relationships between the general practitioners who worked in the five practices during the 1970s as seen both through their eyes and those of the other occupational groups concerned.

PART II

Occupational Relationships and Organizational Forms

3 General Practitioners and Hospital Consultants

In Chapter 1 we referred to the evidence of widespread *malaise* among general practitioners in the 1950s and 1960s. There was also evidence that the division of responsibility for patient care between general practitioners and hospital-based consultant specialist services in the provisions of the National Health Service Act 1946 was either not functioning as it was meant to or had had some unintended and undesirable consequences (Forsyth and Logan 1968). Many health service analysts linked the two phenomena, arguing that the 1946 provisions, however well-intentioned, had had the effect of giving the public as well as both branches of the medical profession the impression that general practitioners, when compared to hospital-based consultants, were second-class doctors (Stevens 1966: 101; Cartwright 1967: 122). It was these kinds of belief which at one and the same time, it was felt, encouraged patients to ask their general practitioners to refer them excessively to specialist out-patient clinics, sapped general practitioners' confidence in their own ability to handle many problems, or soured their views of their role *vis-à-vis* the consultants. Such beliefs could also persuade consultants that they indeed had superior skills to those of the general practitioner (Titmuss 1958: 192). One consequence, it was held, was an undesirable and expensive growth in the demand for consultant services which general practitioners could not or would not hold in check. The latter, it was alleged, were likely to take the view that if the consultants had the prestige they could also have the patients (Fry 1969: 113). Increasing tension and mutual suspicion, if not hostility, between the two branches of the medical profession and the two sectors of the

NHS in which each branch was embedded appeared to follow (Goldthorpe 1963). Soured relationships, it was cogently argued, benefited neither patients, whose welfare often depended on collaboration between hospital and domiciliary-based services, nor the personnel of those services, except in so far as it allowed one or other of the services to attribute failures in care to the iniquitous indifference or inefficiency of others (*BMJ* 1963c: 453).

By the time our study began, a series of measures had been taken at national level aimed directly or indirectly at changing these dysfunctional beliefs and practices. For example, in the 1950s and throughout the 1960s, hospital authorities were adjured repeatedly to allow general practitioners direct access to their pathology laboratories and X-ray departments instead of confining the use of such facilities to their consultants. By the early 1970s most hospitals were doing so even if not all general practitioners took advantage of these facilities (*JRCGP* 1975: 3). The hospitals had also been encouraged to appoint local general practitioners as clinical assistants on a sessional basis, especially where there were difficulties in recruiting sufficient junior hospital doctors (DHSS 1969b: 14). There were of course some cynics who argued that such moves were undertaken to solve the hospitals' manpower difficulties and that it did little to salve any wounded general practitioner pride (BMA 1970: 32); but others were able to point to improved relationships between consultants and general practitioners following such arrangements (DHSS 1972a: 15). The recommendation of the Royal Commission on Medical Education in 1968 (paras 277–79) to make the teaching of general practice a compulsory part of the medical student's training may also have helped to change attitudes to that sector, at least among the hospital-based teachers in those areas where some general practitioners were drawn into the teaching programme.

GENERAL PRACTITIONER VIEWS OF THE DIVISION OF MEDICAL WORK BETWEEN HOSPITAL AND GENERAL PRACTICE MEDICINE

How did the general practitioners in our study see their own position in relation to hospital consultants? Was there any evidence that they felt themselves to be in any way inferior in status or knowledge? Were they conscious of any patient assumption that their own competence was limited, and that patients wanted to be referred to hospital for the care of conditions which the general practitioners felt themselves capable of providing for? Were they aware of any changes in the division of medical work between hospital and community?

The short answers to these questions were, first, that none of the doctors in these practices in their interviews with us were prepared to accept that their knowledge and skills were any less profound or less socially valuable than those of the hospital specialists; second, that almost without exception they felt that the division of work between themselves and hospital specialists was changing and that the direction of the change was towards an enlargement of their own role; third, that the control over the division of medical work lay more in their hands than in those of consultants or patients; and fourth, that the expansion of their role was welcomed by most of their patients. At the same time, although they all gave us many examples of the satisfactory character of their present relationship with consultants, they all, to a greater or lesser extent, were critical of some aspects of the past and present accommodation reached between general practice and the hospital sector, or of the behaviour of some consultants. We now report these findings in more detail.

'DIFFERENT BUT EQUAL'

When asked to compare their own role with that of the hospital consultant the majority of the doctors in the study concluded that they were 'different but equal'. They saw general practice as in itself a specialist branch of medicine warranting post-graduate training and qualification just as much as did the hospital-based specialties. To them, primary and secondary care services were complementary, 'two arms of the total situation with a continuous overlapping movement between them'. The differences which the general practitioners pinpointed fell roughly into three categories: work content, approach to the task, and relationships with patients.

Where the content of work was concerned they recognized a common area in that the hospital specialist was presented with problems, symptoms, and conditions which patients first brought to the general practitioner. But the general practitioner, they claimed, also dealt with problems for which there were no hospital departments, facilities, or expertise. Their image of the hospital doctor was of someone likely to concentrate on a limited range of conditions or to confine himself to the ills of particular parts of the body, while the general practitioner dealt with the whole person, that is not only with physical ills but with conditions which had no identifiable physical basis. The Health Centre doctors also argued that their spectrum included 'difficult' patients, many of whom had been given up by hospitals and other institutions: they instanced the drug addict, the drop-out, and the psychopath – 'those who were so embarrassingly at variance with everything medicine stood for'.

As far as approach was concerned the practice doctors submitted that theirs was 'holistic, problem-solving, and open-ended' in contrast to the specialist's which they saw as narrow, specific, and closed. In addition to diagnoses based either on physical or on psychological symptoms, they – more often than hospital doctors – needed to take both into account, as well as social situations. 'Ideally in general practice', one doctor reflected, 'each patient is recognized as a unique distillation of his physical, psychological, and social experiences.' This approach, they suggested, was in contrast to the 'ready-made' service provided by hospital consultants. General practice, they claimed, was tailored to the needs of each patient.

Whole person medicine in its turn required continuity of association and repeated interaction because these permitted the accumulation of personal, social, and psychological data. Such continuity was possible in general practice where patients could consult when in need and without waiting for long-delayed appointments. It was impossible in hospital-based specialisms. This continuity provided the general practitioners with one of their most important diagnostic assets, the possibility of monitoring even small changes in the health and happiness of their patients. Continuity also fostered the development of personal and friendly relationships on which trust between doctor and patient could be built.

They pictured hospital doctors, on the other hand, as having only single consultations with patients in premises likely to alienate the latter. The consultation might be longer and more detailed than that in general practice, since the specialist would not have available the accumulated knowledge based on repeated contacts, but it would also be less personal and more formal. They attributed this formality in part to the lack of continuity, in part to the more specific role of the specialist, and in part to the nature of the hospital hierarchy. One doctor instanced the awe and respect accorded specialists by nursing and junior medical staff which would very easily, he claimed, be transmitted to patients. Even if the consultant wanted to practise 'whole person' medicine he was expected to focus on those technical diagnostic and therapeutic procedures which general practitioners could not handle. It followed, in the view of some of the general practitioners, that there might paradoxically be an inverse relationship between the extent to which a doctor could respond to a patient as a total human and social being and the degree to which the patient's condition was imminently life-threatening.

So, in contrasting the role of hospital doctor and general practitioner, the doctors appeared to characterize their own service as more humane than that of the hospitals. This idealized picture of their own role and its marked contrast with that of the hospital-based specialist helped to legitimize one of their goals – the maximum containment of patient care within the practice setting. Indeed, some of them argued that primary care needed at times to protect patients from over-exposure to specialist institutions and from some interventions which could not easily be seen as promoting health (T.F. Fox 1956).

How then did the general practitioners view the present division of work between themselves and hospital doctors?

FLEXIBLE AND SHIFTING BOUNDARIES

Most of them stressed that the boundaries drawn were not static and clear-cut but individualistic, situational, and constantly changing. They argued that each general practitioner defined his own boundaries in terms of his own appreciation of the limits of his wisdom, knowledge, and competence. The combination and spread of skills, abilities, and techniques necessary to prosecute first-class medicine across the board, Dr Erickson suggested, were so enormous that nobody could possess them all. When their skills were the equal of anyone else's general practitioners were free to do what they could without seeking help; but, equally, they had to recognize limitations and areas of incompetence and seek help appropriately. Situational factors would also play a part in the boundaries drawn. For example, in London, surrounded by people with greater competence in many fields, a doctor could and should take advice more often than if he were working in the outer Hebrides. 'There', said Dr Alexander, 'I would have to feel omniscient in many fields.' Boundaries were also seen as shifting constantly in response to the interplay of many factors, including their own mood-swings and those of patients and consultants. Dr Alexander concluded:

> 'We would do more to expand our role were it not for the squeeze on the one hand by patients, who feel the need for specialist advice, and, on the other, by consultants holding on to patients for whom we could care.'

Nevertheless, the majority of the general practitioners in our study considered that their boundaries with the consultants were determined in the main by themselves and their patients rather than by the consultant, by virtue of their control over the initial decision whether or not to refer. Once a patient had been referred, however, they recognized that the consultant was in a relatively strong position to decide on patient care, and in particular on whether to retain the patient, return him to the general practitioner, or collaborate with the general practitioner in this care.

As far as their own decisions on whether or not to refer were concerned the doctors claimed, not surprisingly, that it depended usually on whether they felt they could or could not provide the help a patient needed. But they agreed that other factors were relevant. For example, some of their patients were reluctant to go to hospital, and for them they would do more in the way of investigations in the practice than they would for others with less reluctance. Other patients reacted to illness with generalized anxiety and wanted to go to hospital, and in such instances the general practitioners agreed they would often refer without doing the usual preliminary tests.

A considerable proportion of referrals, probably most, the doctors thought, were for the diagnosis of symptoms or conditions about which they were puzzled or unsure. But for their own or their patients' reassurance they frequently referred for a second opinion or for confirmation of diagnoses they had already reached.

They also referred for investigations or treatments which could be given only in hospital, either because the patient needed to be admitted for them or because equipment only available to hospital consultants was required. A referral could also be used as a psychological strategy in the constructive management of a case:

'The other day I saw a patient with a skin condition with which she is probably stuck for life. I knew it was unlikely that the hospital consultant would be able to do much more than I could, but the patient has the right to the best possible opinion and I made the referral because I thought it would be constructive in the long-term management of the patient.'

Infrequently a doctor would send a patient to hospital for tests, investigations, or second opinions because he was difficult and he, the doctor, needed a respite. Dr Adams freely admitted, however, that patients too might need a change:

'We have always held that we would not refer patients who would get better on their own or those suffering from being young, married, or old, but would soldier on. Nor would we refer those who could not improve, but sometimes, for the patient's sake as well as our own, they need to see new faces, hear new voices.'

We asked the general practitioners whether the present division of the medical task between them and the hospital-based consultants was about right or whether it should be shifted in one direction or another. Most of them were eager to do more in general practice, both by limiting referrals further and by regaining control of the referred patient's care sooner. Such job enlargement, they felt, would make the general practitioner's role more interesting and give greater job satisfaction. But there were a few doctors in our study, not confined to any one practice, who did not feel the need for such an expansion, either because it had never been their aim 'to do advanced technical medicine', or because they felt they already had enough on their plate.

Whether or not they had aspirations to enlarge the scope of their work, they all were of the opinion that, in recent years, their boundaries with hospital consultants had shifted outwards, that is, that they were containing more of the care of patients within their practices than formerly. They attributed the change on the one hand to their better access to hospital diagnostic facilities and to advances in treatment procedures which could be given on an ambulatory basis, and, on the other, to organizational changes in the practice and improved accommodation. An example of what the use of hospital X-ray and other investigative equipment meant to them was given by Dr Erickson:

'For instance, if I suspect a kidney stone I will have all the investigations done and only when I have located the stone do I refer the patient. I then put the patient on the surgeon's list and he does the operation.'

Similarly, as several doctors pointed out, the advent of new and more powerful drugs and simplified treatment techniques had made it possible for them to treat conditions which previously they had had to refer:

'We would always diagnose things like hypertension; we can treat it now. We can even treat myocardial infarctions and other things like that without referral to hospital.'

Membership of a group practice and even of a partnership was clearly seen by the doctors as a factor in reducing hospital referrals. Doctors in both group practices told us that when in doubt they would often ask a colleague to have a look at the patient, discuss the problem informally, or present it at one of their bi-weekly practice meetings when all the health workers would be present. They claimed that the scale of their practices meant a greater range of interests, knowledge, and competence on which to draw. Availability does not necessarily imply use; but at least they felt they were able, within their respective practices, mutually to support each other and pool their various expertise. In contrast, Dr Osmond, in single-handed practice, for example, said that if there was anything he felt unable to handle he would refer to a hospital consultant. Dr Erickson told us that, when on his own, he asked for domiciliary visits more frequently than since entering into partnership.

After their respective moves all the doctors believed that their new accommodation had increased their capacity to care for their patients within the practices. The treatment areas in particular were seen as enabling greater containment. Doctors in one group practice and those in the smaller practices were able to work with a practice nurse for the first time. They claimed the result was a reduction in the number of hospital referrals thus saving the casualty department a lot of work and patients a lot of time. As Dr Edmunds said:

'The nurses are doing things in the practice which otherwise wouldn't be done here. Very often a general practitioner with a busy surgery hasn't the time to dress a wound and the patient would have to go to hospital.'

Dr Bennett of the Barr practice reinforced these views with a story from her morning surgery:

'A chronic arthritic lady now needs anti-coagulants as well. She should be seen regularly at an anti-coagulant clinic for tests, but the nurses persuaded me not to send her to the clinic. They said "She can come here and have her tests done and you'll phone the hospital clinic once a week and find out what drugs to give her. She can walk here and come whenever it suits her."'

Health Centre practitioners felt that bringing consultants into the work of their practices enabled them further to extend the scope of their own work. They learnt as a result of their frequent discussions with the attached consultants. As their knowledge of the consultants' specialties increased, so did their confidence in dealing with problems which they might not otherwise have felt competent to handle. And finally, as Dr Adams put it: 'As we get older and more experienced and cynical, we refer less to consultants purely for opinions.'

All the doctors, as we have already noted, acknowledged the influence that individual patients could exercise on their decision whether or not to refer. The doctors in the Health Centre practices, however, noted that there had been a change in patient attitudes. They thought that patients were less, not more, likely than formerly to want a specialist opinion. Not very long ago, Dr Bourne said, many patients assumed they got better care in hospital and 'they let you know'. This had been hurtful. Today their patients increasingly recognized that they could frequently provide as good a service as that given in the hospitals, and consequently put less pressure on them for hospital referral. He attributed the change in part to an increasing tendency for patients to be sceptical of science. 'There has been a general turn against science', he said.

By contrast, the smaller practice doctors made no such references to their patients' attitudes and wishes. The practice differences could, however, have reflected class and other differences in their patients, the group practices having a higher proportion of younger and middle-class patients. (see Chapter 2) We draw attention in Chapters 15 and 16 to some systematic differences in attitudes of patients registered with different practices.

While the general practitioners expressed considerable self-confidence in their ability to handle a larger share of the medical work, at least some of them were conscious that many consultants were not as sanguine as they themselves were. Four of our study doctors, for example, complained that many consultants were still not aware of the level of general practitioner skills and held on to patients beyond the point at which they could be safely discharged to general practitioners with advice about their treatment. Dr Bennett stressed that it was 'essential for the comfort and welfare of patients' that hospital doctors be convinced that there were general practitioners 'able and willing' to 'follow up' patients on early discharge.

Some doctors, on the other hand, reported recent 'positive' changes in their relations with hospital consultants, especially with those in the teaching hospitals serving the neighbourhood. They attributed such changes in part to a move among many consultants towards whole person medicine. The group practice doctors also thought that their own increased involvement in the teaching of medical students had helped to improve these relationships:

> 'Since we became a teaching Health Centre I have found it easier to get a genuine consultation with a professor of surgery or medicine. It's not inherent in the building – it could have happened at the old place – but the space here makes teaching more feasible and it's the fact that we are teaching that has improved our status with the consultants.'

CONSULTANT SESSIONS IN GENERAL PRACTICE

Objectives

We have already indicated in Chapter 2 that the leaders of both the Avesbury and the Barr group practices had developed closer links with some hospital-based consultants than was common in the early 1970s, and that each separately had been able to arrange for a consultant psychiatrist to give them one session weekly during which the consultant would see patients and discuss with practice members both the handling of specific cases as well as matters of general interest. Furthermore, both group practices had felt that they wanted to extend such sessions to other specialties after their move to the Health Centre. They expected that this would be feasible because it would be worthwhile for a consultant to see patients referred by doctors from both practices and to attend joint sessions open to all the doctors, staff, and attached workers of the practice.

Group practice doctors undoubtedly considered that the attachment of consultants to their practices would extend the care they were able to offer their patients within the practices. This was so, first, because the consultants could provide an assessment service at the Health Centre instead of in the more distant hospital; and second, because, in observing the consultants at work, discussing cases with them, and having them lead discussion on topics in their field, their own knowledge and expertise would expand. As a consequence they felt that they would become more skilled, knowledgeable, and confident, and that their standing *vis-à-vis* that of the consultants would improve.

The attachments too seemed to have a symbolic significance, in the sense that they appeared likely to enhance the status of the general practitioner. Many of our study doctors were sure that they would help, first, to demonstrate the shift in the relative importance of general practice and hospital services, and second, to underline general practice's centrality in the health care system and its role as the bridge between the patient and the hospital.

They perceived other likely gains too. At a day-to-day practical level, they thought that the links forged through the attachments would facilitate communication and further mutual understanding of the administrative and organizational needs and problems of each branch of the service. They also thought that seeing consultants in the general practice setting would help transform the image of the hospital as a somewhat remote, austere, and frightening institution into a less formidable one for their patients. They expected too that consultants would benefit from the attachment. Working in general practice would provide them with greater insights into the relationship between social and environmental

factors and the condition they were dealing with. The imagery of
Dr Amery was at least vivid, even if his metaphors were a trifle
mixed. He put it this way:

> 'The consultants benefit by coming from their marble halls
> through the portcullis of the hospital into the jungle of general
> practice where they see nature in the raw, people as they really
> are.'

While expecting mainly gains from the attachment, some of the
doctors felt that there was a potential danger of the Health Centre
becoming a branch of a hospital, and that, in creating links
between their practices and the hospital, they risked a takeover.
Instead of underlining the centrality of the general practitioner's
role, the attachments might serve to displace them, turning the
Centre ultimately into a polyclinic of somewhat the same kind
as that providing ambulatory-based care services in the Soviet
Union. The danger arose because to achieve their own educational goals the doctors needed to provide 'clinical material' for
the consultants.

To resolve these conflicting requirements and to turn a potential
zero sum into a positive one, that is, to further their educational
objectives while avoiding a polyclinic model, the doctors adopted
a formula whereby two categories of patients only could be
referred to the consultants at the Centre: first, those with conditions about which consultants' views would be of interest to all the
doctors and other health workers in the practices; and second,
those who would benefit particularly from being seen initially in
the practice rather than in a hospital setting. These latter would be
patients who were extremely anxious or fearful, or, for other
reasons, resistant to going to hospital. The formula also laid down
that, whenever possible and appropriate, the referring doctor
would be present at the consultation.

Results

How, in the event, did the attachments work out from the general
practitioners' viewpoint?

Two years after the move to the Health Centre there were four
consultants holding regular sessions there. One of them, an
obstetrics and gynaecology consultant, took one of his regular
hospital sessions monthly in the Health Centre instead, during

which he saw patients from both group practice units as well as having a lunch-time meeting with the doctors and practice staff. A paediatric consultant did likewise. Each practice, however, had made its own arrangement with different consultant psychiatrists, who each held a weekly session for patients from that practice, followed or preceded by an informal lunch meeting with the practice staff.

Taking first the consultant sessions in obstetrics and gynaecology, Mr Stimson held an academic post in a teaching hospital. He kept rigorously to the agreed formula in respect of the patients he saw, which meant that it was sometimes difficult to find enough eligible patients for him to see to at the once-monthly session. His comments on individual cases at the lunch-time meetings were appreciated; but because there were comparatively few cases to consider, the meetings were normally devoted to such general topics in his field as pregnancy terminations, obstetric problems, and breast-feeding. As a result the sessions with Mr Stimson were seen as more didactically educational than those with other consultants. The general practitioners had found these educational sessions helpful in the first months of the attachment, but by the time we interviewed them some of them felt that they had begun to exhaust the topics which could be of use specifically to them. They had begun to think, therefore, that it might be useful to phase out this particular specialist attachment for a while and replace it, also for short periods, by attachments of consultants in such specialties as dermatology or physical medicine.

A shortage of eligible patients constituted no problem for the paediatric consultant, Dr Jones. The general practitioners also found it helpful that, in addition to discussing cases referred to him at the Health Centre, he would regularly inform them about those of their patients who were attending his hospital out-patient clinics or admitted to his wards. They felt that his accessibility made it easy to liaise with him when he discharged patients back to their care. One doctor felt that Dr Jones had a tendency to inform rather than consult in the lunch-time meetings and another commented that, although excellent on the organic aspects of paediatrics, he was no better than his general practitioner colleagues on the psycho-social aspects. In the majority view, however, his attachment was of great value to them and their patients. And Dr Ashton, paying him the greatest possible compliment, suggested he had all the qualities of a 'splendid general practitioner'.

The relationships which developed over time with the consultant psychiatrists, Dr Smythe and Dr Stevens, were more complex. Mental illness and emotional disturbance in all their variety were so frequently the essence of the problem with which patients presented that there was a constant need for further understanding. There was also an understandable desire to 'off-load a difficult patient, even if for just a little while'. The attachment of consultant psychiatrists helped to meet these twin but sometimes conflicting needs.

The potential conflict between these twin needs was expressed by some doctors at the Barr practice. All the doctors at this practice had emphasized the value to them of the reassurance their consultant was able to give them that they had done all that could be done. As Dr Bourne said:

> 'Smythe is very experienced. He has been through the thick of things so that when he says "There is nothing more you can do, I couldn't do better," he understands so well how we feel and assists us to resolve our feelings of helplessness and hopelessness.'

Dr Barrett referred to his usefulness as a 'resource-man', his extensive knowledge of appropriate places to which patients might be referred. And Dr Bennett said, 'Often we find we can manage a problem after he has given us fresh insight.' But three of them were less happy with what Dr Smythe termed his 'truly consultative role' than with the assessment service he provided. They acknowledged that sometimes, even when he offered them very good ideas on how to cope with a patient, they might not want to hear them. In short, they were suggesting that at times what they really wanted was temporary respite from difficult patients rather than advice on how to deal with them.

No Avesbury doctor expressed criticism of Dr Stevens, the psychiatrist attached to that practice, nor of the kind of service she provided; they all felt she had increased their capacity to deal with psychiatric problems. As Dr Adams put it:

> 'She has been a great help and support especially when I have felt I might be out of my depth. I've either asked her to see the patient or discussed the patient with her and usually she has just

reassured me: "This is to be expected" or "You're doing OK."
But sometimes she hasn't, she has said "For God's sake admit
him" or "Get someone else to see him" or "I'll see him".'

In general, then, the general practitioners considered that they
had certainly obtained the educational advantages for which they
had hoped from consultant attachments:

'It's an ongoing learning experience for ourselves and the
students who are about. We are kept up-to-date with new
developments and methods. We also find out where the gaps in
our diagnosis and management are.'

Equally, to the degree that the attachments provided assessment
services, these too had met the general practitioners' needs:

'The knowledge that there are other sources of advice and
support and people to whom one can say: "Am I doing it right?
Is this the right approach? Is there another agency which I could
or should approach, or can I handle it with or without support in
the practice?" All this can be answered by the attachments.'

All but one of the doctors believed that their practices' referral
rates to hospitals or other external agencies had decreased as a
result of their increased knowledge, confidence, and, consequently, greater ability to care for patients within their practices. As Dr
Bennett put it:

'Having consultants come to the Centre is very valuable and
special and has built up our confidence to deal with problems
ourselves.'

Dr Alexander spelt out how the attachments had helped to
produce this end:

'Being able to talk face-to-face with people I have come to know
and trust and to whom I have easy access has made it possible
for me to continue holding and supporting patients I would
otherwise have had to refer to a hospital clinic.'

Turning to their other objectives, they considered that the
attachments had succeeded in improving communication between
the practices and the teaching hospital and that this gain, together
with the others already discussed, had improved their service to
their patients. They believed too that there had been direct gains

for their patients from seeing a consultant on their premises: 'It makes them feel very comfortable.' They were less sure how much the consultants had learnt from their exposure to general practice. 'Not an awful lot,' guessed Dr Adair, adding: 'We don't keep the academically interesting accounts.' Indeed, three of the twelve doctors thought there was little that general practitioners could teach consultants, and at least five others felt that the consultants had perhaps failed to use their opportunities to learn as much as they could from general practice. Others considered that at least one consultant had gained in knowledge and understanding as a result of this attachment, but interestingly each had a different consultant in mind.

CONSULTANTS' VIEWS OF THEIR GENERAL PRACTICE ATTACHMENTS

Like the general practitioners the four consultants saw the purposes of the attachment schemes as educational, as an assessment service for selected patients, and as a way of strengthening links and improving communication between the general practices and the hospital.

When we interviewed them both Mr Stimson, obstetrics and gynaecology, and Dr Jones, paediatrics, felt it important for consultants to know how general practitioners worked and equally for general practitioners to understand consultants. Mr Stimson believed that good personal relations with general practice had been relatively easy to achieve in the north of England, where he had once worked, but more difficult in London. Dr Jones used a medical metaphor to express his goals. Attachment for him was a way of 'detoxifying' the relationship between consultants and general practitioners, since, to his amazement, even experienced general practitioners manifested awkwardness when dealing with hospital consultants. The two kinds of doctors needed to rediscover each other as fellow citizens instead of regarding each other as foreigners.

Besides a belief that better relations between the two branches of medicine meant better medicine for patients, both Dr Jones and Mr Stimson admitted to a degree of self-interest in the attachment. The former did not doubt that he was motivated to some extent by a desire to 'nobble' patients at the Health Centre for his own hospital rather than have them go to alternative rival hospitals:

> 'Its not elegant or attractive, but a fact of life in London that if one hospital doesn't get the Centre patients the others will, and I don't want my department closed down. So it's important I satisfy the practices with the services I provide.'

Mr Stimson made the same point. His attachment was in part at least a public relations exercise – 'empire building' he called it – to ensure that demand for the services of his obstetrics and gynaecological unit remained at a high enough level to ensure its viability.

'Empire building' was not a requirement for the consultant psychiatrists. Their problem was how to cope with the growing demand for psychiatric services. Dr Smythe favoured attachments because he was convinced that the future of psychiatry lay not so much in hospitals and other specialist psychiatric units as in the community. He felt that many patients were unwilling to accept referral to a psychiatrist at a 'madhouse', but were prepared to see one in the general practice setting. There too the general practitioner gained by greater involvement in the psychiatric care of those patients referred to a consultant and were less likely to feel they had dispatched their patients elsewhere. The psychiatrist also gained because it made the work more interesting:

> 'It extended my work enormously. After all, 95 per cent of overt psychiatric illness in general practice remains under the sole care of the general practitioner, and a psychiatrist sees only 5 per cent of declared psychiatric illness. So when he sits in his clinic he really has a very, very tip of the iceberg view.'

Dr Smythe was keen that his attachment should not simply mean a transfer of his consulting room from his institute to the Health Centre. He saw his main function as being a resource to general practitioners not only in the transmission of psychiatric knowledge and expertise but also in helping them to gain insight into their own behaviour. For this reason, in addition to seeing patients, at least half his time at the Barr practice was set aside for consultations with individual members of practice staff, including doctors, nurses, social workers, and receptionists. He saw this as a means of helping the health workers directly, and their patients indirectly. He explained the process as follows:

'Why are patients referred from general practice to a clinic? Crudely, there are two reasons: one is because it is felt that the clinic can provide something the practice can't. Perhaps 50 per cent of referrals are for that reason. But the other 50 per cent are made because of some problem in the doctor/patient relationship. The doctor feels the time has come for him to obtain extra support, particularly if he is dealing with a patient who acts and talks in a way which leaves the doctor feeling anxious, confused, angry, or helpless.'

It was in these latter kinds of referrals that things so often went wrong:

'The patient gets to the clinic and the psychiatrist feels he has nothing to offer, precisely because he has missed the cue that the problem arises from the patient's relationship with the referring doctor. So he writes a lengthy learned report to the GP about the patient's background and symptoms, all of which the general practitioner probably knew better anyway – and this helps nobody.'

If, however, the framework existed in which the general practitioner could simply say to the psychiatrist, 'This patient makes me feel utterly helpless,' the former could be helped to deal with the feelings the patient aroused in him and, as a result, provide better care.

All the consultants told us that they enjoyed working with the practices very much and felt that the experience had been fruitful, but the reasons they gave for assessing it as a 'success' were various. For example, Mr Stimson mentioned that his efforts with the biggest practices in his hospital catchment area had 'paid off' in that his unit, unlike many others in London, remained viable. Dr Jones said his 'modest undertaking' had achieved 'a modest success' and, like Mr Stimson, thought it had helped his department to capture a sizeable proportion of patients who might otherwise have been dispersed to other hospitals. Dr Smythe said he had been able to do what he set out to do, that is to help general practitioners support difficult patients. Dr Stevens, in a rushed interview on the eve of her departure for Australia, said she thought her attachment had been interesting and worthwhile.

They were all of the opinion, however, that part of the success was due to the fact that they were working with 'above average' practices. In Mr Stimson's words, 'You're dealing with extremely good doctors'; and Dr Jones described the practices as providing 'good parenting', giving the support and sustenance needed by parents and children alike:

> 'The treatment of organic illness could be done just as well at a faceless casualty department. It's the extra these general practitioners give in the shape of personal care.'

Dr Smythe considered that in general the Barr doctors were highly sophisticated, alert to psychological undercurrents in their patients' problems and having a great deal of insight and psychiatric experience. He commented too on the high quality of the work performed by the health and social workers at the practice, their sensitivity to psycho-social strain or pathology in their patients, and their detailed knowledge of the social and economic circumstances of families. Similarly, Dr Stevens thought the doctors and other health workers in the Avesbury practice were very experienced and sustained a higher proportion of patients who were psychologically sick and bizarre than had anyone else with whom she had worked. She thought they were extremely good at finding out what was really wrong with the patient who presented with a different symptom each week:

> 'This isn't something they've acquired by book knowledge or seminars, but purely by experience; and they handle their patients' problems very well. But the moment these problems are given psychological labels, they begin to get worried and doubt their capabilities.'

All four consultants felt that it was difficult to judge how much the general practitioners had learnt from them in terms of knowledge and skills. Dr Smythe's assessment of his attachment in terms of this measure was perhaps the most positive of the four: he thought the Barr doctors had increased their capacity to contain the care of their disturbed and difficult patients. 'We are reducing the export of patients to specialists.' He gave as an example a very distressed patient whose doctor feared she might attempt suicide. Although the latter thought she should receive specialist treatment he was afraid she might see the referral as a declaration that he could no longer help her. Dr Smythe in commenting on the relationship said:

'It seemed to me they had got stuck. The girl was trapped in a situation in which she felt she could no longer cope and the doctor was grappling with apprehensive feelings she had stirred up in him. We talked it over and he decided to carry on. A few weeks later he reported improvement in their relationship. He had been able to help her bring out her despair and give her the experience that there was somebody who really understood the intensity of her feelings and could tolerate them. Gradually she talked her feelings out so it was an enormous relief to the doctor that he had been able to do this.'

He thought too that for this doctor the experience of being supported in this difficult task would have a 'ripple effect', and that the doctor would feel more confident the next time he faced similar problems.

Dr Jones thought he had been able to educate the general practitioners in some technical aspects of paediatrics. He added modestly, however, that there were not many areas in which his technical knowledge was superior to theirs. Answering our question, Mr Stimson jokingly said that at least he had taught them how to make proper use of some of the Health Centre's facilities:

'I'd say to them, "Have you looked at this vaginal discharge?", something they dealt with frequently in general practice, and generally they hadn't. So I'd lead them by the nose to their microscope in the back room and we'd look at discharges. No special skills were required to make the diagnosis right away.'

Dr Stevens had neither seen her function at the Avesbury practice as a proselytizing one, nor as one of interpreting for the doctors what they were 'doing to each other'. Because the doctors and other workers had been together for a long time and worked well together, she deliberately 'soft-pedalled on them'; she saw no gain in disturbing their relationship. In any event, the doctors had made it clear to her that they did not want their own behaviour analyzed. They had said, 'You're not going to do a "Balint" on us,' and 'We don't want any of that analytic mumbo-jumbo,' even though they knew she was a psychoanalyst. On a few occasions, she had introduced at their request discussions of specific topics, such as depression:

'They sometimes wanted more formal things in order to feel

there really was "the answer" that came from the psychiatrist, and if only you did it, it was all right.'

Like Drs Smythe and Jones she rated the reassurance she frequently gave as at least as important as the transmission of knowledge.

Dr Jones was the only one of the four consultants to mention his attachment in terms of what he had learnt from it about how and with what symptoms patients tended to present, and the ways in which the practitioners had responded. Practice doctors, he found, placed greater emphasis than hospital consultants on what the patient wanted and less on reaching a diagnosis. He concluded that 'in general practice the style is all important'. He liked this approach when sensibly and cautiously used; it worked well with patients who would get better anyway and also with those with terminal illness, but it could 'fudge the issues on the rather uncommon border where specific treatments were essential for recovery'.

The four consultants felt that the assessment aspect of the attachment had worked well, 'breaking the ice for patients requiring hospital attention but afraid to go there'. Dr Stevens, for example, explained that what she and the Avesbury doctors had achieved was:

'To make it easy for someone to be seen fairly quickly without having to go through the rigmarole of going to a clinic that's called psychiatric; so that people could be picked up fairly quickly and dealt with promptly in the hope of averting more serious pathology or more prolonged treatment.'

Mr Stimson had found it easier to provide an assessment service at the Health Centre than at the hospital, at least for the selected patients. They were more relaxed than they would have been at the hospital where there was always a crowded waiting room. Dealing with fewer patients at each session made it possible for him to say, 'Tell me all about it,' whereas at the hospital he would frequently consciously decide not to encourage information from a patient which he would not be able to follow through. This was not, however, Dr Jones's experience. He saw new patients for about forty minutes each at the hospital, but at the Health Centre they were booked in at twenty-minute intervals. Furthermore, he rarely saw a patient with a referring doctor or health visitor, although this had been one of the intentions of the attachment. Had it not been for the discussion at meetings, he would have learned little more than at the hospital about patients' personal or social circumstances. 'To my regret,' he said, 'ultimately, as with referrals to me at hospital, I am left carrying the can.'

The three consultants who had teaching hospital appointments thought their attachments had helped to improve communications between their departments generally and the Health Centre practices, and hence to reduce referrals. The consultants also felt that when things happened at the hospital which disturbed the general practitioners, they had been able to clear the air and diffuse resentment. There was yet another 'spin-off' from the attachment according to Mr Stimson. The informal colleague relationship he had developed with general practitioners served as a model for trainees and students who would see him in the general practice setting.

THE RESEARCH TEAM'S ASSESSMENT

In reviewing the several major strands affecting the general practitioners' views on their place in the division of medical tasks, we concluded that, in general, the group practice doctors exuded confidence about the place of general practice in the Health Service, both in the present and for the future. This confidence was already great before the move to the Health Centre or enlarged practice premises: the moves enhanced it further. Our study doctors did not consider or act as though the Health Service, of which they were a part, was hospital-centred. They looked upon the hospital as a resource available to them in the provision of care to their patients. They were aware that there were many consultants who did not share their views, but believed that in time they would come to do so.

Within this broad consensus, however, there were some individual differences in attitudes. In each practice there were general practitioners actively concerned with enlarging general practice territory still more and with enhancing its status, while others appeared less ambitious in both these respects. The former were more likely to see hospitals as institutions against which to protect their patients; the latter as positive resources which could give as much to patients as they themselves could.

With one exception, the smaller practice doctors did not want to shift their role boundaries outwards by extending their work into areas previously dealt with by consultants. They appeared less committed than group practice doctors to the principle of patient containment in the practice setting, and less involved in exploring ways of enlarging their role. What they were currently doing absorbed their time and energy. Among them there was an element of resignation, a tendency to be less sure of their worth in the eyes of the public and of their status *vis-à-vis* consultants than were their peers in the group practices. They were more prone to show that they were not altogether happy with a role which they felt gave them less recognition and esteem than the consultant. Only one was fully positive and confident of his own worth.

Consultant sessions conducted regularly in the Health Centre, but not in the premises occupied by the smaller practice units, may have helped to reinforce the differences we observed between the group and other general practitioners in this regard. The attachments had laid down and strengthened the groups' channels of communication with hospital departments. They had enabled the general practitioners to obtain some respite from difficult cases without abandoning them by permanent off-loading. They had facilitated learning from consultants and hence increased self-confidence. Some of the muted fears expressed earlier by some of the group practitioners that the sessions could lead to greater subservience to the specialist had not in their later view materialized. The group practitioners emerged after two or three years' experience of attachments with their views of an expanding and central place for general practice in groups and in Health Centres confirmed, and with their belief in the equality of status and the social worth of their own roles reinforced.

We should note, however, that the limited evidence we have of the extent to which the doctors in the different practices actually referred patients to out-patient departments, before and after the move to the Health Centre, does not seem to support their claim to greater containment of patient care within practices. Comparing, for example, the attenders' reports of whether or not their doctors had or were intending to refer them to a hospital out-patient department, we found that in 1972 Avesbury patients were more likely to be referred than those of the other three practices (see *Table 2*). By 1975, the Avesbury referrals had fallen into line with those of the rest; but there was no indication that the group practices differed at all from the smaller ones. Moreover, only the Avesbury use of the hospitals for these purposes seems to have diminished.

Table 2   *Percentage of attenders referred by their general practitioners to hospital out-patient clinics after their general practice consultation 1972 and 1975*

practice	1972		1975	
	%	N = 100%	%	N = 100%
Avesbury	15	(272)	9	(269)
Barr	9	(306)	8	(283)
Cox	10	(134)	9	(86)
Erickson	10	(140)	12	(191)

We were also able to obtain from our home interviewees an idea of how frequently in the twelve months before both the 1972 and 1975 interviews patients had been to hospital on their own initiative, that is, without first consulting their general practitioner (see *Table 3*). Most of such visits were for what the patients called emergencies and were probably therefore to the accident and emergency departments. Once again, the rates for each practice do not provide a clear picture of differentiation between different sizes of practice. In 1972, it was the Barr practice patients who had

Table 3   *Percentage of home interviewees reporting visiting a hospital in a twelve month period in 1972 and 1975 on their own initiative as an emergency or otherwise*

practice	1972		1975	
	%	N = 100%	%	N = 100%
Avesbury	6	(151)	15	(118)
Barr	17	(132)	14	(111)
Cox	12	(102)	10	(71)
Erickson	6	(118)	9	(171)
Osmond	–		(1)*	(35)

* Number too small to percentage.

taken themselves off to hospital more commonly than the rest. In 1975, these patients resembled those from the Avesbury group whose rate had surprisingly doubled. In that year both the larger groups had apparently more patients using the hospital services on their own initiative than did the smaller practices. We feel that these figures illustrate well the need to exercise caution in drawing conclusions purely from the accounts which any set of individuals may give of their patients' patterns of utilization.

The responses of the four consultants most intimately involved with the group practices to our questions about the attachments did not basically challenge the group practitioners' views. They were willing to concede that these general practitioners could and should expand the part they played in the division of medical care and were willing to assist them in doing so. They were not uncritical of every aspect of the general practice they observed; but, by and large, they expressed admiration for the skills they saw demonstrated by the general practitioners and their attached and employed health workers, and tended to assume that these were unusual. Finally, it should be noted that one of their own reasons for being prepared to conduct sessions in the Health Centre was a recognition that, at a time when hospitals in central London were seen to be competing with each other for a diminishing number of patients, and hence of resources, they needed the goodwill of standard-setting general practitioners.

4 Principals as Partners and Colleagues

In describing the philosophies of the doctors who led the practices we studied, we showed in Chapter 2 how their past experiences of and attitudes to the practice of medicine had helped or not helped to orient them to the idea of forming partnerships with other doctors. In later chapters we deal with the relationships between doctors and other health workers employed or attached to their practices, with the doctors' relationships with their patients, and with the functioning of the practices as organic work units. In this chapter we confine ourselves to an examination of the relationships which existed between partners within the study practices, and of those which developed between doctors in the separate practices which came together after the moves to the Health Centre and the group practice centre.

The foci for this chapter were chosen because we were aware that as the exhortations to general practitioners to form groups and enlarge partnerships grew in the 1960s and early 1970s, some practitioners who were held in high regard by their peers had begun to question what they saw as the new but untested conventional wisdom (Barber 1974; Hopkins 1974; Sowerby 1974). They suggested that there were dysfunctional aspects of group practice, for both doctors and patients, serious enough to merit a cautious approach to either practice enlargement or the sharing of common premises by separate practices. Some of their reservations related to the idea of the multi-disciplinary primary health care team located in general practice, and it is not with those aspects of the work setting that this chapter is concerned; but it was also hinted that not all partnerships were happy liaisons, that conflicts could and did arise between doctors over issues affecting practice policy and organization. Moreover, it was clear that relationships between partners could be of very different kinds, varying from the close and equal on the one hand to the formal and unequal on the other. We did not, however, take it upon ourselves to consider or discuss the business arrangements which the general practitioners in the partnerships made amongst themselves; nor did we ask them about the financial rewards of the work or about their relationships with the Local Executive Committee (later Family Practitioner Committee) through whom they made their contracts to enrol patients and from whom they received their *per capita* payments and other income. We did not do so first because this was not part of the brief we had received from the DHSS or the practitioners themselves, but second, while recognizing the potential interest of the financial arrangements, we had enough to enquire into without raising such matters ourselves. Furthermore, rightly or wrongly, we did not think that the business arrangements the practices made were likely to be a major bone of contention or determinant of their professional practices or relationships. It is with issues of this last kind that we now deal.

THE FRUITS OF ASSOCIATION

Colleaguely cover

All the general practitioners in our study held that there were benefits to be gained from some form of co-operation with other general practitioners and in particular from sharing practice premises. They drew attention in their replies to our questions to the kinds of advantages for them which official and professional reports had predicted would accrue from group practice (Ministry of Health 1954: 17; 1963: 115; DHSS 1971).

For example, whether they were members of the two large group practices which entered the Health Centre or members of the smaller practices which from 1974 together occupied common practice premises, all the doctors mentioned such advantages of their situation as the relative ease of colleaguely cover. This enabled them, they felt, to have more care-free leisure as well as opportunities for extra-practice activities while meeting their contractual obligations to patients. 'Now every alternate week-end

is a mini-holiday', as Dr Erickson put it after forming his partnership with Dr Edmunds.

It was nevertheless clear that the doctors differed in what they
thought colleagues could and should do for each other by way of
cover. The Avesbury and Barr practice doctors both wanted more
legitimated time away from their practice commitments, and felt
more strongly that this should be achieved totally by colleaguely
co-operation than did the doctors at the smaller practices. The
latter all made use of commercial services for late night calls, an
arrangement which Dr Erickson felt was 'perfectly reasonable and
the best of both worlds'. The two solo practitioners used these
services most extensively but after their move to shared premises
provided cover for each other until 11 p.m. at night on alternate
weekdays. It seems that we have here an example of the way in
which individuals both trim their expectations to their current
situations and strive to justify their procedures by reference to its
ethical basis. Evidence has begun to accumulate, however, to
suggest that commercial deputizing services are less acceptable to
patients than those based on voluntary rotas of practice partners or
neighbouring doctors (Cartwright and Anderson 1981: 38).

Load sharing

Another advantage of shared premises to which all the doctors
drew attention was the possibility of equalizing patient loads.
Within the group practices this was formally achieved by operating
appointment systems, supplemented by a duty doctor arrangement
whereby each doctor in turn was available to see patients who
arrived without appointments and who, it was felt, should not be
turned away. Their systems had not evolved without some conflict
and were recognized as having their problems, one of which could
be the creation of tension between doctors. When under pressure,
it was not altogether surprising that the pace of work or the poor
time-keeping of a colleague could be held to be the main and
remediable cause. Remedies were often sought through collective
discussion at practice meetings for deficiencies which were tactful-
ly raised, often by receptionists as those who had to bear the main
brunt of patient discontent with long waits; but it was the view of
the research observers at these meetings that the civilized discussions of cause and remedy often concealed latent criticism if not
condemnation of a principal's behaviour. At the Avesbury, in

particular, some doctors felt that some of their number tried to avoid a fair share of the work and particularly of the home visits. They called it, in fact, 'the Avesbury disease' and felt it was growing, perhaps because, as one partner maintained, 'We are older and running out of steam.'

In the smaller practices, there were no appointment systems. After their move to common premises, however, an informal system of equalizing patient loads developed. If at the end of a morning or evening surgery there were still patients waiting for one of their colleagues, the others were willing to see them, provided of course the patients themselves were happy. To ensure that such an informal arrangement did not lead to 'patient pinching', however, the doctors all agreed that they would not take on to their own lists, patients registered with another doctor in the premises. All the doctors assured us that, backed by this agreement, the informal arrangement had enabled some general load sharing without creating organizational problems or personal tension.

What did appear to distinguish the doctors' relationships with each other in the groups from those in the smaller practices was the ability of the former to off-load on a temporary or permanent basis the medical care of patients they found either emotionally tiring or professionally baffling. We deal more fully with this issue in our later chapter on doctor-patient relationships (Chapter 14). Here we want merely to make the point that sharing patients, on the initiative of either doctors or of patients who showed a preference for one doctor rather than another, did not appear to arouse feelings of jealousy amongst most of the doctors. It may of course be that the doctors were well protected by their training and experience from showing any signs of such frailty, but if it were merely a sophisticated cover-up, we would have expected it to apply too to expressions of professional or personal inadequacy. We found no reluctance on their part, however, to acknowledge the superiority of others in either knowledge of particular areas of medicine or in capacity to tolerate patients with certain kinds of problems or personalities.

We felt it possible to deduce, therefore, that group practice of the kind we observed allowed practitioners genuine scope for developing colleaguely, non-competitive relationships in the personal care of patients to an extent which was not possible in either solo or small partnership practices within shared premises. It also permitted what was denied to the doctors in solo practice, the ability to develop some degree of specialized interest in their work. The two-man partnership of Dr Erickson and Dr Edmunds had been able, however, to evolve a limited range of special interests. Dr Erickson ran the practice's well-baby clinic, and Dr Edmunds, by virtue of his clinical assistantship in a hospital otorhinolaryngology (ENT) department, was seen by his partner as a useful man to consult when he was puzzled by ear, nose, or throat problems.

Pooling resources

Doctors in the smaller practices, in explaining their reluctance to work in a partnership at all or in one of more than two members, foresaw the possibility of conflict with partners on financial matters and of disputes about such aspects of practice organization as the employment of support staff and the purchase of furniture and diagnostic equipment. It was from a sense of necessity rather than choice that they decided, on the initiative of Dr Erickson, to share premises with each other when redevelopment of the streets in which their old premises were situated made a move of some kind essential for all of them.

In the event their common occupation of a practice building inevitably involved them in the need to consult with one another on many matters and in decisions to pool resources to meet some expenditures. For example, they jointly employed a married couple as resident caretakers and contributed to a common fund from which supplies of such domestic items as towels and toilet paper were met. They met monthly to discuss the management of the building and evolved an arrangement whereby each in turn took responsibility for a month for dealing with contingencies and paying accounts.

The occupation of a single building also made it possible for them to share the services of the health visitor, geriatric visitor, and nurse whom the health authority agreed to house in the premises. Moreover, on the initiative of one of the practitioners they were all able to make use of the services of a voluntary marriage guidance counsellor who had previously worked for only one of them.

All the doctors expressed general satisfaction with these limited arrangements for pooling resources; but none of them wished the collaboration to be extended into the much closer comprehensive relationship involved in partnership. Neither Dr Erickson, for example, who had initiated the move, nor his partner wished to extend that partnership; and the two solo practitioners, Dr Osmond and Dr Cox, while appreciating the existing degree of co-operation, were adamant that they did not want to enter into any formal contractual partnership with each other or their fellow tenants. They believed that they had all the possible advantages of group practice without its possible disadvantages.

By contrast, the Avesbury and Barr doctors saw only advantages in the larger partnership groups to which they belonged. They all expressed the belief that having a partnership of five or six members had enabled them to obtain the back-up resources of employed and attached staff which they had come to regard as essential for the general medical practice they wanted to do. They expressed no resentment at any curtailment of their personal freedom which membership of a collectivity such as the partnership might involve.

It was clearly theoretically possible for the two group practices to become a single partnership of eleven or twelve practitioners after their common move to the Health Centre. What in fact deterred them? Was it some shared belief in the diseconomies of scale once a partnership had grown beyond a certain point? Was it a matter of the members perceiving the incompatibility of their rather different ideologies and approaches to the provision of service, an incompatibility which could wreck their capacity to provide patient care in the way they wanted to? Was it simply a desire to hold on to an association which had been meaningful to them and to retain an identity which would be lost were they to merge into a larger group? It would seem it was all three.

SHARED PHILOSOPHIES: THE BASIS FOR COLLEAGUELY COLLABORATION

We have some evidence that the doctors of both the Avesbury and Barr practices recognized that partnerships as large as theirs had each grown to be could create difficulties for doctors and for their patients. The Barr practice doctors in particular, at about the time of their move to the Health Centre, seriously considered reorganizing themselves into two groups each of three doctors who would interact more intensively with one another on clinical matters, leaving the six-person formal partnership to deal primarily with the financial and business aspects of their association. The suggestion, which was only partly acted upon for a short period, reflected some general shared unease at the difficulties of maintaining close professional relationships across an expanding primary health care team.

Equally, we believe, however, it was an intuitive feeling on the part of both the Avesbury and Barr doctors that successful partnership rested upon a shared approach to the medical task which led them all to reject any suggestion that they might merge into a single partnership. None of the doctors belonging to the Avesbury group wanted that group to lose its identity by amalgamating as a partnership with the Barr partnership; and the Barr group doctors, for their part, were unanimously as determined to retain their separate partnership existence.

The two groups had many aims in common, sufficient in themselves to facilitate amicable agreements to collaborate with each other in many common activities once they had occupied the Health Centre. Moreover, they were all willing to accept that they had something to learn from the other practice about good patient care; but they all had some major reservations about the approach of the other group which kept them at a certain distance from each other and made the close relationship involved in partnership a non-starter. The Barr practice was even against forming a common rota system for covering patients outside normal working hours for home visits.

Some indication of the nature of the differences has already been given in Chapter 2 where we discussed the philosophies of the senior members of the practices. In later chapters we point in more detail to these differences in so far as they related to relationships between the doctors and other workers employed in or attached to the practices and to relationships with patients. Here we want to consider only one kind of ideological difference between the Avesbury and Barr doctors which bore directly upon their relationships with one another. It concerns the question of leadership.

EQUAL PARTNERS? THE ISSUE OF LEADERSHIP

The age-old insistence of the medical profession that the accountability of a fully qualified doctor is first and foremost to his patient, and that to serve the patient the doctor must have clinical autonomy free from any outside interference, can be shown to have been breached in many ways (Klein 1973: 63; Committee of Enquiry into Competence to Practice 1976: 25). For example, legislative measures taken both before and after the creation of the National Health Service protect the patient in what must often of necessity be an unequal relationship and hence open to abuse by the practitioner. They give him not only the right of final recourse to the law; he is also able to bring his medical advisers to account for their action before their peers. In the hospital today, too, thanks to the development of powerful and hence dangerous diagnostic and therapeutic procedures, the dictum of clinical autonomy applies only to the consultant doctor, who is outnumbered by the juniors he leads and for whose work he is responsible.

In general practice, however, it is still largely assumed that fully fledged principals are accountable for their clinical work only to their patients. Entry into partnership arrangements is not intended to disturb this fundamental principle. Nor is there any evidence from our study or any other known to us that it does. Clinically, as far as we could tell, each principal in our study practices took full responsibility for his or her diagnostic and therapeutic decisions, while remaining free if puzzled to ask for a second opinion or advice from his partners.

Nevertheless, it is probable that as long as partnerships have existed they have as often been between partners who have been unequal in some respects as between those who have been equal. Since general practice partnership is a business run by independent contractors, if not for profit then at least to make ends meet and provide a reasonable income for its members, it is not surprising to find that the individual who has founded the practice and asked others to join, has been the longest-serving member, or has invested the most capital in the building it occupies, may expect and be given some recognition in the form of a larger share of the residual income or a greater say in decisions affecting the work of all its members. By the same token, the last to join, the youngest, or those with no capital tied up in the practice property, may well receive a smaller share of the monetary proceeds or be accorded less voice in policy or organizational matters. And even if these kinds of inequalities do not exist and the partners are seen and see themselves as co-equals, the different personality attributes of the partners may result in a degree of dominance on the part of some, and of subordination on that of others, when organizational decisions are taken.

As we have earlier stated, by tacit agreement with the general practitioners in our study, we did not explore the financial or business aspects of their practice arrangements. We did, however, question the doctors about their relationships with each other and in particular as to whether they felt that one or other of their number could be described as a leader and if so in what sense. We were also able to observe the behaviour of the doctors to one another, mainly in their regular weekly meetings.

It is data of these kinds which helped to form our own impressions as to the character of the relationships among the partners in the group practices. We had no comparable opportunities of observing relationships in the smaller practices. It is worth noting, however, that three of the four doctors involved in these latter practices claimed that no one of them was a leader in the sense that his opinion carried more weight than that of the others. The fourth, however, believed that it was he who most commonly took the initiative and insisted on reaching and recording decisions. This accorded with our, admittedly limited, observations.

Leadership in the Barr practice

All the doctors at this practice agreed that a unit such as theirs needed a leader, that Dr Bourne undoubtedly performed this role, and that he was well suited to it. A leader, they agreed, was necessary for several reasons: first, to represent the practice to the outside world; second, to serve as a focus for patients wanting to lay complaints or make criticisms; third, to steer the group to a consensus; and fourth, to see that decisions were implemented. The quality required was 'a skill in bringing people forward', in encouraging them to state their views, and in orchestrating those views to reach a consensus. The leader's role, they believed, had to be filled by someone who could set high clinical standards, delegate responsibility, and help other workers to realize their potential.

Dr Bourne was regarded by all the other doctors as having these qualities. He had a wide range of interests, was in touch with what was going on in the outside world, and was open to new developments in medicine. He was interested in post-qualification and medical student education in general practice and active in research. In relations within the practice he was sensitive to the needs of others and appreciative of their skills and expertise. There was something about him which caused people to regard him deferentially if not reverentially. 'He functions on a higher plane than other people,' Dr Bridges told us. There was no challenge to his leadership from any of the other partners.

Dr Bourne, for his part, was conscious of the dynamics in the group as well as in the wider practice team and the part he played in them. He maintained that the hierarchy within the group was always potentially fluid, nearly all the partners being capable of leadership in several fields. However, opportunities for them to realize these capabilities had had to wait on the development of his own:

'In the first year after Peter Barr retired, I tended to run everything. I had to learn how to do it: only then could I begin to delegate.'

In recent years he had made space for others by giving the responsibility for a number of concerns to other partners. For instance, one had responsibility for the practice's teaching activities and another for its financial affairs. Yet another had taken his place as practice representative in an action research project conducted by an independent psychotherapeutic institute.

He admitted, however, another reason for releasing his hold. 'If I hadn't,' he said 'I would have had a rebellion on my hands: some of the others were getting restive.' He found it difficult not to dominate the discussions and organizationally was still the 'king bee'. Moreover he still felt uncertain about just how far to go, and about how much to delegate without abdicating ultimate responsibility. He feared that the spirit of the times could take democracy too far until eventually what would be lost would be not just authority but 'personality'. Mother and father figures, not just figureheads, to whom people could relate and, in doing so, feel secure and free to develop themselves were still needed. 'So I remain responsible and am seen by others as responsible.'

Leadership among the Avesbury partners

In describing in Chapter 2 Dr Adams's philosophical approach to general practice, we recounted his belief that primary health care services should ideally be delivered by a salaried team of doctors, nurses, and others with special skills who would have outlived the hierarchical assumptions of authority at present vested in the doctors. A group partnership which would rent rather than own its premises was the nearest he could get to this ideal, given the organization of general practice services under the National Health Service Act 1946. The partnership would be forced to act as a business; but, because doctors were not trained for management and needed to de-emphasize their legal status as employers of nurses and receptionist staff, they would employ a practice manager to whom the partners would voluntarily cede a good deal of their formal authority for practice administration.

These egalitarian tenets were shared by the other partners. When we first interviewed them they were at pains to stress the absence of any hierarchy between the partners. The image which they wanted to project was of the partnership as a family, bound by affectional ties strong enough to provide unconditional support to any of its members who might be facing difficulties of a professional or personal kind.

Our own observations certainly confirmed the informal family-like intimacy among the Avesbury partners, especially when contrasted with the more business-like though friendly relationships we observed among the Barr partners. Nor could we discern the degree of deference paid to the senior partner, Dr Adams, that we observed at the Barr practice for Dr Bourne. Nevertheless, our strong impressions were of a group of partners amongst whom Dr Adams was dominant. By 1976, however, and possibly partially as the result of an interim report from the research team in which we drew attention to differences between the doctors' and our own perceptions of relationships in the Avesbury practice, the partners acknowledged what they had earlier denied; namely the existence of leadership in their practice – that of Dr Adams.

Dr Alexander in 1976, reflecting on the group's erstwhile belief that they were a leaderless group, laid responsibility for the perpetuation of the myth at the door of Dr Adams's socio-political principles, which called for 'a leaderless democracy'. At the same time, and paradoxically, it was Dr Adams's personal qualities which made him stand out among the others and endowed him, whether he wanted it or not, with the role of natural leader:

'He was so much better than anyone else at running a meeting and whenever he gave directions they were so much better than anyone else's. Also he was always having new ideas which lead us into pastures new.'

Dr Adair, also considering the paradox, felt that there had been no deliberate attempt to subvert or undermine the ideal of the leaderless group, yet

'Over the years it has always been Sam in the sense that all discussions which did not readily solve themselves were resolved by him. He would make an intervention of some sort and people's views would always crystallize in line with his suggestion.'

Another factor which may have influenced this general reassessment by the partners of the nature of their relationships with one another was Dr Adams's partial withdrawal after the move to the Health Centre to become a part-time paid official of a medical organization, which was followed by his retirement from the partnership in 1976, an event which was imminent when we were interviewing doctors for the second time.

There was no doubt that the other doctors saw the partial withdrawal as a loss. Indeed Dr Attenborough likened it to the prolonged terminal illness of a close relative:

'For two years he was around but away from us. The fact that he had been so important to us, that he was still around but that he was not there for us ...'

And Dr Ashton used terms appropriate to the funeral oration of a prominent man:

'There is a gap, but life is full of gaps, and when the mourning is done a new team will arise with the type of leadership appropriate to it. His influence will remain and in one way or another there will be continuity of what he built up.'

It was at the time of Dr Adams's retirement that our own detailed observations ceased. We are not in a position, therefore, to indicate how relationships between the remaining partners developed without his presence. We did, however, see that there was no strong competition for the place he had vacated and no single person emerged with the charismatic authority which he had commanded.

The doctors, too, recognized that what one of them described as a centrifugal process, a tendency for the group to atomize, had accelerated with Dr Adams's departure. However, they did not blame the tendency on that event alone. They saw it also as a function of the move to the Health Centre, of their own ageing, and of changes in their life circumstances. Nevertheless, despite the weakening of their mutual bonds, they felt the group had sustained itself by virtue of the deep, underlying affection each member had for the others and the part played by the practice manager, Jean Armstrong, in keeping the Avesbury partners together at times of great stress. The impact of the move to the new premises and of other contemporaneous developments on the practices as a whole are detailed in Chapters 9 and 10. In Chapter 10 we deal too with the ways in which the two group practices felt they had learnt from each other and the expanding field of inter-practice activities.

THE RESEARCH TEAM'S ASSESSMENT

Returning to the theme with which this chapter opened, we must now ask whether the experience of the doctors in this study in regard to those with whom they had either entered into large or small partnership, or, without such formality, shared common premises, gives substance to the fears of those who were advising caution in extending close working arrangements.

Our view is that it does and it does not. It does in the sense that all the doctors in this study, whatever the size of the practice unit to which they belonged, believed themselves to be in the right size of unit for them and saw mainly disadvantages from any further growth in the number of doctors attached to that unit, or in the number of principals sharing their working premises. It does not in the sense that none of the doctors, all of whom had recently participated in moves involving them in closer working relationships with other general practitioners, regretted that aspect of the change or saw it as essentially dysfunctional. On the contrary, most emphasized its contribution to their ability to deliver the kind of service they wanted to give their patients.

In our final chapter we return to certain of the implications of this conclusion. Here we want merely to suggest that the apparent paradox may be resolved if we recognize that all the general practitioners in the last resort were concerned to protect their identity from outside threats. For some, the outside threat was possibly to their sense of professional competence; protection lay in remaining single-handed. For others, the threat was to their accustomed ways of managing their business, their work schedules, or their relationships with patients; protection lay again in solo or two-man practice. For yet others, the threat was to a more general set of social and professional values, in short, an ideology which informed their whole method of work. For these last, sharing was possible, even ideal, if it were with other like-minded individuals. Enlargement of the unit by the inclusion of others whose commitment to the ideology would be questionable was what had to be avoided. Protection lay in maintaining the identity of a group of like-minded individuals.

In short as a hypothesis or as an interpretation of our findings, we would argue that those who feel comfortable in group practices are those who know they share a common set of social and professional values, among which is the belief that primary health care now has to be delivered in the context of a supportive, multi-disciplinary team of health workers.

5 General Practitioners and Nurses

In this chapter we consider the relationships which were formed between the general practitioners and the nurses whom they employed or who were attached to their practices by the Local (later Area Health) Authority. Here, as elsewhere in this book, we examine mutual perceptions of the 'fit' between the skills and longer-term interests of the two occupational groups, and we examine some limited information on how the nurses were seen by the patients who had used their services. We comment too on the extent to which our data lent support to the views of the advocates of closer working relationships and re-drawn boundaries (Ministry of Health 1954: 14; RCGP 1968: 47) or to those of the critics who, in the 1970s, suggested that placing nurses already working in the community in general practice units was likely to extend the arena in which doctors dominated nurses from the hospital to the community (RCN 1977: 16). At least one doctor indeed claimed that practice nurses had not shared in the increased status enjoyed by hospital nurses (Leiper 1975).

Before giving the views of the doctors and nurses in the study practices, it may be useful to set the scene by reminding readers of the way in which nursing services in the community had been provided in the early days of the National Health Service and of the changes which had begun to take place in the 1960s and were still proceeding when our study began.

AND NEVER THE TWAIN SHALL MEET: HOME NURSES AND GENERAL PRACTITIONERS

It has been pointed out, not infrequently, that the National Health Service itself was not as innovatory in 1948 as much popular and especially overseas opinion believed it to be (Lindsey 1962: ix; Stevens 1966: 91; Abel-Smith 1976: 24). Home nursing services before the National Health Service were provided, in the main, by district nursing associations (PEP 1937: 174) topped up for a minority of well-to-do clients by nurses employed by private agencies or working on their own behalf. The local authorities had only recently acquired powers to employ district nurses themselves (Public Health Act 1936), and these could only give service to a few specific categories of patients, that is, to those suffering from infectious diseases, to children under five with specific illnesses, and to expectant and nursing mothers. The National Health Service Act extended the local authorities' powers either to provide direct services to all those requiring home nursing (section 25) or to reimburse the district nursing associations which continued to provide such services. Thereafter the work of the private nursing agencies in the domiciliary field gradually diminished.

The nurses had to be state registered and often had a district nursing or Queen's Institute of District Nursing Certificate. They were mostly unmarried; in cities they generally lived in hostel accommodation owned by the local authority or voluntary association and presided over by a superintendent nurse who allocated duties to them on a daily basis. Those who were married could work from their own homes, but they too were expected to have the bags in which they carried their supplies checked each morning by the sister in charge. They might never speak personally to the local general practitioners, who would be expected to contact the superintendent, not the nurse, if they wanted help for a patient. In so far as they communicated with the local doctors, it was generally by leaving a note for them on their patients' mantelpieces (Harding 1982). These arrangements reflected the rigidity of the nursing hierarchy and the etiquette of the time. They also reflected the often mutual hostility and suspicion of general practitioners and local authority-employed personnel.

Before the war and the advent of antibiotics the nurses, especially those living in their own homes, could be called out directly by the relatives of patients to deal with the crises which were a common feature of infectious diseases such as pneumonia (Blythe 1969: 200). The doctors, themselves, could be considered too expensive to call in. After the war and the advent of the National Health Service, general practitioners would call on district nurses in such crises; but the latter dealt increasingly with the regular, on-going nursing of chronically sick and handicapped patients, sufferers from long-term illnesses, who were being cared for in their own homes, as well as with mainly elderly people in terminal illness (Baly 1973: 228). These patients, in contrast to those of an earlier generation, would all be registered for free medical advice and treatment with a general practitioner; and it would be the general practitioner or the hospital who would ask for continuing nursing attention for a patient from the district nursing service. Once referred, however, there was still often little or no contact between the nurse and the general practitioner. The former was expected to report tᴄ ner superintendent and not to the doctor (Jefferys 1965: 120; Hockey 1968: 128).

In the 1950s and 1960s, increasingly attention began to be drawn to the dysfunctional consequences of the separation from one another of the two health services which were charged with the responsibility of caring for individuals in the community (*BMJ* 1953b: 144). Particular emphasis was given in a number of reports to the harmful consequences of the chasm which yawned between general practitioners and health visitors (Ministry of Health 1963: 37) (see Chapter 6), and one or two studies also highlighted the disassociated way in which general practitioners and community nurses served the same patients (Jefferys 1965: 122; Hockey 1966: 66).

Responsibility for the separation of the public health services from that of the general practitioners was laid by a number of working parties at the door of the tripartite division of the National Health Service as it was structured in the 1946 Act (Medical Services Review Committee 1962: 158). Some enterprising medical officers of health, however, believed that structural changes requiring legislation for their implementation were not needed to improve the co-operation between their domiciliary-based services and the general practitioners (Swift and McDougall 1964; Warin 1968). At first experimentally and tentatively, and then with increasing confidence, they switched health visitors, district nurses, and domiciliary midwives from caring for people who needed their services in a defined geographical district to caring instead for patients grouped by their registration with specific general practitioners.

By the early 1970s, 77 per cent of district or home nurses were working on this so-called 'attached' basis, either wholly or in part (DHSS 1974a). In London and some other highly urban areas such attachments were much rarer because the local health authorities only felt it feasible to make the switch if the general practitioners in an area either worked in groups of at least three from common premises or had reasonably reliable records and room to accommodate a nurse.

THE SURGERY-BASED PRACTICE NURSE

The existence of a clear-cut functional division between nursing in the home and nursing in the general practitioner's surgery, which had existed universally prior to 1968 and persisted in most practices after that date, including the group practices in our study, is explicable in the light of the way in which general practice itself had developed. Before the war, it was, as we have already stated, carried on essentially by single-handed practitioners, most of whom depended upon their wives or housekeepers to act as receptionists or as chaperons when they examined women. Some wives undoubtedly had nursing qualifications and may well have acted as assistants to their husbands; but anecdotal, often autobiographical, accounts of general practice before the National Health Service suggest that it was only the unusually successful doctor with a lucrative practice, perhaps in Harley Street or its provincial equivalent, who was likely to employ a paid nurse, and in such instances she was still likely to combine the role with that of receptionist (Dopson 1971: 86).

Few general practitioners employed nurses solely as nurses before 1968, as far as we can judge. Cartwright (1967: 160) estimated that 12 per cent had at least one nurse but that she often functioned as secretary-receptionist as well. In 1968, there were only 244 whole-time equivalents distributed among the 20,000-odd principals in England and Wales (DHSS 1974b). Many of these nurses worked on a part-time basis, so that there were considerably more than 244 employed nurses in general practice; but the comparatively small numbers indicate that it was still the very unusual practice who employed them. Thereafter, there was a steady increase in the numbers employed; but, according to Reedy et al. (1976), only 24 per cent of general practice units in 1974 employed any nursing staff, while 68 per cent of them had the services, at least on a part-time basis, of an attached Area Health Authority nurse.

Reedy, who made the only national study of nurses in primary care in the United Kingdom in the 1970s, did not set out to discover why comparatively few practices employed nurses in the early and middle 1970s compared with the much larger numbers with attached nurses. His figures, however, at least indicate that employed nurses were not substitutes for attached nurses. In other words, the practices with employed nurses were most likely to have attached ones as well. He also found that larger practices were more likely than smaller ones to employ nurses. In other words, for most general practitioners, employed nurses were not substitutes for partners or for nurses attached to them by the Local (later Area) Health Authority.

What then lay behind the strong advocacy of both the employment and attachment of nurses from central government and from many members of the Royal College of General Practitioners?

POTENTIAL GAINS AND LOSSES

The major advantage that was stressed by these bodies was the capacity of the surgery-based nurse to take over some routine aspects of medical diagnosis and some simple therapeutic procedures, thus achieving two desirable objectives at one and the same time, namely, reducing the dependence on the hospital casualty department and pathology laboratory and freeing the general practitioner himself to concentrate on those aspects of diagnosis and therapy which only he was trained to do (DHSS 1971: 31; Hodgkin 1967). The value of attachments of home nurses was usually held to lie in the capacity of the latter to inform the general practitioner about the state of health of housebound patients who were receiving regular nursing care in long-term or terminal illness (Joint RCN/RCGP 1974: 14). Some general practitioners, however, saw the possibilities of home nurses undertaking initial or follow-up visits to patients who had requested a home call from a doctor (Weston Smith and Donovan 1970).

While the chorus of voices raised to urge general practitioners to accept attached home nurses or employ surgery nurses sang in almost complete unison, a few discordant notes could occasionally be heard. Some general practitioners, for example, were happier to employ nurses than to accept attached nurses, perhaps because they feared some future inroad into their autonomy. They believed that they could have no say in deciding which nurse was to be attached and that she would continue to be responsible to her nursing superior in the local or area health authority and not to them (Forman 1974).

Other general practitioners sounded warnings about allowing nurses, whether attached or employed, to substitute for themselves in a variety of ways. They pointed, for example, to their own ultimate responsibility for every patient registered with them and the legal ambiguities which could arise were things to go wrong following procedures undertaken by a nurse (*JRCGP* 1975: 157). Still others expressed concern at the possible dilution of the doctor-patient relationship were nurses to undertake tasks the patients expected them to do (Weston Smith and Mottram 1967; Williams 1967).

Nurses' organizations for the most part supported the *rapprochement* with general practice, but some misgivings were also expressed and notes of caution sounded. Some home nurses, for example, valued their independence from direct medical control and feared that this might be lost with attachment and the imposition of dual control of their activities.

Where did the general practitioners in our study practices stand on these issues?

The two group practices had had district nurses attached to them before our study began. The smaller practices' patients were served by a district-based not practice-attached nurse until their move to common premises in 1975, after which they shared the services of two attached nurses, both of whom combined district nursing with work in the doctors' surgeries, the Health Services and Public Health Act 1968 (section 11(2)) having allowed them to do so. The group practices' attached nurses continued their traditional function of only nursing patients in their homes. They did not undertake any nursing tasks in the general practitioners' surgeries. The practices employed nurses directly for this purpose.

DOCTORS' VIEWS OF THE PRACTICE NURSES' WORK

With unhesitating unanimity the doctors in all the practices spoke warmly about the value of the surgery-based nurse's work and the contribution it made to patient care. Those in the Barr and smaller practices who had only comparatively recently worked with one were particularly enthusiastic, and emphasized the difference which having a nurse on the spot made to their own work.

In the accounts which the doctors gave us of the contribution which their surgery-based nurses made there were three main themes, the first having two sub-themes. First, the nurses were described as undertaking work which otherwise would fall to the doctors to do, that is, substituting for the doctor; this they could accomplish either by undertaking work on doctors' orders, or by becoming the patient's primary carer at the latter's instigation. Second, doctors saw nurses as relieving patients of the necessity of going to a hospital for treatment or investigation, that is, substituting for services usually provided by the hospital. Third, nurses were seen by some doctors as providing services which patients might not otherwise receive at all, that is, as supplementing or extending basic primary care services.

Nurse as doctor substitute at the doctor's discretion

In considering the first theme – *substituting for the doctor* – the doctors listed commonly performed procedures like blood pressure testing and throat swabbing and treatments such as ear syringing, injections, and the dressing of wounds. One doctor indeed pointed to the fact that nurses by virtue of their training were better fitted for these tasks than were the doctors. The unsupported general practitioners had had in the past to acquire such skills since there was no nurse available to perform them. Only one doctor expressed any form of regret that the presence of nurses in the practice relieved him of the necessity to do such work himself. He had found that undertaking these practical tasks allowed him some degree of relaxation in what could otherwise be a relentless mental and emotional grind.

None of the doctors suggested that having a nurse undertake such procedures had had any deleterious effect on their relationships with their patients. In fact they implied that lightening their own load of some of the less exacting procedures left them freer to concentrate on that part of the diagnostic work for which they and not the nurses had been trained. Some also claimed that they had more time to perform their psychotherapeutic task of listening, although they did not claim this last as a skill which they alone possessed. None of them suggested that nurses gave them more recreational time. They did not argue either that it was the presence of practice nurses in the team which permitted them to participate in extra-mural medical activities. That ability they attributed to work sharing with other doctors (see Chapter 4).

The only real diversity among the doctors on this aspect of the nurses' tasks was whether the latter should be permitted to undertake such procedures as taking a cervical smear or fitting an inter-uterine device, which were still regarded by most doctors at the time as essentially medical and not nursing tasks. Most of the doctors in the study shared this view, but it was beginning to be challenged in the Health Centre where two of the nurses serving the group practices had attended special courses in family planning and were fitting contraceptive dutch caps. Another had acquired some skill in diagnosing respiratory complaints by learning how to use a stethoscope to listen to chests.

Nurses with their own clientele?

In our questions to doctors we put it to them that the presence of nurses in their practices might lead to a situation where an increasing number of patients chose to consult nurses rather than their doctors, that is, decided to substitute the nurse entirely for the doctor. We wanted to know whether they believed this to be happening and, if so, whether they were at all anxious about its implications for their own authority.

The group practice doctors all agreed that some of the patients registered with them now chose to consult a nurse directly instead of them. Most of them were happy for patients to do so when it was clearly a matter of patient preference. They believed that their nurses would not act irresponsibly and that the nurse's need to obtain the doctor's signature for any drugs prescribed provided an adequate safeguard. One or two were less happy when patients by-passed them at the suggestion of the receptionists and saw the nurse without seeing the doctor with whom they had an appointment. This could happen when patients were faced with a long wait.

There were, however, some differences among the doctors about how far the nurse could or should become an autonomous worker with, in effect, a clientele of her own which seldom or never consulted them, or chose to consult her rather than them for specific reasons.

Dr Adair of the Avesbury practice, for example, in discussing the work of one of their nurses in family planning expressed her dilemma about the extension of the nurse's work in this field:

> 'I don't let them fit caps simply because I'm prepared to make mistakes and take responsibility for a patient getting pregnant; but I and the patient would be furious if the nurse had done it. I don't let them do smears. They can do it; but I think I should look at the cervix and examine breasts. I may be denying their expertise, but that's how I feel about it.'

This doctor, on the other hand, was happy to let the practice nurses have considerable freedom to decide whether patients who consulted them first about physical symptoms should or should not be referred to her, whereas Dr Bridges from the Barr practice insisted that patients seen first by nurses in a new episode of illness should always be referred to a doctor. He told us:

> 'I'm not very happy about nurses seeing sick people and making a diagnosis and their then going away without seeing a doctor. There can be a come-back if something went wrong.'

Not unexpectedly, the doctors in the smaller practices with less experience of working with a nurse were the least willing to allow patients to consult nurses directly. Three of them did not believe it was happening, and felt they would not condone it if it did. The fourth, Dr Erickson, felt that his reluctance to contemplate such independence on the part of the nurse and the patients was partly a function of the length of time he had worked with the nurse. He could foresee a time when he had sufficient trust to make it possible for patients who wanted something like an anti-tetanus injection to go to a nurse directly. However, he went on to say:

> 'I believe the basis of medical training is that you don't accept someone else's word but examine the patient and come to your own decision. I believe in this, not just ritualistically.'

Our exploration with the doctors of the consequences for their own work and authority of an expanding role for nurses in general practice made it clear that there was a recognition, at least on the part of the doctors in the group practices who had the longest experience of working with nurses, that traditional ideas as to what was appropriately doctor's work and what was nurse's work were not sacrosanct. The boundaries were shifting, not merely as a result of their own desires to delegate the work they found less stimulating or less congenial: the nurses too, they realized, were beginning to show a desire to shape their own work and perhaps to prise away from doctors some tasks which the latter had seen as essentially medical. As Dr Balfour put it:

'The interface between doctor and nurse is one in which there could easily be muddles.'

Nevertheless she and the other group practice doctors maintained that there was virtually no conflict between them and the nurses, an absence which Dr Amery attributed to the nurses' good sense:

'They take us for the fools we are and humour us!'

Nurse as substitute for hospital services

The doctors in the two group practices in the Health Centre with their shared central treatment room, which contained a mini-laboratory and was surrounded by cubicles where patients could be seen in privacy, believed that the nurses made it possible for them to have many procedures carried out which otherwise would have had to be performed in hospital. It should be pointed out, however, that by that they did not mean that the nurses had taken on the functions of the hospital's pathology laboratory. The general practitioners had direct access to it as frequently as they wished. The practice nurses did not undertake the analysis of blood, sputum, or urine: their task was to supervise the taking of such specimens, a task which required the kind of skills which a state registered nurse would acquire during her basic training. In other words, they had not extended their role beyond the usual nursing role to take over any part of that performed by the laboratory technician.

The existence of a well-equipped treatment room did, however, enable the nurses to undertake treatments which would otherwise have involved patients in going to the accident and emergency departments of hospitals, where the treatments would have also been carried out by nurses. In such work, they took over entirely from the hospital, in contrast to the more limited role they played in diagnostic work. The doctors believed that many quite serious burns or wounds, as well as skin disorders, which earlier would have involved an inevitable hospital visit, were treated in the Health Centre.

Nurse as extender of services

Some of the doctors, in discussing the practice nurses' work with us, said they also saw them as providing services which genuinely extended the traditional scope of general practice. They were seen as enabling general practice, first, to enter the field of preventive medicine and, second, to support certain dependent patients in an intense form.

The nurses' contribution to preventive medicine in the group practices was through pre-symptomatic screening. As a special exercise, which they intended to make routine, the nurses took the blood pressure of all the adults who had made appointments with the doctors. The purpose of the exercise was to identify those with hypertension who could benefit from regular medication. The occasion was also used to weigh patients and to give those who were clearly over-weight advice about diet and exercise. There was no doubt in the minds of the doctors that such a programme would not have been undertaken without the nurses. The screening was also the basis of some of the epidemiological research in which the practices participated.

It was, however, the capacity of the nurses to support some of the most dependent patients simply by being willing to listen to them quite informally which was most often mentioned appreciatively by doctors. One doctor described the practice nurse as a source of comfort for sick children and for people in pain and discomfort. Another felt some patients confided in the nurse and would tell her things they would not tell the doctor through diffidence or because they did not want to 'worry the doctor'.

'Everyone has this tiny curtain of fear and shyness in relation to the doctor which they do not have with nurses.'

Dr Barrett of the Barr practice gave us an illustration of the intensive support which one of the nurses gave to a schizophrenic patient. The woman in question had daily injections from the nurse who was also willing to see her several times during the day, a contact from which the patient 'seemed to draw comfort and stability'.

Dr Alexander of the Avesbury summed up this aspect of the nurses' work as follows:

'In the long run, the most useful functions performed by a nurse are to do with personal advice, talk, listening – what you might call the social work element of the role, involving attitudes and skills which are not taught to doctor or nurse, and the nurse has learnt as well as the doctor.'

Yet another Avesbury doctor talked about what he described as the nurse's 'integrative function'. There were perhaps two senses in which he used this term. Nurses, in the first place,

'get a bird's eye view and are in touch with a great number of happenings and feelings in individuals and families which individual general practitioners are not, so she can fill them in.'

In the second place, she was also

'a second opinion on all sorts of things, giving the general practitioner a sense of security and making him feel less isolated and less a last-ditch operative.'

THE PRACTICE NURSES' PERCEPTIONS OF THEIR SITUATION

How did the nurses employed by the group practices see their role and their relationship with the general practitioners who employed them? There are many different ways in which we could have answered these questions. For example, the nurses we interviewed, four in all, told us a good deal about their entry into the general practice setting and the contrast between nursing in that context compared with the hospital. We chose, however, to concentrate in this chapter on their views on the issues we discussed with the doctors and, in particular, on the extent to which the nurses saw their work as distinguishable from that of the doctors. We also consider how much they felt themselves to be practitioners in their own right or as working only with the delegated authority of the doctors.

Competence: its expansion

There was no doubt in our minds after interviewing the four nurses that working in the group practices had given them opportunities to extend their areas of competence much beyond those for which their basic nurse's training had prepared them. It had also provided much greater variety and, they believed, much greater responsibility than they could have expected to obtain elsewhere. It was, moreover, from the new areas, those in which their work was most likely to resemble that traditionally carried out by the doctor or by the social worker, rather than from the performance of standard nursing procedures, that they derived greatest satisfaction.

We had two main grounds for feeling able to make this last statement. First, all four nurses said they liked working best with those doctors who did not overload them with requests for routine procedures, who recognized their treatment skills, who consulted them about patients and who did not interfere with what they were doing. Second, they complained about the 10–15 per cent of their time which was taken up with non-clinical, housekeeping activities such as maintaining the equipment in the treatment room, ordering medical supplies, filling in forms for doctors and patients, and dispatching specimens to hospital laboratories. They felt such work could be delegated to a nurse-auxiliary, less qualified than they were, leaving them free to do work of greater clinical significance.

The expansion of their role and its encroachment into areas once regarded as belonging to a doctor or a social worker had come about in two main ways, the one deliberate, the other developing more or less opportunistically out of their more traditional nursing tasks.

As an illustration of the first, the deliberate expansion of the nursing role, Nurse Anstey had taken it upon herself to attend a hospital out-patient clinic to learn more about the cause and treatment of skin complaints, since she had felt that the doctors in her practice were not knowledgeable enough about these conditions and hence were too ready to refer patients to hospital. Nurse Bond and Nurse Denton had opted to attend a special course on family planning and Nurse Denton had begun to learn how to listen to chests in order to play a more active part in the care of children. These were all instances of a consciously contrived effort to develop knowledge and skills beyond those which would be expected of the state registered nurse. Moreover, since their expertise differed, the three nurses could and did refer to and consult each other. One nurse might be seen as an authority on rashes and another on contraception. To varying extents they also saw scope for further opportunities for expanding their expertise, given a little more training. Nurse Anstey suggested simple eye care as one:

> 'So often doctors refer people to the eye hospital whereas we could do something for them here if we knew more.'

The more opportunistic extension of their traditional role occurred by their increased use, in conjunction with nursing procedures, of listening, a method more commonly associated with the stock-in-trade of the psychiatrist or the social worker. breast, about which they said, 'they did not want to bother a realization that:

> 'Many patients haven't come for advice. They have come to tell us something, to get it off their minds; and having told us, they often feel better. That is all they wanted.'

Sometimes, however, that was not all patients wanted. They had worries about potentially serious things, such as a lump in the breast, about which they said, 'they did not want to bother a doctor.' Nurse Anstey felt her willingness to listen meant that in the course of applying dressings or doing other physical procedures, patients would talk about their families, their work, their home circumstances, the everyday substance of their lives. She therefore had the opportunity of acting as a 'sorting officer', performing what might be called a 'triage' function (Brent 1983), establishing their needs and, if unable to deal with them herself, deciding who best could – the doctor, the psychiatrist, the dentist, the social worker, and so on.

In general then, they felt that, because there were several of them and they had space and facilities in the Health Centre, the role of surgery nurse had expanded and would continue to do so in the future:

> 'Now that we are a team, there are, every year, a few more treatments which nurses do which in the past only doctors have done.'

Clinical autonomy and accountability

We have said earlier that the doctors in our study differed on the extent to which they felt the practice nurses should exercise their own discretion when patients chose to consult them, or were pointed in their direction by receptionists who felt patients needed immediate attention and a doctor was not available.

The nurses were aware of these differences. They respected the views of the doctors who wanted to limit their functions and were careful to fit in with their wishes; but it was clear that they preferred working with those doctors who were willing to give them most scope for exercising their independent assessment, and for action.

Nurse Anstey, for example, describing the degree to which she was able to function independently of the doctors, told us that if, after listening to the patient and examining her, she thought a listed drug was needed, she would suggest it to a doctor and obtain his signature on the prescription form. If she felt tests were essential for a diagnosis, she would take and arrange to send a throat or vaginal swab, or a blood specimen to the hospital pathology laboratory and suggest the patient call back to see the doctor when the results were received. The patient could thus leave the premises without having seen a doctor. Similarly, if she suspected a fracture, she might send the patient directly to hospital without referring to a doctor:

> 'Where we know a doctor would say it's safer to have an X-ray, then to save time we write the letter to the accident department ourselves and arrange to get the patient there as soon as possible.'

We asked our nurse informants, as we had the doctors, whether they had a clientele composed of patients who chose to see them rather than the doctors. They were all sure they did and gave us illustrations of the kind of patient involved.

Usually, they said, those electing to see a nurse in preference to a doctor were patients with long-term problems. Nurse Anstey felt she was generally recognized as a person 'able to cope with madness', and mentioned the emotionally disturbed patients who had attached themselves to her. Nurse Bond too saw herself as caring for mentally ill patients, such as the woman with schizophrenia mentioned by Dr Barrett. She also instanced patients with such long-term conditions as diabetes, anaemia, arthritis, and hypertension. Nurse Denton's list included patients who came for regular check-ups on their blood pressure. There were many elderly patients among them and their visits enabled her to check that they were taking the prescribed drugs. She also provided an example of the kind of relationship a patient might build up with her or the other nurses:

'Mrs Pullen was advised by Dr Bridges to have a hysterectomy but was afraid of the operation. She kept coming into the treatment area to talk to one of us. After a number of such visits she seemed to have talked out her fears and conflicts and went off to see Mr Stimson who confirmed what Dr Bridges had said. But she then had to have lots of further talks with us before she underwent the operation.'

Nurse Abbott thought that the patients who consulted her in preference to a doctor included some who had heard about her from a relative or friend. In particular, she said,

'We get a lot of women's problems, young girls with menstrual or sexual problems who won't go to a doctor, but when they know we are here come to us.'

Practice differences

After the move of the group practices to the Health Centre, the doctors agreed that the nurses employed by one practice should treat patients of the other practice if necessary, and in time the two nurses were joined by a third who was jointly employed by the two practices. The shared central treatment area in the Centre made such an arrangement possible. We were curious to know whether the nurses were aware of any marked differences in approach which could be attributed to practice policy and if so how it might influence their own work.

It turned out that the nurses felt there were more differences among individual doctors than there were between the practices as such. Nevertheless they did think there were differences in practice style which affected the work they did for each. For example, the nurses agreed that the Barr doctors were more likely to accede to patient requests for services and to give these services themselves rather than refer the patient to the nurse. Nurse Bond referred to this as 'spoiling' the patients, and suggested that it occurred because they had less experience of working with nurses than had the Avesbury doctors: she considered them to be 'improving', that is, referring patients more often to the nurses. Avesbury doctors, by contrast, were seen as not pampering their patients. Their tendency, if anything, was to over-use the nurses by asking them to do too many routine tests. At the same time, the Avesbury doctors gave the nurses greater scope to exercise initiative.

Not surprisingly, Nurse Anstey, who had worked with the Avesbury practice for many years, preferred their style. Nurse Abbott, the nurse who replaced her, as well as the two others working in the Centre after the move were unwilling to express a preference for one or other style of practice. Nurse Denton perhaps summed up her allegiance to both when she told us:

'The times I feel closest to the Avesbury practice are those when I think the Barr doctors are doing things they probably think are unnecessary just to please the patient. I feel closer to the Barr practice when the Avesbury doctors are loading us with things I feel are unnecessary.'

Nurses as a challenge to doctor authority

Given that all the nurses were anxious to extend their work beyond the traditional boundaries of the nursing role, and given that in doing so they could, at least theoretically, expect to establish relationships with doctors of a different kind from those they would have encountered in the hospital setting, we were intrigued to know whether they felt competitive towards the doctors or resentful of the authority which the latter could command, if only by virtue of their position as employers and as 'possessors' of the patients registered with them. Did they feel that they in any way challenged or constituted a threat to the authority of the doctors?

The simple answer to these questions was 'no'. In a taken-for-granted way, the nurses thought of the setting in which they worked as the doctors' domain and of themselves as there to assist the doctor to do his best for patients. Their function was to relieve the doctors of some of the load by taking over work which they could do as well as the doctors, leaving the latter free to do work which they, the nurses, could not do. They might differ among themselves about what a doctor could do which a nurse could not, but they all recognized some situations which they felt to be within the average general practitioner's competence and outside their own. The dividing line tended to be drawn between the visible and the invisible. Moreover, they were not slow to point out that, in the last resort, doctors could not be held legally responsible for the nurses' actions if done without medical blessing; hence for self-protection they felt they had to consult and defer to their employers. The ultimate responsibility had to rest with the doctor, and they were content that it should be so.

As it was they felt themselves to be in a much more egalitarian relationship with the doctors than they would be elsewhere in the National Health Service. Nurse Bond, indeed, suggested that when she first joined the practice, in the light of her hospital experience, she had been very much in awe of the doctors. It was they who had encouraged her to respond to them as fellow human beings, not as superiors. It was they who provided the scope for her to use her initiative, test her potential, and develop new skills. Nurse Denton illustrated the part they had played in her development:

> 'They will call me into an examination room or bring a patient with inflamed eyes or a rash to me and ask, "What do you think of this?" or "What do you think should be done?"'

Nurse Abbott, perhaps, summed up best the sentiments which we believed they all tried to express:

> 'We are not equal from the point of view of work. Doctors have much more responsibility and knowledge. Otherwise there is as much equality in these practices as is feasible without making the work impossible.'

DOCTORS' VIEWS OF THE HOME OR DISTRICT NURSE

The doctors had much less to say about the work of the attached home nurses and their relationship with them than they did about their employed practice nurses. They made very complimentary comments about the reliability and caring qualities of the nurses assigned to work with their patients, while suggesting that they would have welcomed closer contact and more integration into their team than the nurses appeared willing to have. For example, one of the Barr practice doctors remarked:

'Nurse Bligh may be old-fashioned and resist any change to her long-standing working patterns, but she is an excellent nurse, providing loving care for her patients and deeply involved with them. And, ultimately, that's what matters.'

Although the amount of contact which they had with attached nurses was much less than with other attached workers, the doctors were clear in their own minds that having a nurse attached rather than having to rely upon one assigned on a district, non-attached basis helped to promote mutual trust and was infinitely preferable. For example, Dr Alexander maintained that in the course of casual conversation in the Health Centre he became aware of the attached nurse's particular skills, foibles, and deficiencies and could therefore adjust prescribing and management patterns to take these into account.

Dr Cox, who was anticipating advantages from working with the nurse recently seconded to his practice, described the disadvantages of having to depend upon a district-based service:

'Our practice is on the boundary between two districts of this AHA. So we had to be sure we phoned the office of the right district. Then, depending on where the patient lived, they allocated a nurse; but not even at this level could we always be sure of the same one.'

Among the group practitioners there were several who would have liked the home nurses to have been adventurous enough to expand their work beyond the bedside nursing of patients referred to them by doctors or the hospitals. They hinted, for example, at a future possibility of nurses undertaking first visits to selected patients asking for home calls, but one of the doctors remarked that those attached to his practice were not 'psychologically ready' for this function. Furthermore, he recognized that they had little power to shape their own role since they were subject to the authority of the divisional nursing officers of the Area Health Authority.

We did not interview the home nurses attached to the Health

Centre practices, nor the two attached nurses who, late on in our study, began to perform both home and surgery work in the premises occupied by the smaller practices. We cannot, therefore, give their views on their work and its relationship to that of the general practitioners.

MEASURES OF NURSING ACTIVITIES AND OF PATIENTS'
VIEWS OF THE SERVICES

In this chapter we have discussed the perceptions which doctors and nurses in the group practices had of the nurses' role in patient care and of their relationships with one another. It was clear from their accounts, and our own observations at meetings and elsewhere confirmed it, that both occupational groups felt that they had achieved a satisfactory division of work and hence a mutually satisfying relationship with one another.

It has not infrequently been pointed out, however, that service providers may collude in their own mutual interests and claim that in so doing they are improving the services they render to their clients, without any real evidence that this is so. We need to ask, therefore, in this instance, first, whether there was any independent evidence that nurses were undertaking the work they and the doctors alleged they were doing, and second, whether the practice patients approved or disapproved of the expanded role accorded the nurse.

The evidence we can call upon is limited, but in the main it supports the contention that patients more often received services from the employed nurses in 1975 than in 1972. This, however, was only true of the Barr patients; 24 per cent of the sample of home interviewees in 1975 had had a service from a nurse during the year compared with only 5 per cent in 1972. The Avesbury home interviewees, both before and after the move to the Health Centre, were more likely to have had a nurse deal with them on at least one occasion (40 per cent in 1972 and 39 per cent in 1975). These practice differences confirmed the contentions of the nurses themselves, and an analysis of a three-month record they kept in early 1976 suggested that they dealt daily with about three Avesbury to every two Barr patients (See *Table 4*).

It is more difficult to confirm or refute the other proposition made by the doctors and nurses, to the effect that the latter's work

Table 4   *Procedures undertaken by employed nurses in the Health Centre for Avesbury and Barr patients in the first three months of 1976*

type of procedure	Avesbury		Barr		all patients	
	%	N	%	N	%	N
treatments	35	(1199)	59	(1307)	44	(2506)
taking specimens	28	(1058)	21	(496)	25	(1554)
measuring	30	(1119)	9	(223)	22	(1342)
observing and examining	4	(159)	8	(189)	6	(348)
miscellaneous and unspecified	3	(253)	3	(139)	3	(392)
total	100	(3788)	100	(2354)	100	(6142)

saved many patients going to hospital, since we have only information of what they did in any detail in 1975. The three month record the nurses kept showed that their main activity was providing various kinds of treatment, of which the most common were dressings and injections followed by ear syringing. The rest of their recorded work consisted of approximately equal proportions of specimen-taking (mainly blood and throat swabs and urinalysis) and measurements (such as blood pressure, weight and pulse, temperature).

The records also indicated that there were differences in the relative frequency with which nurses undertook particular kinds of procedure for patients of the two practices. They performed about the same *number* of treatments for each practice but took over four times as many measurements for the Avesbury doctors and twice as many specimens as they did for the Barr doctors (*Table 4*). It cannot be inferred from the comparative figures, however, that the Barr were less likely than the Avesbury patients to have measurements such as blood pressure or specimens for urinalysis taken or that they were more likely to be sent to hospital for diagnostic or treatment procedures. A more likely explanation is the one the nurses themselves gave, namely that the Barr doctors were more likely to perform these procedures themselves than were the Avesbury doctors who had had much longer experience of working with a nurse.

We had hoped to use these records to assess how far the nurses' claims to act as a primary care giver to a large clientele was borne out. The records showed, for example, that nearly all the measurement and specimen-taking procedures were recorded as done at the request of the doctor. However, when we looked at the records of treatments, it was clear that when patients returned directly for dressings or injections without seeing a doctor, the nurses had recorded them as self or receptionist referrals. Only 8 per cent of all the treatments were designated as doctor referred, although many of them must have been initiated at some time by a doctor's referral. We were not able, therefore, to use the records to gauge how far the nurses were seeing a clientele which had not been initially referred to them by the doctors.

In 1975 we asked those home interviewees who had had contact with the nurses at any time whether they had been satisfied with the service. Only one in six had mixed feelings or was dissatisfied. At the same time we asked all the home interviewees whether they always wanted to see a doctor whenever they needed medical advice, or whether they would be prepared to see a nurse on occasions. The Avesbury patients were the most likely to say they were prepared to see a nurse for some purposes (45 per cent of them did so compared to only 31 per cent of the Barr practice home interviewees). The patients of the smaller practices were even less willing to contemplate seeing a nurse as a substitute for a doctor (26 per cent of both the Erickson and the Cox practice patients and only 14 per cent of Dr Osmond's). We felt it legitimate to conclude from these practice differences that experiencing the services of a nurse made individuals more willing to consider their use as a substitute for a doctor, at least for a limited range of conditions which, were no nurse available, they would take to the doctor.

THE RESEARCH TEAM'S ASSESSMENT

Returning to one of the central questions which was being asked during the 1970s, that is, whether there were serious disadvantages in the employment of nurses by general practitioners, we feel that the accounts we obtained from both doctors and nurses in our study, as well as our own observations of their interactions in meetings and elsewhere, provided us with a clear answer. It was that both doctors and nurses in the study practices felt that they and their patients gained from the latter's presence in the practice setting.

The doctors varied in the amount and character of the work they were prepared to ask the nurses to do; they varied too in the extent to which they thought that nurses should become the chief source of help and advice for some patients. Generally speaking, the longer the time they had worked with a practice nurse, the greater the degree of autonomy they were likely to accord to the nurse and the less likely they were to express anxieties of any kind.

The nurses for their part believed that the general practice setting gave them scope for expanding their work, for taking initiatives, and for accepting more responsibility than any other nursing situation. They were prepared to accept the ground rules because these were sufficiently flexible to enable them to vary their own work and negotiate with the doctors if they felt dissatisfied with the volume or character of the work delegated to them by the doctors. In these circumstances, they saw no need to challenge the final authority which they saw vested in the general practitioners, their employers.

We cannot speak with equal certainty about the attached nurses. Their relationships with the doctors were less close and neither side appeared to be pressing the case for a closer one or for a changing function for the home nurse.

6 General Practitioners, Health Visitors, and Geriatric Visitors

In this chapter we first describe the relationships between the doctors and the health visitors attached to the practices and then those between the doctors and the geriatric visitors. As in previous chapters, we have chosen to deal only with those aspects of the relationships which analysts of health services writing in the 1960s and 1970s had suggested could raise difficulties, or lead to discord between the occupational groups concerned. And in order to do this, we start by sketching briefly the general lines of the development of health visiting on a national scale and its relationship to general practice.

SHAPING THE HEALTH VISITOR ROLE

If it can be summed up in a nutshell, the central historical role of the health visitor, since her celebrated origin in 1861, has been to preserve infant life and improve its quality. In the first decades of her existence, if the histories have it right, she was likely to be a capable woman from the skilled manual working classes who had successfully raised a family herself in straitened circumstances (McCleary 1933: 85). With some extra schooling from the benevolent upper middle-class ladies whose voluntary endeavours gave her a small salary, she could go into the homes of the poorest families and, using her own experience, tell women with limited resources how to obtain the best nutrition for their children and how to reduce the risk of infection by improving their domestic hygiene (Nightingale 1893: 353). Although concentrating on the very young, she would indirectly be influencing family health as a whole for the good.

By the third decade of the twentieth century, the role had been formalized. It was only to be performed by those with a basic nursing qualification followed by a further training period and certification (Minister of Health 1925). It had by then in essence become a career for women, most of whom could expect to remain single and childless throughout their lives. They were employees of the local authority under the jurisdiction of the medical officer of health. Their main function was still to visit families with new-born babies and offer advice on infant feeding and hygiene; but they had also acquired some statutory duties under the child life protection legislation which gave them the authority to enter homes where a child's life could be at risk through cruelty or neglect (Children's Acts 1908, 1933). They could recommend the removal of a child from its parents. This 'policing' function did not make them altogether popular with all women. They had also, in many areas, begun to staff infant welfare clinics to which working-class women were encouraged to bring their children to check on their developmental progress.

These developments, although regarded by the Ministry of Health and local government medical officers of health as contributing greatly to both the reduction in infant mortality and the prevention of long-term disability, which were taking place despite much continuing poverty (McCleary 1933: 147), were not viewed with universal approbation by general practitioners. As private entrepreneurs they depended for their livelihood not only on building up a sizeable panel of compulsorily insured workers, for each of whom they received a *per capita* payment; they needed too to be able to obtain some income from treating the dependants of the insured workers. To some of the doctors it seemed that the local authority clinics, while ostensibly concerned with giving advice only on feeding, clothing, and hygiene, were liable to extend this to advice about matters of illness in children and mothers, in defiance of the demarcation agreement which had been voluntarily reached between them and the medical officers of health (*BMJ* 1954a: 125).

INTER-OCCUPATIONAL CONFLICT

It would not be unfair to say, therefore, that at the time of the National Health Service Act in 1946 relationships between general practitioners and health visitors were either non-existent or strained (Ministry of Health 1956: 37). Nor were the terms of the Act and the climate in medical circles at the time immediately propitious to the healing of old sores. The general practitioners came into the new service with somewhat of a chip on their shoulder, feeling that they had lost status to the hospital-based consultants (Stevens 1966: 95). They still feared a take-over by the local authorities from whose predatory excursions they felt they had fiercely to defend their independence. Health visitors belonged to this enemy camp. Although by the terms of the Act general practitioners acquired women and children as well as bread-winners in their head counts, some of them found it difficult to rid themselves of the suspicion that health visitors were invading their territory and pinching their patients, especially when the latter made it clear that they were comparing the advice offered by doctors in the field of child care with that given by health visitors in the infant welfare clinics. In such circumstances they could pull rank, asserting what they felt to be their rightful authority over the members of an occupational group whom they regarded as their professional subordinates. They were not above having sly digs at the health visitor, pointing to the inappropriateness of an unmarried childless woman giving advice to multiparous women on child rearing. The men among them seemed not to have reflected on the irony of their own claim to be able to offer women such advice.

Things were not plain sailing for the health visitors either. By and large they had emerged from the war with a high reputation in the public health field. They had spear-headed the successful campaign for immunization of infants against diphtheria which had resulted in a dramatic decline in the incidence of and mortality from the disease. They had taken on board too the dissemination of information on vitamin supplements and were often in charge of the clinics where supplies could be obtained for the priority classes of nursing mothers, pregnant women, and pre-school infants. Because they had responsibility for such tasks, their clientele had extended far beyond the very poor mothers who had been the main, sometimes reluctant, recipients of their attentions before the war. Many women from better-off classes who before the war would have called on doctors for advice began to find that the health visitors were often more knowledgeable. They could also be supportive in situations where husbands were absent in the forces and female kin far away.

The war-time extension of their role to cover a greater proportion of the population and a broader set of functions was probably the major reason why the framers of the National Health Service Act of 1946 included provisions for her role. The Act designated the health visitor as an all-purpose family visitor and endowed her with the responsibility of visiting all those mothers whose babies' births had been compulsorily notified to the local authority's medical officer of health by the midwife or doctor present at them (National Health Service Act 1946, part III, section 24). These statutory duties gave her protection, if she needed it, against people who might resent her intrusion into their homes, and to an increasing extent her work was moulded around this one task – the obligation to visit the new-born.

UNCERTAINTY IN ROLE DEFINITION

In the decade and a half after the war, however, the role prescribed for her by legislators and medical officers of health was attacked, not altogether disinterestedly, by spokesmen and women of other occupational groups. General practitioners, for example, continued to express hostile comments from time to time, alleging that health visitors were interfering busybodies whose ministrations were disliked by their women patients (Jefferys 1965: 124; Clark 1973: 80). Some suggested that as trained nurses they were desperately needed in hospitals and homes and would have done better to stick to such a last rather than set up pretentiously as experts in health education.

The general practitioner critics of health visiting were joined in such attacks by some social workers, who complained that the health visitor was claiming a degree of expertise and competence in the field of human relationships for which her training had not equipped her. Indeed, some social workers claimed that a nursing background was likely to be counter-productive. They particularly resented the suggestion from medical officers of health that, as the need to give advice on infant feeding and hygiene had diminished with a better informed generation of mothers, health visitors should turn their attention to preventing what was now seen as the major health problem to be tackled, namely social pathology in its many different guises (Hunter 1959).

The attacks by social workers on health visitors' competence were particularly virulent round about the time of the report of the

Jameson Working Party on Health Visiting in 1956. The Working Party itself was set up to try to work out a clearer picture of what health visitors could and should be doing (Ministry of Health 1956). In its recommendations it tried not to offend the social work lobby and spelled out a brief for health visitors which suggested combining basic health education, on an individual or collective basis to people in all kinds of family constellations, with concern for incipient signs of social disorder. It was careful to stress, however, that it did not wish health visitors to become involved in the long-term community care of patients with mental illness or handicap (Ministry of Health 1956: 112).

Shot at from different quarters by professional workers, who the health visitors felt should have been their allies, it was not surprising that morale was reported to be low among many of them in the early 1960s (Jefferys 1965: 86). Uncertainty about what they should be doing and how they should relate to other health workers was rife.

ATTACHMENT: A SOLUTION OR A DELUSION?

In the early 1960s, however, a way out of what seemed to be the professional isolation of a devalued worker was presented. The Medical Officer of Health for Oxford decided to attach some of the health visitors employed by his authority to several groups of general practitioners, to work with their patients instead of on a strictly geographical basis (Warin 1968). He found groups sufficiently unprejudiced to agree to the experiment. Within a few years all the authority's health visitors were so attached and early reports suggested that both health visitors and doctors liked working with each other and felt that in doing so they were providing a better service for the general practitioners' patients than they were by working separately. Other authorities followed suit and in 1971, according to Clark, about 60 per cent of all health visitors in office were attached on some basis, for at least part of their working day, to general practitioners to serve their patients (Clark 1973: 19).

One result of such attachments seemed to be a switch in the health visitor's work from almost exclusive concern with families where there were infants and pre-school children to a more varied clientele, including particularly the very old. While this was a cause for contentment to many general practitioners and social analysts who were conscious of the changing demographic pattern of the country and the health visitor's designation as a family visitor, other commentators were not so satisfied. The Court Committee on child health services, for example, reporting in 1976, believed that the spread of her concerns across all age groups had resulted in her having less time for and expert knowledge of very young children, and especially of those most likely to need attention if lives were to be saved and handicaps prevented (DHSS 1976: 73, 108).

Some members of the profession itself also began to voice doubts about the policy of attachment and the virtual abandonment of district-based work (*Health Visitor* 1975: 252). They suggested that attached health visitors could lose some of the independence which they had enjoyed as district-based health visitors, in the sense that they would be under some pressure from doctors to do crisis rather than preventive work. With some justification they argued that the general practitioner was not oriented to preventive work and would see them as extra hands in helping to deal with sick people. They also felt that some doctors were not above exploiting health visitors to reduce their own work, especially among their elderly housebound patients.

Yet another problem of which there was increasing awareness, especially in cities and other centres of substantial population turnover, was that of coverage. Health visitors believed they were more likely to locate newcomers with young children, who might be the most in need of their help, if they worked on the basis of complete coverage of a district. Several studies had shown that many mobile families, especially those from overseas, did not register with a general practitioner. The health visitor serving only a practice's registered population had to assume that the mothers and babies she saw on her rounds were being visited by the health visitors attached to other practices (DHSS 1976: 76, 110).

A LOCAL VARIANT ON A NATIONAL THEME: GERIATRIC
VISITORS

Before it was abolished in 1964, on the formation of the Greater London Council (London Government Act 1963), the metropolitan borough in which our study practices were situated had had a team of visitors to keep in touch with its elderly inhabitants and try to identify their social and medical needs, in order either to meet them themselves or refer them to other health and social services. These visitors usually had assistant nursing qualifications and were not eligible for district nursing or health visiting posts. At the formation of the new enlarged London boroughs in 1964, the Medical Officer of Health of the borough in which our practices were situated persuaded his council to continue to maintain this corps of visitors, alongside their teams of health visitors and district nurses. They were called geriatric visitors and, in due course, some of them too were seconded to work with practices, including the two group practices in our study.

In this borough, therefore, attachments to general practice did not involve health visitors in such an extension and diffusion of their tasks as it appears to have done elsewhere in the country. By general agreement between all the parties concerned, the geriatric visitors attached to the practices performed the tasks which elsewhere might have fallen to health visitors.

We need to ask, however, what role the doctors saw health visitors and geriatric visitors playing in their practices and whether they felt that their presence was wholly beneficial or raised any problems. Similarly, we discuss the views of the health visitors and geriatric visitors as to their part in the work of the units and their relationships with the doctors.

DOCTORS' VIEWS OF ATTACHED HEALTH VISITORS

The doctors in our study were in no doubt at all that they liked working with attached health visitors. They thought they contributed a great deal to the welfare of mothers and young children, especially when they worked in general practice units. As Dr Balfour of the Barr practice said:

'Before attachment we didn't know what they could do and we frequently didn't use them at all. Nor did they know what we could do. Since we have been together both parties have grown in ability and have learnt to be effective in new fields. Together we have generated new work.'

All the doctors in their replies to our questions showed that they recognized that the focus of the health visitor's work was essentially different from that of their own. They accepted that she was there to give mothers advice on feeding and bringing up children and that her work inevitably entailed screening and assessing general populations, the majority of whom might require little help from her or from them. They saw the health visitors as possessing an expertise in this work which they themselves did not have. As a consequence they were able to recognize her right to visit and advise their patients without their own intervention.

Nevertheless, it was also clear that much of the appreciation they had for their own attached health visitors was for the skills they displayed in helping them to manage patients with multiple difficulties including those of a psycho-social kind. Dr Alexander, for example, describing their work said:

'They go well beyond their purely statutory functions. They are very much involved with psycho-social problems in families and function as psychotherapists and do so very well. They take on a lot and, almost on their own, look after some of the most difficult families in the practice.'

The research team's notes of practice meetings revealed many instances which confirmed Dr Alexander's summation of their attached health visitors' work. For example, we recorded the following from a longer discussion at the Avesbury practice about a patient with an alcohol problem:

DR ADAIR   Mrs Albert seems to be relapsing. I saw her in the street pretty drunk. She seems to feel so hostile to all of us.
DR STEVENS   Barbara was the only one able to sort her out last time, and I must say, she does seem to have stayed off for quite a while. [To Barbara.] Perhaps you would see her again and, for the time being at any rate, all dealings between the practice and her could go through you?

Dr Stevens was, of course, the consultant psychiatrist attached to the practice; Barbara Almont was one of the health visitors.

The involvement of health visitors in families with social and psychological problems suggested that the distinctions drawn by the doctors between their competence and that of the social workers attached to the practices were not clear-cut. Our observations at meetings tended to confirm this impression, and in our questions to doctors we probed to discover what, if anything, they felt distinguished the health visitor's competence from that of the social worker, and the practical consequences of any distinctions they made between the two workers.

It transpired that none of the group practice doctors were prepared to draw a clear-cut dividing line between the competencies of the two types of worker. They all saw the health visitor and not the social worker as the possessor of knowledge and skills relating to physical health. At the same time, they felt the former had some competence in social and psychological pathology, that is, in the field in which social workers' expertise lay. The doctors differed among themselves only as to the extent to which they felt the social workers' knowledge exceeded that of the health visitors in this area.

In deciding, therefore, whether to ask for help from a health visitor or a social worker, doctors' assignments tended not to be taken on the basis of any hard and fast criteria of occupation-based expertise. They usually adhered to an unwritten but mutually understood demarcation agreement whereby the health visitors were invited to intercede where young children or pregnant women were involved, and social workers where there were adolescents or adults only. An earlier study of the work of an attached social worker had a similar finding (Goldberg and Neill 1972: 170).

One of the advantages of calling on the health visitors, according to several doctors, was that no stigma would be attached by neighbours to their visits, since everyone recognized their statutory duty to visit where there were young children. Consequently, if the doctors were worried about a child or family, they would ask the health visitor to 'drop in and check the situation out'. A visit from a social worker, they presumed, might be less socially acceptable to the families concerned.

HEALTH VISITORS' VIEWS OF WORKING WITH GENERAL PRACTITIONERS

The eight attached health visitors whom we interviewed were generally in favour of attachment to a general practice unit as a basis for health visiting. In describing the merits of working from within a general practice unit they said that they found it easier in such a setting to mobilize medical or social work help for families in need. It also enabled them to exchange information more readily and gave them access to relevant medical and other records. It made for co-ordinated strategies of care and lessened the likelihood that their messages to patients might conflict with the doctor's. It made them feel less isolated and more supported. Sharing anxieties about patients and responsibility for decisions about their care with doctors was more comfortable than 'living with the self-doubts' which, they argued, not infrequently assailed health visitors who were working on their own. Then again, they felt that working with doctors had made them more knowledge-able about 'medical things'. It also made it easier to see people who, as Ms Almont put it, 'didn't actually welcome health visitor visits'. Because they could say they were coming from a doctor, some people clearly found their visits more acceptable.

Attachment, they felt, also made possible a different way of working. Their visits, other than those for basic statutory purposes, could be more selective:

'Instead of rushing through everyone in a street as geographic visitors tend to do, we can plan our work to allow more time for patients who need it. It makes the quality of visiting better.'

Of particular value to them was their participation in the weekly case discussions which were also attended by the consultant psychiatrist. This they thought had increased their understanding of psychological and emotional problems and their confidence to deal with them. As a result they were undertaking casework which, were they not attached to these practices, they would have referred elsewhere or left undone. This work, although difficult and demanding, was interesting, absorbing, and rewarding.

On the debit side, however, attachment meant not working a 'patch' or small district in which they knew everybody and all the services and schools. Some of the people they felt they should be serving were not registered with any general practitioner, and could be missed if all health visitors were attached to practices. Dealing with a practice's patients only sometimes involved a visit to one family and, if the family was out, a waste of time since they might not have another family to contact in the immediate neighbourhood. Some health visitors were also conscious that their clients could lose out too. They knew that some people did not want their health visitor to be so closely associated with their general practitioner.

Since attachments had, as they saw them, both advantages and disadvantages the majority of those we interviewed argued that a mix of attached and non-attached workers within each district was best. In the case of large group practices where there were several attached health visitors, they advocated an internal division of labour on geographical lines, in other words a 'patch' approach within a practice's catchment area.

AUTONOMY AND AUTHORITY

As we have seen earlier in this chapter, some health visitors writing in their national journals, as well as other analysts, had argued that, in agreeing to work with general practitioners' patients, health visitors faced the prospect of losing their autonomy, that is, their right to organize and plan their own work, and a risk of domination by the doctors. We therefore tried to explore such issues in our interviews with the eight health visitors attached to our study practices.

When we asked them questions which bore upon the extent to which they were independent of the doctors or had to defer to them, they all felt that they enjoyed day-to-day autonomy both in deciding what work they should do and how they should do it. They recognized doctors as at the apex of the authority structure in the practice teams and 'certainly', as Ms Boston put it, 'as the most valuable or, at least, the most essential members of the team'. They attributed their own freedom from control by the doctors to two factors. First, the health visitors had statutory responsibilities to perform for which they were not responsible to the general practitioners but to the Area Health Authority which employed them. Indeed, Ms Blane, recognizing the duality in her position, so far from feeling that it exposed her to more authority, reckoned it gave her both greater freedom, 'there's no one breathing down our necks', and more support than she would otherwise have had:

'So it's good both ways. When things are going smoothly you can be fully independent. When you need support you get it. If it's worry about a patient, you get it from the doctors or other practice workers. If it's an administrative or legal problem, you get it from your nursing supervisor. If you want to start a slimming clinic, both give you encouragement.'

The second reason, however, was their belief that the doctors with whom they worked were really rather special people who recognized their skills and their right to decide their own priorities to an extent which most doctors would not. When pressed they acknowledged that there were times when a conflict could arise between their own view as to what they should be doing and that of the doctor. Ms Brodie gave us an example of the use of authority by a doctor which she had resented:

'A mum with a baby she was fostering – not one of my clients – had a feeding problem and asked for a doctor. The receptionist asked if I would go. I said she'd asked for a doctor and it should be a doctor. The receptionist phoned back to say the GP was not going and had said I was to. I was very cross. I visited and got a cool reception from the mother, which was natural because she wanted a doctor.'

In general, however, in so far as any pressure was put upon them by doctors, it was to improve their skills in handling psycho-social questions. This was a direction in which they all wanted to go and in which they felt they had much to learn within the context of the general practice unit to which they were attached. They regarded it as encouragement rather than pressure.

OCCUPATIONAL SPECIFICITY

We have seen earlier in this chapter that the general practitioners in our study did not have a uniform view of the distinction to draw between the health visitor's and the social worker's skills in social and psychological matters, and hence adhered in the main to the general rule that health visitors dealt with the families where there were young children and social workers with those where there were only adults or adolescents.

The health visitors in our study raised no objection to this way of allocating work to them and showed no signs of rivalry with social workers for a greater or lesser allocation or for more or less esteem in the eyes of the doctors. In short, we could find no evidence in the group practice unit of the kinds of competition, suspicion, and ill-feeling which had characterized some of the exchanges between the two occupational groups in the 1950s and 1960s.

The health visitors, when asked to discuss the distinctions they drew between themselves and social workers, acknowledged the blurred boundaries between health and social problems and between preventive and ameliorative efforts. They saw social workers as mainly concerned with crises, while they supported families through everyday problems. They also said they would cheerfully refer their families to social workers if 'things needed a lot of sorting out', or where there was evidence of deep emotional problems, serious family discord, or economic or housing eligibility difficulties. In some instances, the referral would be undertaken merely for load-shedding purposes: working with case loads of thirty and not three hundred, social workers had more time for intensive exploration. In other instances, however, they referred because they felt the social worker attached to the practices had special counselling and psychotherapeutic skills. They had grave doubts about referring to the local authority's social services department because the family might well be put in touch with someone less skilled than themselves in dealing with emotional problems.

The health visitors also saw a great deal of merit in the policy of the area health authority for the locality whereby the geriatric visitors took over responsibilities for the aged which elsewhere would have formed part of the comprehensive duties of the health visitor. They were aware that the National Health Service Act 1946 called upon them to provide health education and support in *every* phase of the family life cycle, but they argued against this idealistic notion, maintaining that, in practice, interests, needs, problems, and solutions differed in each phase of the cycle, and consequently what a family visitor needed to know and do for young families was not the same as what she needed to do for older families and individuals in later life. They were therefore in favour of a distinct occupational group of trained nurses concentrating on the problems of the elderly while they concentrated on the young.

MEASURES OF HEALTH VISITOR ACTIVITIES

In the nature of things it was not possible for us to check many of the claims which health visitors and doctors made about the former's work and their mutual relationships. In particular, we obtained virtually no information from the recipients of the health visitors' services about how they viewed them or what they thought their role should be. As we have said in Chapter 1 we did not have the resources to explore the work of the Family Health Clinics as we had originally intended to, and only 2 per cent of our sample of home interviewees in 1972 had had any direct contact with a health visitor in the year in question.

However, the health visitors, both before and after the moves to the Health Centre, made detailed, if incomplete, records of the kinds of visiting they undertook over a limited period of time. These records were kept, moreover, by the district-based health visitors lodged in the Health Centre as well as by the practice-attached health visitors. It was, therefore, possible for us to evaluate, if only to a limited extent, some of the claims which the attached visitors made about the nature of their work compared to that of the district-based visitors.

The records for 1972 show no consistent differences between district-based and practice-attached visitors, either in the age of the individuals who were being seen in home visits and in the health visitors' own office, or in the type of questions discussed at the visits. In other words, there was little evidence from the records that the practice-attached health visitors were engaged in a great deal of crisis intervention at the behest of the doctors. The practice-attached visitors, however, appeared to spend rather more of their working hours in home visits and less in administrative duties associated with clinics than did the district-based visitors (see *Table 5*).

Early in 1976, the health visitors kept even more detailed records for us of the families they visited during a three-week period. These showed that there were systematic differences in the visiting patterns of the health visitors situated in different organizational units. However, the differences were not associated with whether or not they were practice-attached or district-based. The visiting patterns of the health visitors attached to the Avesbury group were more like those of the district-based visitors, while those of the Barr group were more like those of the health visitors working with, but more loosely attached to, the smaller practices now occupying the same new practice premises.

A further, more detailed analysis of these data which sought

Table 5   *Percentage distribution of time spent in various activities by health visitors in 1972*

activity	district-based	practice based		
		Avesbury	Barr	Cox and Erickson
	%	%	%	%
home visits	25	35	34	42
clinics and health education	15	11	13	15
all other professional work including case conferences	14	24	17	13
office work	42	24	27	23
miscellaneous	4	6	9	7
total hours = 100%	(7147)	(3227)	(2776)	(1678)

explanations for these variations found that the Avesbury health visitors and the district-based Health Centre visitors were more likely to be visiting 'vulnerable' households than were the Barr- and Cox-Erickson-based workers. In this analysis, we created an index of vulnerability for households based on the presence or absence of six characteristics, including, for example, single parenthood, and an unemployed head (Bedford College 1979). We were not able, however, to explain why the Avesbury and Health Centre visitors had visited a higher proportion of vulnerable households than their counterparts elsewhere. It was not a finding which we had been led to expect from differences in our interviews with the health visitors concerned.

THE GERIATRIC VISITOR

Doctors' views of the role

Unlike the health visitors, the geriatric visitors had no statutorily imposed duty to visit; nor, unlike the district nurses, were they charged by the doctor or hospital to carry out specific nursing procedures. There was, moreover, no nationally based service or recognized occupational career which could guarantee widespread unquestioning acceptance of their work by the population at large and the elderly population in particular. The role had not been created initially by general practitioners or by nurses; it had been the brain-child of medical officers of health, the predecessors of the present community medicine specialists. In detail, it had to be fashioned experimentally by the geriatric visitors themselves.

As with the health visiting service, the Area Health Authority had some district-based geriatric visitors and some attached to local general practices. How did the general practitioners view the role of those attached to their practices?

At first glance, the description of the geriatric visitors' work given to us by the doctors did not seem to differ much from that they had given of health visiting except that the former dealt with the old instead of the young. Their functions, they thought, were to visit patients, mobilize services for them, keep a constant check on their health, and alert the doctor if necessary:

'She's our alarm system and well-equipped by her nursing training for the task.'

Nonetheless, they recognized that fit old people might resent a visit from someone called a geriatric visitor. They would not assume, as most mothers of young children would, that such a person had a duty and a right to call on them. The work therefore called for endless tact, and hence neither nursing qualifications nor health visiting training were sufficient to make a good geriatric visitor. Even health visitors, they said, acknowledged they could not deal unrelievedly with geriatric work. It required a different attitude of mind, an interest in the 'failing organism' as well as special knowledge of services and resources for the elderly. One doctor admitted she thought their job a terrible one, and was extremely grateful there were geriatric visitors who did not think so.

The doctors differed somewhat in their views of how the geriatric visitor's work affected their own. Just over a third saw it as a substitute for it. Were she not there, that is, not attached to their practice, they would again perform much of her work, as they had before her attachment:

'They take the load of social visiting that I used to do and I am jolly grateful. I know they will let me know when I am needed.'

Another third, however, suggested that the geriatric visitor supplemented their own work by arranging services and procuring equipment for the elderly, tasks which they themselves had never had the time to do. The remaining third felt the role was basically complementary, a new one 'serving the community in a unique way'. Among these was Dr Cox who considered that her advent had had 'a marked beneficial effect on his old people' which he noticed when he now visited them. An Avesbury doctor who, with others, regretted that their practices did not have sufficient resources to provide coverage for all the old people on their lists, attempted to pin down the special contribution they made:

'Besides the logistics involved in crisis intervention and in finding aids and equipment, their work is to wave the flag and let the elderly know that somebody knows and cares who, where, and what they are.'

Finally, there was no doubt in the minds of the doctors that the value of a geriatric visitor with nursing qualifications was greatly enhanced by attachment. Commenting on the recent attachment of one such visitor to work with the patients of the three smaller practices, Dr Cox compared the value of her work as he saw it in the before and after situations:

It's so much better than having to get in touch with anonymous persons at the other end of the phone.'

And Dr Bowen at the Barr practice claimed:

'I would find it very difficult now to work in a practice without a geriatric visitor. To me she is perhaps the most valuable of the "paramedics". She probably saves me more work and increases the standard of care of old people more than any other worker does for any group of patients.'

The geriatric visitors' views of their role and of attachment

The six attached geriatric visitors, when questioned about the advantages associated with attachment as against a district-based visiting system for elderly patients, made very much the same points as the health visitors had done. One of them, however, made an additional point which bears upon the size of the practice to which the visitors were attached. It was to the effect that, while gaining from close association with a multi-disciplinary team, they also felt a need to communicate frequently with at least one other member of the same occupational group.

Closer co-operation with the doctors was the main reason why all the attached geriatric visitors were overwhelmingly in favour of attachment. They recognized that working on a non-attached basis could make it easier to become familiar with a district, but they felt that this advantage was far outweighed by the benefits of easy access to the patient's doctor, availability of medical records, and easier liaison with other health personnel. Even if the doctor had to be 'nobbled in the corridor', knowing that he was available for consultation and would shoulder responsibility if necessary seemed to provide them with a feeling of security in work which, some of them acknowledged, was too unstructured and in which they would have liked more authoritative guidelines.

In contrast, the district-based geriatric visitors at the Family Health Clinic, whom we also interviewed, were strongly in favour of non-attachment. They voiced the fear that attachment simply meant greater exploitation by doctors – 'being at their beck and call':

'They can't come up to me at five-thirty and ask me if I can visit so-and-so because they're too busy. I don't mind being part of the service, but I don't want to do a doctor's job.'

With their clients distributed among a large number of general practitioners, relationships between them and the local doctors tended to be distant and communication mainly by telephone. The multiplicity of workers involved and the absence of personal contact, they recognized, called for diplomacy on many occasions; but they still felt the balance lay in favour of a district patch rather than a practitioner's list.

The fear that the geriatric visitor could be exploited by the doctors and less autonomous in arranging her own work was not borne out as far as we could judge by the experience of the attached workers in the two practices. They did not report back on referred cases unless there was good reason to involve a doctor further. Having once referred a patient, the doctors generally left them free to determine their own course of action. Indeed, the attached visitors, rather than complaining of doctor interference, more commonly grumbled about the difficulty in involving the doctors enough. They appreciated joint visits to clients and would have liked to see more communication with and more feedback from the doctors.

We invited the attached geriatric visitors to comment too on aspects of their working relationships with other members of the practice teams and with their clients. It must be said first that, with one exception, the geriatric visitors were not accustomed to analyzing their relationships in the ways in which we asked them to think about them. Although trained nurses, they had not had a health visitor's training, which at least encouraged some analysis of relationships in which they might be involved. They had mostly learned 'on the job'. In so far as the practice setting was concerned, they tended to accept it and to adjust themselves emotionally to it without asking how it should or could be changed.

When pressed, however, two of them were prepared to admit that they were frequently made the recipients of work which others, and especially the social workers, did not want to do, and we detected an element of resentment in this admission. For these two visitors, there was also some recognition that their status with their clients was not as great as they felt it should be or as that of other health workers. They attributed this paradoxically to the need for informality in their relations with old people if they were to fulfil their role of part counselling and part monitoring. As a consequence, they were often not accorded the status and authority of professional workers but were regarded as friends, and they felt somewhat ambivalent about this image. These two geriatric visitors were more career-oriented than the others and, indeed, they left geriatric visiting during the course of the study to train as health visitors. The others appeared to be unconcerned about their occupational status and its image and stressed the intrinsic satisfactions they found in the job of trying to make life worthwhile for their old people.

In contact with their clients, the geriatric visitors felt they had considerable freedom to interpret their role and define its boundaries. One of them described it as concerned with both the social and the medical, but at least one of them was clearly not too pleased to be seen by clients as merely concerned with the former:

'I seem to do a lot of social work. Lots of the clients think we're just social workers. They call me the social welfare lady.'

Another in the same practice said that she regarded herself primarily as a nurse and preferred dealing with the medical side. She, as well as most of the others, felt ill-equipped to deal with frank mental illness and steered clear of such cases if she could:

> 'I once refused a referral, although I found it very difficult to say "no". The social services department tried to refer a depressed person under pensionable age. I happened to know the background of the case and as far as I was concerned what was needed was a GP – it was a medical problem ... the person committed suicide later. Straight mental health problems worry me stiff. Depression – I can't cope with that!'

They felt, however, that they could cope with many confused elderly people, even if the situation proved frustrating and distressing at times. One of the research team who accompanied a geriatric visitor on a visit described a client who had been frequently visited by the geriatric visitor during the previous six months and who did not remember who the geriatric visitor was.

Geriatric visitors' records

The geriatric visitors kept some records of their visits throughout the period of our study, and we examined and analyzed a sample of them in 1972 and again in 1975–76. Like those kept by the health visitors, they were imperfect, but showed that there were differences in the clientele of the geriatric visitors in different organizational settings. These did not always appear to be associated with whether the visitors were district or practice-based. For example, in 1972, the Avesbury group visitor had a considerably higher proportion of clients aged seventy-five years or more than did the Barr attached worker or the district-based geriatric visitors in the Family Health Clinics (83 per cent at the Avesbury compared to only 61 per cent at the Barr and around 70 per cent at the Clinics). The Avesbury visitor averaged about forty visits per week compared to only twenty-nine by the Barr visitor and by those at one clinic and to twenty-six at the other. On the other hand, the Avesbury worker made the smallest number of referrals to agencies other than the general practitioner service itself (2 per cent of all the Avesbury visits resulted in a referral compared with 14 per cent of the Barr's).

The referrals themselves were to a wide range of statutory and voluntary agencies, but, in view of the emphasis which the doctors and visitors themselves had put on the latter's preventive work, we were interested to find that only 1 per cent were to a hospital or audio centre for hearing loss. No referrals were recorded for dental treatment. It was also interesting to discover that only 1 per cent were referred to the incontinence laundry service available in the borough.

Without satisfactory measures of need for preventive and supportive services in the population served, it is, of course, impossible to infer deficiencies in the services given by the visitors to their clientele. Taken at their face value, however, the bare statistics suggest that, at the time, the geriatric visitors were concerned with monitoring an essentially healthy population of elderly people who, at most, required assurance of potential social and medical support should their health deteriorate.

In 1975, there were fewer discernible differences in the visiting patterns at the two practices and we did not examine those of the district-based visitors then. There appeared to be a tendency for the visitors to make fewer but longer visits and to revisit a smaller clientele more frequently. It was not clear, however, whether such changes were a result of a deliberate policy decision and if so where it was taken, or whether they were associated with the change in personnel which had happened at both practices during the study period.

THE RESEARCH TEAM'S ASSESSMENT

In returning to the questions posed at the beginning of this chapter, we felt confident as to how we should answer them. The doctors in these practices saw virtually no difficulties of a professional or personal kind for them in attaching health and geriatric visitors to their practices. The arrangement constituted a very definite plus, not a zero sum. From their point of view, these health workers brought a new dimension, a new capability, to the work centred on general practice. In particular, they enabled the practices, if only marginally, to reach out to potentially vulnerable populations instead of having to play the purely responsive role of waiting for their patients to consult them. The extent to which the practices utilized this new capability, however, was more questionable and a matter to which we return in Chapters 12 and 15.

From the perspectives of the attached health visitors and geriatric visitors, the siting of their work in the practices rather than on a district basis was also regarded as positive. The health

visitors, however, were conscious of the debit side to the arrangements and believed that district-based work must continue alongside practice-based health visiting if the service was to reach all
those who could benefit from their expertise. They were also
aware of the pressures which could be exerted on them by doctors,
given the latter's authority, to engage them in the care of
individuals and families with multiple difficulties, at the expense of
that part of their work which was concerned with the promotion of
healthy ways of living in the general population.

Finally, there was unanimity among doctors and visitors as to
the advantages to be gained from the work of a group of
nurse-trained workers concentrating entirely on the needs of the
elderly, leaving health visitors to deal with those of families in the
earlier phases of the life cycle.

7 General Practitioners and Social Workers

Our two previous chapters have dealt with the relationships which developed between general practitioners and workers who, while having different roles to play in the practice setting, had a nurse's training and a hospital background in common. This last they shared with the general practitioners whose units they were joining as either employed or attached staff. Most of them also shared with the majority of general practitioners in our study a rejection of the hospital as the setting in which they wished to exercise their skills. These shared experiences, albeit from distinct positions, are likely to have given the general practitioners and the nurses who worked with them a feeling of familiarity, of mutually agreed expectations, of fit between each other's work, and hence a sense of security in working together in the general practice setting.

In this chapter we deal with the relationships between the general practitioners and the members of an occupational group who did not share a common background or a set of ready-made mutual expectations of how they should relate to one another. Furthermore, the past history of relationships between the medical and social work professions as a whole had not been smooth and flawless. It is against this general backcloth as well as against a more specific local experience that the relationships which we observed between doctors and social workers must be seen.

CONFUSED EXPECTATIONS – THE LEGACY OF THE PAST

It is probably true to say that until the 1960s the average general practitioner would have had no direct contact during his professional career with anyone calling herself or himself a social worker. He may have known about a person called a hospital or lady almoner who worked in some of the bigger voluntary hospitals, but he was likely to be vague about her duties and to assume, only partly correctly, that she was there merely to help poorer patients whose hospital stay might be causing financial or other difficulties for their families. He would not necessarily be aware that members of this occupational group, in line with their expanding and changing function after the creation of the National Health Service, had officially changed their name to that of medical social worker (Snelling 1954). He might also know that some mental hospitals had a person called a psychiatric social worker whose function it was to obtain information about the social circumstances of patients with mental illness. (Hunnybun 1954; Irvine 1978).

Most general practitioners would also have come across people called duly authorized officers (later mental welfare officers) and know that they had a statutory role to play as guardians of mentally handicapped people in the community. They, as well as families, could call on such people if someone had to be compulsorily removed to a mental hospital (Ministry of Health 1959: 49). The mental welfare officers were often older men who had had experience in the army or police before taking up their duties in the health or welfare departments of local authorities (Jefferys 1965: 26). They would not have had much in common in training or social background with psychiatric or medical social workers, most of whom would be university-trained women.

General practitioners might also be aware that the local authorities, under welfare state legislation (National Assistance Act 1945 and Children's Act 1948), had acquired considerably increased powers and duties to make domiciliary and residential provision for the old and frail, the chronically sick and disabled, the blind and the deaf, and children at risk of neglect, corruption, or cruelty in their own homes. They would also know that a host of different occupational groups under a variety of titles including the words 'visitor', 'social worker', or 'officer' had grown up to deal with the social needs of each such group. At the same time, voluntary associations with household names such as the National Society for the Prevention of Cruelty to Children and the Family Welfare Association continued to function and to employ a mixture of paid and voluntary workers to deal with the special needs of their clients (Jefferys 1965: 248–98). General practitioners could also claim with justice that the general public was likely to be as confused as they were by the multiplicity of workers with varying qualifications and of agencies with broad or narrow social welfare functions.

THE REBIRTH OF SOCIAL WORK AS A UNITED PROFESSION

By the mid-1960s, however, the general practitioner who was considering the possible advantages of group as opposed to single-handed or two-man partnership practice, and of health visitor and district nurse attachments, would probably have begun to be aware that two kinds of parallel moves were afoot in the social welfare field. The first was a move which received an impetus from the Report of the Younghusband Committee in 1959 (Ministry of Health 1959) and the establishment of a Council for Training in Social Work in 1962 (Health Visitor and Social Work Training Act 1962), to bring into existence a basically unified social work profession whose members would share a common basic training much as doctors did, specialize after that common training, and have as assistants those who might or might not train later, but who in the meantime would undertake the more routine or simpler tasks involved in meeting social needs. The second move was designed to simplify the local government structure in which social workers were employed by unifying those departments or parts of departments mainly concerned with meeting needs for personal social support and placing the unified department under the control of a qualified social worker. This latter move was achieved by the creation of social services departments in 1970 (Local Authority Social Services Act 1970) a step which had been recommended in 1968 by the Seebohm Working Party on personal social services (Committee on Local Authority and Allied Personal Social Services 1968).

It would be fair to say that both these moves were greeted with some ambivalence by many members of the medical profession. Those who had complained that the plethora of different occupational titles and welfare agencies made it difficult for them to know to whom to refer patients requiring social help had logically to welcome the simplification involved in both moves. On the other hand, the consolidation of social workers – at least in the statutory social services – in a single department which they themselves controlled meant that they were no longer under the direct aegis of those members of the medical profession who had previously been held responsible for their activities – namely the medical officers of health or the hospital consultants. Indeed, the medical officers of health were facing other challenges to their authority at the same time: community-based nurses were making a bid for self-management and the various forms of environmental control were sliding slowly but surely into the hands of engineers, housing managers, and public analysts in local government (DHSS 1972b: 7). In retrospect, it is not difficult to see that hospital consultants were not in such imminent danger of losing their authority to other occupational groups in the hospital setting; but they disliked arrangements whereby hospital-based social workers were employees of the local authority social services department merely on secondment to the hospital (Local Authority Social Services Act 1970). Such arrangements could be and were interpreted as lessening the authority of the hospital to determine who it could allow to work within its walls and over the work that could be asked of the social workers.

MUTUAL ACCUSATIONS

General practitioners, as independent contractors outside the bureaucracies of hospital and local government, would not have been so directly affected by these challenges to the authority of their profession; but many of them undoubtedly shared a widespread belief that those who called themselves social workers were either untrained 'do-gooders', likely to be fooled by cunning and unscrupulous clients, or alternatively pretentious meddlers with dubious theories of human behaviour who complicated unnecessarily the simple, common-sense task of separating the deserving sheep who needed sympathy from the undeserving goats who merited discipline. This is not in essence far short of the caricature of the social worker drawn by those general practitioners who participated in the Annual Representative Meetings of the BMA, or in that organization's Council when relationships with social workers were discussed (Barnett 1971; *BMJ* 1972: 189).

At the same time, the views commonly expressed by social

workers of the medical professional were no more flattering. They were apt to draw a picture of a profession more concerned to defend its authority and its privileges than to consider the welfare of its patients in the broadest sense (de Gruchy 1970; Huws Jones 1971: 14). It was seen, moreover, as putting obstacles in the way of developing a genuinely egalitarian sense of teamwork and common purpose by emphasizing such contingency issues as leadership and confidentiality, issues which, given goodwill and trust, could be easily overcome (Committee on Local Authority and Allied Personal Social Services 1968: 199, 214).

AN EXPERIMENTAL *RAPPROCHEMENT*

Professions are not, however, monolithic bodies composed of individuals who share all the beliefs which broadly characterize the profession at a particular epoch. During the 1960s, there were some general practitioners who recognized that many of their patients faced social or psychological difficulties occasioned by a life event such as a bereavement, or by more persistent disturbed family relationships, or inappropriate life styles, and who felt that these patients might be more effectively helped were they to have direct assistance from a social worker closely associated with them. Similarly, there were some social workers who saw general practice as a setting from which they might be able to work more effectively. This was so because, they argued, many of those requiring social services presented first or only on the general practitioner's premises and because social stigma was less likely to attach to a referral to a social worker situated there than to one in a labelled social work agency, which could be associated with poverty and charity.

As a result a number of general practitioners and social workers in various parts of the country began to find ways of working together. Their arrangements were not experiments in the strict scientific sense of that word, but they gave the general practitioners and social workers concerned the opportunity to explore the problems which might arise in closer working and ways of sorting them out to their mutual satisfaction. Some of these experiences were reported in books and periodicals (Collins 1965; Forman and Fairbairn 1968; McCullough and Brown 1969; Brandon 1969; Goldberg and Neill 1972; Ratoff, Rose, and Smith 1974).

One of the first general practice units to provide facilities for a social worker within their premises was the Avesbury practice. A charitable trust in 1966 agreed to pay the salary for a period of four years of a social worker who had had previous experience in a voluntary family welfare agency. It also agreed to support a research worker employed in a national institute concerned with social work to help describe and analyze the experience.

By common consent, the experiment was deemed a success and when it was over the Avesbury doctors asked the local authority social services department to second one of their staff to work from their premises with their patients. After some negotiation, in which the Barr practice also joined, the local authority agreed that one of their social workers should work half-time at the Avesbury and half-time with the Barr. This was the situation when our study began. Five years later, this social worker had resigned and her place had been filled by two social workers each working part-time at one of the practices and part-time in one of the local authority's social services department's area offices.

AVESBURY DOCTORS – THE PIONEERS OF SOCIAL
WORKER ATTACHMENTS

As members of a group which had pioneered the idea of social worker attachment to general practice, the Avesbury doctors not unnaturally adopted a rather proprietary stance when asked to discuss the work of their attached social worker. They felt that, together with Jane Atkin, the first social worker to be with them, and her research colleagues, they had virtually invented the idea and mapped out a suitable role for an attached social worker. Briefly, it was, first, to provide a consultative or diagnostic assessment service on psycho-social problems for doctors and other practice workers: second, to undertake short-term crisis intervention and counselling: third, to liaise with external social service agencies. They had been led by Jane Atkin to accept that they could not refer all those patients needing material help or long-term social support to her, and they conscientiously refrained from doing so with her successor, Margaret Dalby. Such patients were referred directly to the area office of the social services department.

There was no doubt in the minds of any of the Avesbury doctors that having a social worker attached to them was a success. They did not feel that she abused any confidences they placed in her or that she challenged their own sense of professional security. The gains were variously described. Dr Adair mentioned that she was particularly useful in what she termed 'the grieving business', or when people's lives had been upset and they could not see a way forward. The social worker could spend an hour with each patient and achieve much more than a doctor with his seven-minute consultation. But it was not only that she had time on her side: she also had 'things at her fingertips to enrich people's lives'. Another doctor believed it was her presence on the doctor's territory which made her advice and help acceptable to some patients who would never consider seeking help from a local authority or voluntary welfare agency because they would see it as stigmatizing.

Despite their commitment to a social work attachment to their practice, the comparisons most Avesbury doctors drew between the three social workers who at one time or another had held such a position indicated that they tended to regard its usefulness as variable, depending on who filled the post. The individual who received most praise was described as 'someone special', someone whose contribution to patient care was beyond that which they felt they could themselves make. 'She's just too good,' said Dr Amery, 'she is psychologically as well as socially trained in a way doctors aren't.' He confessed she alone of the social workers had not made him feel competitive. We attributed the particularly favourable comments the doctors made about her to her ability to increase their sense of security by conveying to them that she knew what her role and its boundary with medicine were. Her strengths were variously described as 'not leaving situations open-ended', as 'not mucking about', as coping well in a 'very difficult psychothera-peutic area,' as 'keeping us well-informed'. By implication, other social workers had not possessed these abilities, at least in the same measure. The selection of these specific qualities to praise may say something about general practitioners' needs for positive help rather than for a magnification of the uncertainties inherent in their work.

That this last interpretation may not be far off the mark was also evidenced by the comments of some of the Avesbury practitioners about the local authority social services department in general. One of them suggested that in separating themselves from the health services they were seeking to build their own empire and had 'put themselves out on a limb'. Another was critical of the policy which had led to the replacement of specialist social workers, such as psychiatric social workers, child care officers, and blind welfare visitors by generic workers with responsibility in a geographic area for meeting all kinds of social needs, whatever their origins or the characteristics of the client. Two or three of the Avesbury partners particularly regretted the passing of the mental health officer, who they felt had been a great strength in helping them handle seriously disturbed patients. Today they alleged they were frequently as concerned for the safety of the young inexperienced social worker called to certify an involuntary admission to hospital as they were for the welfare of the patient. And Dr Amery, who was medical adviser to an old people's home, was angry at what he saw happening there and attributed it to the social services rather than the health services:

> 'The social services have fallen flat on their face and will have to re-examine their role in the care of the elderly. They are arrogant and full of anti-professionalism while the care of the elderly in the Home has become horrendous.'

Nevertheless, despite these criticisms, the Avesbury doctors frequently referred patients directly to the local social services office. A part-time social worker providing a mainly consultative service, they said, could not possibly cope with all the needs of their patients. Those referred directly to the local office were generally patients already known to the social services, those with material needs only or those with a multitude of problems requiring lengthy sorting out. Given their understanding with their own social worker they would only occasionally first discuss with her the advisability of the referral.

THE BARR DOCTORS – A CASE STUDY IN AMBIVALENCE

Six years after the part-time attachment of a social worker to their practice, all the Barr doctors expressed some reservations about social work or uncertainty about its place in general practice. None of them was opposed to an attachment and all of them were able to point to at least one advantage of such an arrangement; but to varying degrees and for varying reasons their views displayed less than total enthusiasm. What were the reasons they gave for their somewhat ambivalent stance?

The arguments for the attachment of a social worker given by the Barr practice doctors resembled those of the Avesbury doctors. Basically, they preferred to refer patients to a known individual with a room in the same building as themselves than to an unnamed, and hence impersonal, source in an area social services department. Dr Balfour made the point that the latter course risked her losing touch with what was happening to the patient:

> 'Of all workers, the social worker in the area office is perhaps the most autonomous. When she is looking after a patient, we have very little contact. Liaison between us is poor.'

Nevertheless, none of the Barr doctors expressed the hostility to social services departments that several of the Avesbury doctors had voiced. Two even maintained that they had good relations with individual workers in the local area offices, having attended case conferences there.

Where doubts were expressed about social work they seemed to us to stem more centrally from the fuzziness of the boundary between their own work and that of the social worker. All of them acknowledged that since they were themselves committed to counselling their patients on emotional problems originating in their social relationships, there was bound to be some overlap between their work and that of the social worker. To Dr Bennett the overlap was large but did not matter much:

> 'It's difficult to work out our boundaries but it doesn't matter much if we go over the same ground. Different facets of our patients' problems and personalities are brought to light.'

But for others, the absence of a clear-cut distinction between their own skills and that of the social worker, in an area in which they claimed some expertise, may have created unease. One frankly acknowledged an element of competition: 'I don't think doctors should give it all over to them.' Psycho-social counselling was one of the most rewarding aspects of his own work which he did not want to lose.

Two recognized an area of social work expertise not shared by doctors, mobilization of social resources or, as they put it, the social component of social work:

> 'Besides discussing problems with her, she helps people over crises by arranging financial help, finding accommodation, helping them cope with problems ranging from handicapped children to pregnancy terminations.'

It was for these sorts of practical help that the two mainly referred, although one of them wondered whether in providing practical help social workers might not do more harm than good. 'Might not patients,' she speculated, 'eventually sort out those aspects of their lives themselves?' She seemed to be wondering whether social work might not create an undesirable social dependency on the part of its recipients. She recognized that medicine too might create dependency in its patients (see Chapter 12); but perhaps for her dependence on chemo- or psychotherapy dispensed by an independent medical practitioner was more defensible than dependence for material support on a social worker as an agent of the state.

At the same time, and not without paradox, the Barr doctors were pleased that the second social worker to be attached to their practice was prepared, unlike her predecessor, to become involved with patients on a long-term, not merely a crisis, basis. This kind of help from someone who obviously liked carrying people was what they looked for from a social worker. Working with her helped to lighten the burden of caring for the long-term dependent or of maintaining difficult and disturbed patients in the community.

THE VIEWS OF DOCTORS WITHOUT ATTACHED SOCIAL WORKERS

None of the doctors in the smaller practices had had the experience of working with an attached social worker. One of them would have liked such an attachment: the other three were not pressing for one. Dr Erickson had, however, secured the voluntary help of a marriage guidance counsellor and was enthusiastic about the work which such an individual could do from a general practice setting. When he and Dr Edmunds moved to premises shared with Dr Cox and Dr Osmond, the latter two were also able to utilize the counsellor's services on behalf of their patients. We were unfortunately not able to explore reactions to her work either with the doctors or with her.

In the absence of an attached social worker, Dr Erickson and his partner Dr Edmunds referred all the patients with social difficulties to their attached health visitor, relying on her to contact the social services department where necessary. They were happy with this arrangement and claimed the health visitor was too. Dr Osmond dealt directly with the social services, an experience which was not always a happy one. Nevertheless, if he were to be offered an attachment, he thought he would not want to complicate his practice organization further by accepting it. It was Dr Cox who would welcome an attachment as a way out of the complications he currently faced. These are worth quoting at some length:

'The day of contacting the individual social worker is long gone. As I earlier explained, if we wish to contact a district nurse, we have to do so at one of two offices. If we need a social worker, there are five offices and it depends where the client – not now the patient – lives. Not only do we not contact the individual worker we happen to have got to know in one of the five offices, we contact the intake team, the people in which are always different. They then decide whether it is going to be a short case to be dealt with by the intake team or a long case, in which case they will assign the client to another social worker. Eventually the client has his or her social worker and will see that social worker each time, which, provided the social worker doesn't leave, is a good thing. But it has become very difficult for the doctor to get in touch with the social worker to find out what has happened to the patient. Generally, when the doctor is not involved in surgeries, the social worker is out or at a case conference.'

Like the Avesbury doctors, the smaller practice doctors regretted the disappearance of specialist workers and their replacement by generic workers. 'We're now dealing with people who haven't the same expertise in child care or acute mental illness as they used to have.' Moreover, they felt that some of the statutory powers of the social worker should rightly belong with other workers. Dr Cox again:

'A geriatric visitor had for many years been visiting an old lady who was a patient of mine. The day came when the geriatric visitor thought and I agreed that the old lady could no longer look after herself and would benefit from Part III accommodation. The geriatric visitor could not make the application for this accommodation herself; she had to get a social worker who had never known the lady to do it. I think this is quite wrong; the geriatric visitor should have the power to handle such matters.'

THE SOCIAL WORKERS' VIEWS OF THEIR OWN WORK AND THAT OF OTHERS

When the study started, the sole social worker, Margaret Dalby, had been attached to the two group practices for two years and remained there for a further three. Joan Audrey and Mary Bancroft, who replaced Margaret Dalby, the first to work part-time with the Avesbury and the second part-time with the Barr, had been with the practices for approximately a year-and-a-half when the study ended. Our data come from these three social workers.

The main objective of their work according to all three attached social workers, and expressed in the words of one of them, was 'to help people to modify their behaviour – to look at what they are doing'. This involved them in three overlapping functions: first, diagnosis and assessment; second, casework, that is the process of helping the client to gain insight into her or his own behaviour; and third, the mobilization of resources on behalf of the client.

There was, they acknowledged, some overlap too between their functions and those of other workers in the primary care field. They had no difficulty in distinguishing their expertise and contribution from those of others; but they were less sure that others always saw the differences as they did. In their view, the differences related, first, to the breadth and depth of understanding of human behaviour; second, to the approach to clients' problems; and third, to the techniques of management, including knowledge of the resources available and how to obtain access to them. These were more important than the statutory powers which they alone possessed to deal with certain kinds of problems such as the taking of children into care.

Dealing with each of these distinctions in turn, the social

workers recognized that their expertise was confined to a more limited area of human needs than that of doctors, nurses, and health visitors. Comparing themselves with general practitioners, for example, Ms Audrey said:

'There is considerable overlap in that we are both trying to see what the problem is, but obviously they are more oriented to physical problems than I am. Theirs is a much wider spectrum. They try to make a whole diagnosis including the psycho-social and psychiatric aspects, aspects of the area in which I work. Compared to theirs, mine is a relatively small area.'

They claimed, however, that because the whole of the social work field was only a part of that of others, their knowledge and expertise in it was more profound. What others referred to as 'the grey area of psycho-social problems' was for them the focus of their work: 'somewhat less grey, more in relief'. Within that area, their own exploration of the problems went considerably 'deeper' than that of other workers. They tried to 'break down' the problems and identify and deal with their strands and elements, 'get the client to focus on them one at a time'. Rather than deal with 'global' conditions such as depression, or even with their manifest causes, the social worker's task was:

'to help people work out what is happening to them and to understand the relationship between their feelings and their difficulties – whatever they are – in the different areas of their lives; in short, to help them work through their problems.'

Working through problems and helping clients towards greater insight, fortitude, and self-dependence was, they felt, the hallmark of their profession. Contrasting social work treatment with that provided by doctors, one put it this way:

'They have all sorts of treatments which I haven't got. I've only the relationship to work on. The relationship is obviously a part of their work too; but they have drugs and a lot more referral agencies that can help in their treatments.'

Then again, they argued that their style of working was less 'interventionist' than that of the doctors. The latter they suggested handed out advice and suggested steps that might be taken and, coming from them, it was often acceptable: they could be and were much more directive than social workers. Social workers, however, believed in the therapeutic value of allowing clients to make their own decisions, to plan their own way forward. Acknowledging that health visitors also adopted a non-directive style, the social workers maintained that they did so 'less penetratingly'. Health visitors or geriatric visitors' relationships with their clients were usually on-going and supportive. In times of crisis they used the relationship to show they cared and to ease the family burden in practical ways. However, while they might gently encourage change, they did not, as social workers did, attempt radical modification or reconstruction of behaviour patterns.

It was, in their view, in the mobilization of social resources that there was least overlap between their work and that of others, and in particular of doctors. It was a social work function, they claimed, to apply for aids which made life more tolerable for the chronic sick and disabled, such as a telephone for a housebound angina sufferer. They too could try to secure rent rebates and heating allowances for partially sighted and other handicapped people. It was they who would arrange for a patient recovering from a mastectomy to have a recuperative holiday, secure a nursery place for a child whose mother was under strain or in poor housing, make an application for an educational grant for a would-be student, or find somewhere to live for a homeless person. Much of this aspect of their work consisted of 'liaising with other agencies or helping clients to contact them', a job for which they had been trained while others had not.

All three social workers compared their own attached role in general practice to that of a social worker in an 'intake' team in an area social services department office, as that role had developed since 1970. Like intake team workers they were to receive clients, assess their difficulties, and provide short-term or 'crisis' intervention if that was judged to be all that was required. If more was wanted they had to refer their clients to others for long-term support. At the Avesbury practice it worked out that way. At the Barr practice, after the arrival of their second attached social worker, Mary Bancroft, it tended to have more of an element of long-term supportive as well as intake work.

THE PRACTICES COMPARED

Towards convergence

Although attached to the two practices, Ms Dalby, the first attached local authority social worker, said that until the move to the Health Centre she had felt herself 'more an Avesbury than a Barr person'. She was housed in the Avesbury practice premises as was her secretary who was still financed by a research fund project: 'I am the only worker in either practice with a personal secretary and personal phone.' She felt that this was one reason why she tended to identify more with the Avesbury and less with the Barr. There was no permanent accommodation for her at the Barr practice and her sessions there were conducted in a doctor's consulting room. Boxing and coxing in this way provided little opportunity for meeting the partners.

Another and more important reason, however, was the way in which the two groups viewed the role and related to her. At the Avesbury practice, where the role was established before her arrival, the doctors' conceptions of it accorded well with her own. They referred to her for her opinion or for intensive treatment, practical help or referral to another agency, or for a combination of all three reasons. They did not attempt to use her as a substitute for long-term care available at the local social services department or elsewhere.

Initially this was not the case at the Barr practice. That practice, she thought, had asked for a social worker attachment for two main reasons: first, so as not to miss out on a scheme which, from all that they had heard, was a success, and second, to help them deal with patients with chronic social problems for whom, without an attached social worker, they would have sought external help. Two years later, and before the move to the Health Centre, Barr doctors, she believed, still viewed her role as an 'aid to containment'; she had not convinced them that 'her approach to its use was the best'.

Although allocating the same number of sessions to each practice, she received considerably fewer referrals from the Barr doctors than from the Avesbury, and more of them were for long-term support (see p. 153). Moreover, whereas there was little difference between the referral rates of individual Avesbury doctors, referrals from two Barr doctors, both amongst the youngest, accounted for half her Barr practice caseload. The older Barr doctors not only referred less and mainly for practical help, but 'communication with them tended to break down' whenever she entered 'the psychotherapeutic process'. She found it difficult and frustrating to 'compartmentalize' herself and offer only practical help. As she put it, she was unable with their patients 'to fully fulfil' her function.

There were differences too in her status at the two practices. Avesbury doctors, she felt, viewed her as a colleague. Their referrals to her were 'lateral', to someone with skills different but equal to their own. At the Barr practice her position was somewhat 'nebulous'. She could not quite define it. Her appointment had, however, brought about some general restructuring of relationships in that practice. The fairly rigid division between the doctors and the other professional staff, symbolized in the use of surnames, began to give way when the Barr doctors, following the Avesbury example, called her 'Margaret' from the start. Thereafter, they addressed their health and geriatric visitors by first name with the tacit invitation, not always accepted, to reciprocate.

Once in the Centre, her relationship with the Barr doctors improved. In part she attributed the change to the location of her offices in the new building. It was neutral territory not within that part of the premises allocated to either practice. Moreover, she was now as available to Barr as to Avesbury doctors and doctors at each were equally accessible to her. But most important in the 'levelling process' was the change in Barr doctor attitudes which she thought had not so much to do with the move *per se* as, following the move, with her attendance at their weekly meetings devoted to the discussion of patients' psycho-social problems. At these meetings the practice psychiatrist frequently involved her in the discussion and recommended referrals to her for assessment or casework. He both made the doctors aware of 'the social work potential' in their midst and endorsed her definition of the role. The change in doctor attitudes increased the scope of her role and improved her standing at the Barr practice, bringing it more into line with her position at the Avesbury. Because she had her own office and because of the convergence of her role at the two practices she came to see herself as 'one cell in a large unit', rather than as a member of two group practices:

'I have a full-time job instead of two part-time ones. I am a social worker in a large organization and sometimes forget which practice referred the patient.'

Nevertheless, as sole representative of her profession surrounded by relatively large numbers of members of other occupations she began in time to feel increasingly isolated: 'virtually out on a disciplinary limb'. Although she enjoyed the job and gained a great deal from it, she began to feel she needed 'to re-stoke her social work self and skills'; with this in view she left the job for one in a local authority area office.

Renewed divergence: short-term intervention at the Avesbury

The decision to replace Margaret Dalby with two workers each working part-time at the Health Centre and part-time in a local authority area office seems to have been influenced by her experience of isolation. It was based too on the argument that workers attached to general practice needed to have first-hand knowledge of community services and resources and be well acquainted with the personnel administering them.

Joan Audrey who joined the Avesbury practice found it very much to her liking. It suited her way of working and gave her as much freedom to work in her own way as she could find anywhere. When she first joined the prctice the level of the responsibilities doctors transferred to her had caused her considerable anxiety. She was unused to it for, at the area office, she was answerable to someone higher up than her in the hierarchy. As she became familiar with the work at the practice and more confident of her contribution to it, she found she liked responsibility:

'I think it is good that I am left to handle the problems they refer to me in my own way. I couldn't now imagine working here in any other way.'

Once problems were referred to her, responsibility for dealing with them was entirely hers:

'You are not directly answerable to anyone and don't get the feeling that you have to tell the doctors or anyone else what you are doing. Yet you know the doctors carry on with the medical care and are always there for the patient.'

She especially valued the practice policy decision, taken well before her time, not to refer to her people whose problems went on for ever and ever or those who, if sent away for a week to sort themselves out, would get better without any intervention at all. She had always preferred short-term work. She had never been happy doing long-term work: 'staying with a family for years and years and becoming part of its way of coping instead of a resource for problem solving'. Her style was to set goals and, as far as possible, decide in advance how much work was needed. She would say to a client: 'Let's give ourselves three, four, six interviews and see how it goes.' Setting limits helped even those with chronic problems to focus their minds and frequently brought unexpected results:

'There are people with lots of problems. I help them with specific areas and tell them to come back if they need more help or even say "Come back in three months' time when we will look at another of your difficulties."'

Such short-term 'contract' work was justifiable if there was a 'really open-door policy' and people knew a 'closed case' did not mean they would not be seen again.

Problems referred to her at the practice were mainly depressions, anxiety states, and other kinds of psychological and emotional problems, with just a trickle of practical problems, a rather different mix from her caseload at the area office. The doctors generally invited her to meet the patient in their consulting room. The latter, therefore, usually had a clear understanding of what it was she was to help them with and, she believed, rarely failed appointments. She liked this specificity in regard to the referral. Talking about one of the Avesbury doctors she summed it up:

'He knows exactly what he wants from a social worker. He rarely wants assessment. He has generally weighed it up for himself and decided a specific type of help is needed – marital help, help to separate or reach another kind of decision.'

Lastly, she liked the general atmosphere in the practice which enabled everyone to participate in decisions:

'As an organization the Avesbury is pretty democratic. Obviously, the doctors carry more weight in decision-making.

They are always involved in decisions, whereas everybody else is selectively involved. But everyone contributes what information they can.'

Ambivalence at the Barr

Mary Bancroft, who replaced Margaret Dalby at the Barr, did so in part because she wanted to 'fly the flag for area social workers', feeling somehow that doctors maligned them and thought more highly of those social workers more closely identified with psychiatric and medical services. A job split between community and general practice seemed the right vehicle to achieve this objective. However, after eighteen months in the post she felt that, although she was accepted and appreciated by the doctors, she had made little impact on their views of area-based social workers. In *accepting* her, the doctors at the practice also *excepted* her. They would say: 'Oh yes, you will do that, but they don't do it at the area office.' Her cause was not helped by the area office's not infrequent inability, because of pressure of work, to respond promptly to requests made to them:

'When I have persuaded doctors to refer to the area, they have to wait and wait for the matter to be dealt with.'

Nor could she persuade the doctors to attend case conferences as often as she would have liked, although they were quite good about doing so if the conference was at the Centre. Of late, however, she was less sure about the necessity for conferences:

'At first I used to think: "We've got to talk about it." My discipline requires that we sit and talk and talk. When I think about it, we do love talking. Doctors don't.'

There was a real need, she felt, for more sharing of responsibility in the community as it was shared in the practice. In the community, decisions such as whether or not a child should go into care were frequently left to the social worker with doctor and health visitor simply nodding: 'It's up to you, ducky.'

Competition

Ms Bancroft believed that, especially when she first joined the practice, there had been an element of competition between her and some of the doctors as to 'who had the best magic wand'.

There had been no discussion with the doctors about her role or clarification of her function. She had anticipated that her practice caseload would be made up predominantly of short-term clients, but in practice this had not been the case. Initially, at any rate, the doctors referred few patients to her and most were patients who, had she not been there, would have been referred for long-term support or for practical aids to the area office. They seemed to want to give as much help to patients within the practice as they could. Even after eighteen months when, either because she was too busy or thought a problem might be better dealt with elsewhere, she recommended a referral to the area office, the doctors were likely to say: 'Oh no, we don't want to do that. If you can't take him, we'll leave it for a bit.'

It was some time before they referred patients to her who needed psycho-social help to tide them over crises, since the doctors saw it as part of their own role to help such patients. A few, however, when really hard pressed themselves, used her to ease the pressure on them:

'It had very much to do with what they had on their plate at the moment. When there was a crisis – someone wanting to be seen immediately and no doctor available – it was over to me.'

She also recollected a doctor referring a patient to her and then actually taking him back saying:

'I think I can deal with it now.'

She was, however, very prepared to acknowledge that the slow initial rate of referrals was due to a correspondingly slow build-up of doctor confidence in her. She admitted that she may at first have tried too hard to assert her professional authority, to establish the way she would work in the practice. She recalled attempting a firm stand:

'Dr X thought the problem should be handled one way, I, another. I felt I was being told, "This is what I want you to do." It may have been that I was new, but basically I was not going to do anything I didn't think was in the client's interest.'

She did not see the patient again. Dr X and a health visitor dealt with the problem as they thought fit.

A year after her arrival, however, she felt that all the doctors were involving her in patient care in ways which were helpful to the patients and gratifying to her. They were recognizing her skills and utilizing them. She no longer had time on her hands. A doctor would say: 'I am referring so-and-so to you. I think there is something going on which I cannot get to. Could you find out what it is?' And frequently she did. Or she would receive a referral note such as the following:

'I would be grateful for your help with this rather lonely isolated girl who I've always found it difficult to communicate with. The problem is ambivalence re pregnancy termination.'

Having gained the doctors' confidence, however, she was not certain she wanted as much responsibility as they were then prepared to give her. She would have liked 'more sharing' – opportunities to voice her anxieties; and she wished that, when she voiced them, the doctors would not merely blandly reassure her with, 'We think you're doing fine.' They seemed fairly sure she was coping and would scream if anything went terribly wrong. From time to time they asked how *their* patients were getting on; so she assumed that, at the back of their minds, they believed they had final responsibility for the patients.

Finally, Ms Bancroft recognized her own part in carrying a larger proportion of long-term patients in her caseload than her counterpart at the Avesbury. She confessed to difficulty in establishing therapeutic relationships which did not entail 'transference' or strong patient attachment to her:

'So many people in the vulnerable state in which they come, share so much with you that it is very difficult to detach them, and perhaps I don't leave enough time in a session to deal with that.'

She felt too that there were some people who interpreted a limited contract as a reflection of their effect on others: 'Am I so awful that she can't bear to see me more than three times?' There was also the problem of new material emerging towards the end of a contract. She was not under any obligation to extend the contract, but mostly she did. One of her difficulties was not being able to discipline herself to say 'no'. Furthermore, while all forms of social work were stressful for her, seeing new people all the time, as she had to do in short-term work, was particularly so.

Again problems might, in the course of treatment, manifest themselves as more complex and deep-rooted and as needing more time than at first appeared. She felt that in such instances she should be referring elsewhere; but often patients did not want to be referred; nor, she reiterated, did their doctors want it. Even were she to overcome doctor and patient reluctance to seek outside help, it was not always possible to procure the kind of help needed, so she would end up thinking 'What have they got if they don't come here?'

SOCIAL WORK RECORDS

In addition to interviewing doctors and social workers, members of the research team were able to observe their interaction in practice meetings and to analyze the records which the social workers kept of the clients they saw in the course of twelve months in 1972–73 and 1975–76. We asked the home interviewees whether they had had any services from an attached social worker during the year prior to the interview. Not surprisingly given the small number of people the part-time workers saw each week, none of them had. We did not approach any of the patients they had seen to see how they felt about the service.

Our observations at the practice meetings did not contradict anything we had been told by the doctors and social workers themselves. Their exchanges were cordial throughout and, as time went on, the social worker who had half-time appointments in both practices appeared to be more at ease in the Barr group meetings. Like her, we saw the consultant psychiatrist as an important agent in securing a change of attitude towards her from the majority of previously polite, but rather distant doctors. Her replacement towards the end of our study had also to work herself into the group before her contributions began to be valued. At the Avesbury, the interchanges were much less formal, in keeping with the practice's style, and the second social worker was quickly drawn into the proceedings.

The records too in general confirmed the picture that the social workers and doctors had given us of the clients referred to the former. For example, in both 1973 and 1976, the Avesbury doctors referred more patients than did the Barr. In both cases, however, the numbers who were accepted by the social workers as clients (that is, who had a file opened and at least one service proffered) was very small. For example, the average monthly rate in 1976 at the Avesbury was 12.6 new clients and at the Barr only 4.2. A few of these individuals, fewer than we had been led to expect by the social workers themselves, were referred by a non-medically qualified member of the team, especially at the Barr. The number of referrals from particular doctors also confirmed that, although all the Avesbury doctors referred with about the same frequency, some of the Barr doctors made very few referrals in 1973. By 1976, the spread of referrals had become more even. The records also indicated that, contrary to Ms Audrey's own impressions, a not inconsiderable number of those referred to her by Avesbury doctors failed to keep the appointment (15 per cent, according to our calculations in 1976).

Unlike general practitioners, social workers, in assessing their work output, generally discuss the size and character of what they call their caseload (Holme and Maizels 1978: 125). This can be variously defined, and analyses make little sense unless it is clear what is referred to when the term is used. The analysis which we made was of the clients who were served by a social worker at least once in two twelve-month periods during 1972–73 and 1975–76. We do not claim that it adds much to the picture built up for us by the social workers themselves. The analysis showed that the majority (two-thirds at the Barr and three-quarters at the Avesbury) were women. Ninety per cent were first-time referrals during the year. They were more likely to be single, divorced, or widowed than the population of the borough in 1971 and less likely to be currently married. The Barr social workers' clientele in 1976 were more likely than the Avesbury clients to have been referred with practical problems and other difficulties associated with long-term illness and anxiety. The latter were more likely to be thought to have personality or relationship problems. They were also more likely to be middle class.

THE RESEARCH TEAM'S ASSESSMENT

We began this chapter by drawing attention to the differences between the historical relationships which the medical profession had had with nurse-based professions on the one hand and with the social work profession on the other. Our interviews and our observations in the group practice settings suggested that, despite differences in approach and background and in the cultures of medicine and social work (Huntington 1981: 1), the practitioners in the group practices had learnt to work with social workers and to value the help they gave to patients.

Appreciation of their services was more marked at the Avesbury than at the Barr practice. The Avesbury partners had been pioneers in attaching a social worker to their practice and had a commitment to multi-professional teamwork based on general practice. They needed it to succeed and in their eyes it had. Nevertheless, the unflattering comments about social work outside general practice from some of the partners indicated that for them, at the general level, tensions of a kind still existed between the two professions. Their social worker, rather than social workers in general, had passed the test.

The Barr doctors also displayed some ambivalence to social work in general. They wanted an attached social worker to enable them to contain the total care of their patients within the practice. To begin with, except at times of great pressure, they did not want a social worker to form an intense therapeutic relationship with a patient which would supplant or even supplement their own. The social worker, it seemed to us, was seen as a possible competitor in an area of professional expertise which they wished to retain and develop. They later modified this position, but in our view some of them remained ambivalent to the end.

Each social worker was aware that, initially, she had been under scrutiny. As time went on all of them, to varying degrees, felt that good relationships and mutual trust had developed between them and most of the doctors. They were able, despite being situated in a doctor-controlled environment, to do work which they found professionally satisfying and which gave them as much autonomy as they wanted. It may even have enhanced their opportunities for successful work with clients.

Nevertheless, both doctors and social workers were aware of some continuing inherent tensions and dilemmas not only for them but for the patients referred to the social workers. A doctor who decided to refer a patient could give that individual the impression of 'passing him or her on', to a professional person whose work in the recent past, if not in the present, was associated with poverty or delinquency. It might have taken the doctor time to establish the true nature of the patient's problem and in the process a relationship could have been built up between them. The doctor might then he loath to withdraw and allow another worker to take over. Moreover, to the patient a referral might imply that the doctor rejected him or her as an unacceptable person. In short, referral to social workers for psychotherapeutic casework, albeit within a primary care team, is a delicate process, easily hindered by misconception or lack of understanding on the part of any of the individuals involved.

8 General Practitioners, Receptionists, and Administrative Staff

Sir John Brotherston, one-time Professor of Social Medicine at the University of Edinburgh, described general practice in the immediate post-war years as still basically a cottage industry (Brotherston 1967). With few exceptions, general practitioners at the formation of the National Health Service essentially ran small family businesses in more senses than one. Not only did they purport to provide services *for* families; they also involved members *of* their *own* families in the running of their practices.

Most general practitioners practised from their homes and relied on their wives to receive patients, take messages, chaperon female patients, and protect them from excessive demands on their time and energy. Wives were often responsible too for the small amount of secretarial work, book-keeping and form-filling which the business entailed (Lewis 1955; Cardew 1964). The exceptions to this pattern were likely to be the very successful men who combined general practice with quasi-specialist consulting and those in industrial towns who practised from shops or commercial premises close to their working-class patients rather than in their homes (PEP 1937: 143). The latter often had difficulties in earning a reasonable living and would not ordinarily employ anyone to perform the receptionist or nursing duties which, were they practising from their homes, would in all probability be carried out by their wives (Inter-departmental Committee on the Remuneration of General Practitioners 1946). They could genuinely be described as single-handed, although they might still call upon their wives at least to answer the telephone and keep track of payments made to them.

The correspondence columns of the medical weeklies and the reports of the British Medical Association's annual representative meetings suggest why, during the 1950s and 1960s, general practice was becoming less commonly a family business and more commonly an embryonic association of formal business partners, employing others to do work previously done by wives. First, general practitioners were becoming aware of a general trend to a shorter working week and may have felt that it would be easier to achieve for themselves, were they to separate the locations of their professional and domestic lives (Subsachs 1960; Finnerty 1961). Second, more employment opportunities were developing for women, and wives may have begun to resent the assumption, accepted by their predecessors, that by marrying a general practitioner they automatically became an unwaged assistant (Lewis 1955; Rolfe 1956). Third, partnerships were increasingly between equals who may have tried to avoid possible conflicts involving family members by, in terms of an old cliché, 'not mixing business with pleasure'. Fourth, despite the picture which general practitioners liked to paint of their impoverishment, the National Health Service had given them a guaranteed income which enabled them to pay for some ancillary staff (Titmuss 1958: 159).

As we have pointed out in Chapter 5, it is likely that the helper employed by the single-handed general practitioner in the early days of the National Health Service was expected to play the undifferentiated role of helpmeet to the doctor, much as a wife had done for his predecessor. Wives not infrequently had nursing experience of some kind and anecdotal accounts suggest that this was also true for a good many of the paid receptionists who began to be employed in increasing numbers in the 1950s and 1960s. Indeed, working as a doctor's receptionist on a part-time basis might well have been regarded as suitable employment for married women with nursing experience who did not wish to accept the full-time hospital posts which were still commonly the only health-related jobs available to them. In this connection it was interesting to note that, before their move to the Health Centre, one of the Barr practice's receptionists was a nurse. The move to enlarged premises with a purpose-built nursing area enabled her to function thereafter entirely as a nurse and to give up her receptionist duties.

Cartwright found that by 1964 just over three-quarters of all general practitioners worked in practices which employed at least a secretary or a receptionist (Cartwright 1967: 159). The proportion was much higher, as one would expect, among doctors who worked in groups. It was the single-handed practitioner who was the most likely to have no help of any kind. A further boost to the employment of individuals who would act as receptionists, record clerks, and secretaries came in 1966. Implementing the Family Doctors' Charter, provision was made for general practitioners to reclaim 70 per cent of the salaries paid to such staff (Review Body 1966). The practitioners were also encouraged with an additional allowance to form a group practice, a unit which would be large enough to employ several workers with differentiated tasks such as reception work, record filing, typing, fixing of rotas, and the management of premises. Such units would give doctors the opportunity, if they so wished, to delegate some of their managerial functions for staff and premises to those employed specifically to manage, instead of having to fulfil these functions themselves.

RECEPTIONISTS' GROWING VISIBILITY

Closely related to the increasing employment of receptionists was the growth in the use of appointment systems in general practice. In the early 1960s it was relatively uncommon for practices to arrange to see patients by appointment. Cartwright found in 1964 that only 37 per cent of doctors operated any kind of appointment system (Cartwright 1967: 152). The rest expected patients to be seen on a first-come-first-seen basis during fixed surgery hours, the almost universal practice before World War II.

Whether the doctors who instituted appointments systems in the 1960s and early 1970s did so as a result of real or perceived pressure from patients, of exhortations from the profession's leading figures, or of a new perception of self-interest, is immaterial (Ministry of Health 1954: 16; Stevenson 1967). The point we wish to make here is simply that an appointment system virtually dictated the employment of receptionist staff. By the same token, it was the development of appointment systems which directed the attention of the public to the importance of receptionists who *inter alia* appeared to control access to the doctor.

Seeming to control access to doctors brought in its train the possibility that receptionists might be blamed by those patients who were unable to see their doctor as soon as they wanted to. And indeed, from the late 1970s, there appears to have been an escalation of complaints against receptionists, most of them alleging that they prevented or at least discouraged patients from seeing their doctors in the surgery; that they put unacceptable pressure on patients who wanted home visits from their doctor to come instead to the surgery; that they gave unsolicited advice on health matters and suggested remedies; that they were unsympathetic or rude (Klein 1973: 115).

We recognized, therefore, that the receptionist's role of intermediary, a role which sociologists have likened to that of a gatekeeper, was one which simultaneously endowed its incumbents with some power and yet left them vulnerable to scapegoating. In questioning the doctors and the receptionists themselves about the latter's work and in observing them both systematically and from time to time throughout the study, we were primarily interested in seeing how far such inherent tensions were recognized and, in so far as they were, what steps were taken to resolve or reduce them.

THE RECEPTIONISTS' WORK

Views of the doctors in the small practices

The four doctors in the smaller practices gave us the feeling that they did not see anything particularly controversial in their receptionists' work. They maintained that the latter had been well-briefed by them as to what they were required to do and what they must not do. In the absence of an appointments system they had merely to find the records of patients who called to see the doctor, write out prescriptions for those who only wanted a repeat one, and take telephone calls from those who wanted a home visit. None of these tasks required the exercise of much discretion, and the doctors insisted that they did not permit their receptionists to make any clinical decisions, give advice, or determine whether or not a home visit should be made.

Reception work in their practices did, however, entail some decision-making which the doctors were prepared to leave to their receptionists, giving them merely general guidelines as to how they should act. For example, Dr Erickson expected his receptionist to direct obviously sick or infectious patients to him ahead of their place in the queue. In other words, she was given authority to make what amounted to a clinical judgement and to exercise discretion in the light of her decision. He was satisfied with the way she did it and was not aware of patient complaints about her.

Questioning the doctors on other aspects of their receptionists' work also revealed that they implicitly delegated some authority to their receptionists to determine who had access to them and in what circumstances. For example, while they had not explicitly instructed them to discourage certain kinds of would-be patients from joining their lists, they tacitly condoned their actions in telling 'hippies, drop-outs, and drug-outs' that the lists were full (see Chapter 12). Or again, Dr Cox, talking about the induction of a new receptionist after the move to shared premises, admitted that she was trying to modify his patients' requests for home visits by bringing them more into line with that of the other practices:

> 'She is trying to cut down on home visits for me. Traditionally, because of Dr Charlton's response to home visit requests, my practice gets more home visit calls than the other practices and she is being influenced by the other receptionists to cut them down. My patients think she is being tough, but she is just acting this way because the other practices do. But I don't really think she has ever deflected a visit.'

Dr Cox's incidental comment was the only indication we obtained from any of the doctors in the small practices that carrying out their delegated authority might put the receptionists into the firing line between doctors seeking to reduce demands upon them and patients seeking to obtain as much access as they wanted.

The Barr doctors' views

The doctors in the Barr practice acknowledged that the role of receptionist in their practice was a 'confused one' and that the confusion stemmed from their own conflicting needs to be as available as possible to patients and to pursue other external activities which, they believed, ultimately made them better doctors. Consequently, as one described it, the receptionists in their practice were 'the defensive part of the set-up'. They had:

'To skate somewhere between two functions, protecting workers from patient demands and encouraging and welcoming
patients and being friendly to them.'

They were aware too that the receptionists were often not only
'umpires', but also 'buffers' between doctors and patients, on
whom the latter vented irritation and frustration at long waits.

Another important receptionist function was to make the practice's appointments system work. This often meant 'sorting out the
very sick from the less sick', a task they had to accomplish quickly,
having little time in which to make decisions. It fell to the
receptionists too to deal with difficult patients. One doctor praised
their capacity in this respect: 'They are always tolerant and
even-tempered and take account of the particular needs of individual patients.' Another suggested that they contributed vitally to
the image which patients formed of the practice as a whole.

In general, then, the Barr doctors were conscious that receptionists were cast in a role which could make them the scapegoats
for decisions for which the doctors, not the receptionists, were
responsible. As a result, they felt it was up to them to support their
receptionists whenever possible, to be their 'back-stop'. We were
told that the most frequent reason for the removal of a patient
from the practice lists – itself a rare occurrence – was rudeness or
other abusive behaviour to a receptionist. They admitted, however, that they were not always as supportive as they should be. Dr
Bennett suggested that receptionists sometimes took a good deal
of flak from patients because they over-protected doctors. She and
her colleagues could 'convey that we are pressured and perhaps
have more important things to do than listen to them', and at times
of stress treat receptionists as 'instruments instead of people'.

Awareness of the strains which could arise when patients'
expectations of being able to consult their doctor within a few
minutes of the appointed time could not be met, led the Barr
practice doctors to try to devise special machinery, whereby
receptionists could not only express their frustrations but convince
doctors of the need for better organization. The receptionists
themselves seemed rather unwilling to raise issues or voice their
opinions in the weekly practice meetings; so one of the partners
was deputed to meet them at regular intervals and to discuss with
them ways in which their work could be eased. At a later stage,

the decision of the group to appoint a half-time manager was prompted in part by the hope that such an individual would be able to help them resolve difficulties which, they recognized, hit the receptionists hardest.

The Avesbury doctors' views

Without exception, the Avesbury doctors felt that the role of receptionist in their practice was an exceptional one. This was because, unlike most general practitioners, they held that all members of the practice team, whatever their particular tasks, were involved in patient care, and because, acting on this tenet, all team members including receptionists must be treated as equals. As a result, the Avesbury doctors used rather a different imagery for the receptionist role from that of the Barr doctors. To the former it was not 'the practice's defence', 'the intermediary', 'the umpire', 'the buffer': they saw it as 'the front line' of patient care. 'It's the very important and sometimes difficult one of first contact with patients,' said Dr Attenborough. Dr Adair's comment was even more pointed:

> 'This receptionist is the number one diagnostician. This is normally so in all practices. The only difference here is that we give explicit recognition to this function.'

Other Avesbury doctors concurred. One maintained, for example, that their receptionists performed what amounted to a social work function: 'A lot of serious work – talking, advising, listening, getting to know patients well.' Another claimed that they were 'the eyes and ears' of the practice, learning things about patients which doctors and other team members had not and which might be relevant to treatment.

The Avesbury doctors believed too that the practice employed fewer receptionists and that they were better integrated into the whole primary care team than was the case in other practices of comparable size. They thought that there were fewer latent tensions between them and their receptionists, mainly because the latter did not feel 'they had to be reticent or could not be frank if one or other doctor had been the cause of somebody's upset'. They acknowledged too the extent of their own dependence on the 'good mood' of the receptionists:

'Doctors can't function well if the receptionists don't function well. Each can make life difficult for the other.'

The receptionists' views

There were thirteen receptionists employed in the five practices we studied. Four of them worked in the smaller practices where they manned the desks during morning and early evening surgeries. Because there was no appointments system and fewer patients in at each surgery session than at the group practices, they also took charge of work which, at the latter, fell to nurses, record clerks, secretaries, and, at the Avesbury practice, the practice manager. For instance, the senior receptionist at the Erickson and Edmunds partnership completed vaccination forms and saw to the supply of syringes, dressings, stationery, and whatever else the doctors needed for surgery use. She typed letters for hospital admissions and arranged ambulance transport.

In contrast, the nine receptionists employed at the group practices, eight of them on a half-time basis, spent their time almost entirely at the reception desk. They dealt with requests for surgery appointments and home visits made by telephone or in person; with patients who turned up with or without appointments; with telephone requests to speak to the doctors and other health workers; with the registration of new patients; with requests for repeat prescriptions; and with a myriad of patient enquiries and complaints.

Divided loyalties: buffers, umpires, and front liners

The differences which we did observe in the extent to which receptionists at the study practices saw themselves as principally there to serve the doctors or to serve the patients seemed to us to be at least partly a function of the presence or absence of an appointments system. They could also, however, have been associated with differences in the size of practice, in the number of receptionists, in the range of functions, and in practice philosophies.

On the whole, the smaller practice receptionists saw themselves as there to 'lighten the doctor's load', to take work off his shoulders, to be his handmaiden in the traditional sense. This did not, of course, preclude friendly relations with patients; but there was no doubt in their minds as to whom they were accountable: they were after all employed by the general practitioners.

The six receptionists at the Barr practice were more aware of actual and potential conflict in the orientation of their work and less certain about where their own loyalties should lie when they had to act, as they often did, as a buffer. One of them, for example, felt certain that her main task was to protect the doctors from excessive or unreasonable demands on them. The stances of the others veered from one side to the other depending upon whom they felt was to blame for the situation, or on what they thought was reasonable. One of them, for example, said she tended to side with patients where surgery consultations were involved but with the doctors in dealing with requests for home visits. She recognized that she might be seen by patients as an 'angel' in the first instance and as a 'dragon' in the second. The senior receptionist at the Avesbury practice maintained that her first responsibility was to the patients. Her duty was to safeguard their interests in obtaining the professional help they needed. Another of her colleagues, however, said her priority was 'protecting the doctors' while the third said hers was 'helping both'.

The simile which most of the receptionists preferred for their own part in situations which involved conflicts between doctors' and patients' interests was 'umpire'. Umpires were expected not to take sides but to try to enforce the agreed rules of the game. They recognized that, on occasions, this would not endear them to either side, but they held that if they remained calm, courteous, and kind, they could also remain firm. All the same, the rules of the game ensured that it was the doctors who could break them in the last resort. When doctors did not play fair, they had no other recourse but to make it as clear to the doctors as they could that patients as well as they, the receptionists, suffered. The 'umpire' or final arbiter imagery itself broke down.

Exercising discretion

Our interviews with the receptionists persuaded us that they were all delegated some authority to exercise discretion on quite a wide range of issues, and that they all used it. Those with the longest experience, not unnaturally, felt happiest with this delegated authority. They had had more opportunities of testing out their own capacity and were more certain that they would be supported by the doctors and other team members if the way in which they exercised their discretion was questioned by patients.

There were three main kinds of requests on which they were most likely to have to use their discretion: for emergency consultations, for home visits, and for repeat prescriptions. Whether they operated a queuing or an appointments system, all the practices had a policy for suspending normal rules and labelling certain kinds of patients as constituting an emergency and hence requiring that they be given priority. The categories included the very sick, those with infectious diseases, the recently bereaved, and the very distressed or disturbed. At the smaller practices, patients in these categories were allowed to queue-jump and see a doctor ahead of those who had arrived before them. At the Avesbury practice, if the duty doctor, there for precisely such emergencies, was away on a call, patients were 'squeezed in' between appointments. At the Barr practice where 'squeezing in' or 'double-booking' was not encouraged by the doctors, the receptionists not infrequently faced dilemmas which they found difficult to resolve. Their system seemed to favour those who were not actually ill and made appointments ahead of time. In the words of a Barr receptionist: 'It has been said this practice is good for well patients but not for sick ones.'

The policy at the smaller practices and at the Avesbury was to restrict home visiting by discouraging requests for it. At the Barr practice there was no such explicit policy. On the contrary, many of the doctors felt they had a duty to respond as far as possible to such requests. Yet the receptionists at all the practices adopted the view that home visits were only unquestionably acceptable if it was difficult or dangerous for the patient to come to the surgery. In dealing with such requests, they routinely asked questions about the nature and duration of the patient's condition and the patient's age. They generally asked too whether the patient had access to transport to the surgery. Their aim was to convert a home visit into a surgery consultation whenever possible. If they thought any individual request should be so converted, but the patient continued to insist on a home visit, they would leave the decision to a doctor. In effect, their exercise of discretion stopped short of ultimate decision-making if their judgement was challenged. They gave us the impression that it seldom was.

At all the practices, repeat prescribing without seeing the doctor for varying lengths of time was regarded as permissible for patients who were stabilized on specific drug regimes. Equally the doctors felt under an obligation to keep their repeat prescriptions under review. In practice, the receptionists recognized that they had considerable responsibility in this regard, since it was they who prepared the scripts for the doctors' signatures. The doctors relied upon them to indicate if the prescription had not been reviewed for some time. One receptionist, for example, said that on her own accord she would attach a note to the script reminding the doctor that a patient on sleeping pills had not been seen by a doctor for an awfully long time: 'I like every patient to be seen by a doctor at least every six months.'

In all these ways the receptionists were involved in exercising discretion. From their own accounts of the criteria they took into account in doing so, it was clear, as the Avesbury doctors recognized, that they were making clinical judgements. They and some of the other study doctors might well have denied it if we had suggested as much.

Rewards of the work

All the receptionists told us that they enjoyed their work and got a great deal of satisfaction from it, although it was not without its difficulties. For example, at the Avesbury practice, when the doctors were very busy, the receptionists occasionally had difficulty in arranging for a doctor to undertake a home visit. There seemed to be general agreement, however, that the most stressful part of the work was dealing with demanding or unreasonable patients, and they described the variety of ways in which they had learnt to cope with them. Only four of the thirteen, including three at the Barr practice, claimed that they had had guidance from the doctors as to how to handle difficult patients. All these four believed that it was the doctors' explanations of why patients behaved as they did which they found the most helpful.

The rewards of the work were variously described. The receptionists at the smaller practices were more likely to mention the satisfactions they felt in helping doctors and patients to achieve their objectives. The group practice receptionists, and particularly those at the Avesbury, were more likely to talk about the intrinsic rewards of establishing informal, often intimate, relationships of trust and confidence with patients, and 'working friendships' with doctors and other team members. Our own observations made it clear that some patients undoubtedly treated the receptionists as their special confidantes and justified the latter's claim to have their own 'following'. The number of patients who sought and received reassurance that someone cared about them may well have been small; but it certainly included some patients who might otherwise have put a good deal of pressure on doctors or other team members, or have left the surgery without solace. In short there was justification for the claim of some receptionists that they were a source of comfort and support for some patients.

Patients' views of receptionists

In the light of the fear expressed in a variety of quarters that receptionists could utilize their position to reduce patients' pressure on the doctors and increase their own sense of authority, we asked home interviewees in both 1972 and 1975 a number of questions about the service at their practice.

It was clear from the responses we received that in both years most home interviewees saw the receptionists either in a neutral or a favourable light. Less than 10 per cent in either year said they were dissatisfied in any way with the receptionists, except at the Barr where 13 per cent in 1972 and 15 per cent in 1975 were less than satisfied. The same proportion in 1975 at this practice, but not elsewhere, alleged that the receptionists appeared to make it less easy rather than easier to see the doctor. However, a majority in this practice, as elsewhere, saw the receptionists as positively assisting the process rather than merely regulating it. The proportions who made this kind of judgement in the different practices ranged from 60 to 77 per cent.

Both the doctors and the receptionists had told us that the latter often befriended individuals and in that sense acted as primary care givers. At the same time, the receptionists were anxious to deny that they gave advice on medical matters. The home interviewees on the whole confirmed that the receptionists did not offer advice except on rare occasions; but between 11 and 19 per cent at each practice said that they had had help from a receptionist. Sometimes this turned out to be just fitting them in to see the doctor when they had not made an appointment or making out a prescription script when they did not want to see the doctor; but in

Table 6   *Percentage of home interviewees who described their practice's receptionists as kind and understanding, and as efficient, in 1972 and 1975*

quality	practice									
	Avesbury		Barr		Cox		Erickson		Osmond	
	'72	'75	'72	'75	'72	'75	'72	'75	'72	'75
	%	%	%	%	%	%	%	%	%	%
kind and understanding	67	67	55	46	71	67	82	73	–	82
efficient	81	74	83	73	83	74	88	86	–	89
N = 100%	(135)	(103)	(109)	(93)	(84)	(57)	(102)	(159)	–	(28)

most instances the help took the form of answering their questions or giving them information, and was clearly appreciated.

We also asked the home interviewees whether they would describe the receptionist(s) at their practice as kind and understanding, efficient, both or neither, and we found some considerable differences between the responses of those from different practices (*Table 6*). They suggest, once again, that, for whatever reason, the receptionists at the Barr were not seen as kind and understanding as commonly as those working in the other practices. It may, of course, be not unconnected with the doctors' own admission that they were not as available to patients as they recognized as desirable. (See Chapter 14, p. 273). The figures also suggest that the home interviewees in three of the four practices were likely to be more critical of the receptionists' efficiency in 1975 than they were in 1972.

ADMINISTRATIVE WORKERS: EXPANDING RESPONSIBILITIES, EMERGENT ROLES

We have already pointed out that, in the smaller practices, the receptionists undertook secretarial work and the general housekeeping chores of the business. In the two group practices, these tasks were done by workers with more limited and discrete functions. For example, both practices employed record clerks whose job it was to search for records of patients attending the surgeries or requesting home visits and to file correspondence concerning patients in the record folders. The practices also employed secretaries, but the history and significance of the 'secretariats' at each was very different.

As part of his philosophy and programme for transforming post-war general practice from a cottage industry into a service capable of meeting primary health care needs, Dr Adams had argued for the separation of professional and managerial functions in general practice. He had maintained that health workers had not the training, time, or energy to attend properly to the latter function. Hence as soon as he and two colleagues founded the Avesbury practice they employed a secretary to help with its organization and attend to administrative matters. The person engaged was someone with a great deal of political acumen and organizational experience who shared Dr Adams's ideological position and objectives. Starting *de novo* she shaped her role into that of practice manager with executive as well as secretarial functions. She left the practice in 1962 and her place was taken by Jean Armstrong.

Although initially a part-time worker only and somewhat diffident about fulfilling all the functions undertaken by her predecessor, Jean Armstrong extended her hours and her responsibilities as time went on. By the time of our study she was the acknowledged manager of the practice. Little by little she had been encouraged to accept the authority the partners wanted to delegate to her for organizing the expanding staff, maintaining the practice premises, ordering supplies, arranging their own timetabling and undertaking the financial management of the practice. She participated in partners' business meetings and helped to decide such matters as the size of the practice lists and the number of principals.

There is no doubt that the Avesbury partners assigned much significance to the part played by Ms Armstrong in the life of their unit. They came to rely on her not only to supervise the running of the practice as a viable organization: they also leant increasingly on her to sustain their morale when individually or collectively they faced crises or periods of frustrations and indecision. This occurred particularly after the move to the Health Centre when Dr Adams took on outside work and reduced the time and energy he could give to the practice, and when, as a consequence, the remaining partners appeared temporarily to falter (see Chapter 4). She was variously described by the partners as the practice's leader, the cement which held it together, a mother figure.

The authority which she, a non-medically qualified person, possessed was, we have reason to think, a relatively rare if not a unique phenomenon in general practice at the time. It was possible, we believe, because the professed philosophy around which the practice had been founded envisaged a team made up of individuals with different qualifications and capacities in which leadership would be either shared or, if individual, emergent and appropriate to the circumstances, not pre-ordained by virtue of professional qualifications.

Ms Armstrong, for her part, saw that her responsibilities had expanded; but modestly she seemed to think that anyone with average intelligence and commitment could handle them. She had learned the job on the job, and her 'know-how' came simply from experience, from trial and error. She did not feel that she had a greater share of responsibility than others: a team of their size could be managed as 'a collective', without a leader. She herself she described as 'co-ordinating' not 'leading':

> 'My task is to keep the daily work ticking over, to liaise, not to lead.'

As a member of a collective, she felt she had a great deal of autonomy in carrying out her tasks; but it was no greater, in her view, than the autonomy accorded to other workers within their assigned tasks. She instanced here the freedom given to the receptionists to do their work in the way they wanted, just as the doctors, health visitors, and social workers practised in their own ways. Possible conflicts on matters of principle surrounding the work could be resolved by the democratic method of discussion. 'Individual psychotherapy' could help where clashes were between individuals.

Besides Ms Armstrong, the Avesbury 'secretariat' included Stella Aldiss. Already in 1964, it was recognized that, if Ms Armstrong was to fulfil the managerial function, a secretarial assistant was needed. Stella Aldiss joined the practice as a school-leaver and began doing the more routine filing work, but with the encouragement of the doctors she had taken a year's course as a medical secretary and returned to work for them.

Apart from dealing with general correspondence, she acted as a receptionist on the desk if they were short-staffed and towards the end of the study was informally understudying the work of the practice manager. She too was satisfied with her work in the practice and the opportunities for further development which she was offered.

At the Barr practice, their secretary, Joyce Bryce, began as a part-time shorthand-typist in 1967: by 1970 she was working a thirty-eight hour week with responsibility not only for all the doctors' correspondence, but for the day-to-day management of the practice's finances, including the payment of employed staff, claims on the Local Executive Committee (now the Family Practitioner Committee) for the remuneration of doctors and trainees, income tax, and so on. She stood in as receptionist on every fourth Saturday morning.

Ms Bryce described herself as something of a handmaiden to the doctors, 'there to do their bidding'. Her relationship with all the doctors was 'easy'. Nevertheless it was with Dr Bourne, the senior partner, that her relations were most satisfying, because he did discuss practice matters more generally with her at a regular weekly session. It was this recognition of her potential contribution to the practice which made her feel the work was worthwhile. The other partners often asked her opinion about this or that, but she did not feel they always took it seriously.

In short, as the Barr practice expanded the scope of its work and the number of its partners, employed staff, and attached workers, its need grew for someone to take charge of the day-to-day management of resources and personnel. However, during the period of our study, the partners retained most managerial functions themselves and did not seek to include their practice secretary in policy decisions. Indeed, they did not give her the title of practice manager. In the closing stages of our enquiry, however, they had come to the conclusion that there was a need in a practice of their size and kind for at least the part-time services of a person who would carry more responsibility for staff management problems than they had given to their practice secretary.

THE RESEARCH TEAM'S ASSESSMENT

None of the practices in this study was the simple family business which still characterized much general practice in the early days of the National Health Service. When we first began to study them they all employed at least one part-time receptionist; the groups had already a number of individuals performing distinct roles designed to regulate the flow of patients to see the doctors and facilitate the measures which the doctors took to meet their patients' needs. This administrative support staff continued to expand and the structure of roles became more elaborate during the course of the study, especially at the group practices.

Our interviews and observations suggested a close rapport between the doctors and those undertaking the receptionist and other administrative chores. The latter felt that they were there to help the doctors provide services for the sick; they identified in general with the underlying philosophies and approaches to patients which characterized the practices. The partners, for their part, were confident that their staff would pursue their objectives and were therefore content to give them considerable freedom to decide how they should work. The close identification of the receptionist and administrative staff with the practices may well have been due to the method of selection. Almost all those who joined the larger practices were introduced by existing staff as people already known to them and likely to fit in with the team.

In the course of our casual and systematic observations of receptionists we saw no examples of receptionists acting in a way which might be seen as an abuse of the power over patients which their position gave them. They were courteous, kind, and considerate and obviously distressed when patients had long waits. They questioned telephone callers who wanted home visits with great tact and were often able to persuade patients themselves to reconsider their request. Only on the assumption that every such request should unquestionably have been granted could their conduct have been faulted.

We noted, at the two group practices, that the flow of patients through the waiting room to the consulting room was considerably more rapid and without incident at the Avesbury than at the Barr practice. Receptionists were less frequently beset by patients asking 'How much longer will I have to wait?' at the former than at the latter. Our measurement of the average length of time waited by patients before a consultation in practice waiting rooms confirmed these observations (see Chapter 16). It may well have been these long waits which resulted in a higher proportion of Barr practice home interviewees than of the home interviewees of other practices who were not prepared to describe their receptionists as kind and understanding.

We witnessed only one instance of the potential extent of the receptionists' power. It was an instance when the wishes of the doctors, not those of the patients, were overridden, and it occurred at the Avesbury practice.

All the doctors working at the Health Centre had agreed to participate in a screening programme which involved receptionists asking all the patients in certain age groups to see a nurse to have their blood pressure tested and their weight measured. It only seriously got under way, however, at the Barr practice where the doctors had no difficulty in obtaining their receptionists' co-operation as well as that of the nurses, who were also committed to the scheme. At the Avesbury practice, the doctors had been lukewarm and had taken no steps to persuade the receptionists and nurses to carry the programme through. In the event, it was the receptionists who brought the scheme to a premature end by failing to steer patients in the direction of the nurses. They did so without informing the doctors who only discovered at a staff meeting that it no longer operated when a nurse asked why they were no longer being sent patients. At this meeting one of the receptionists announced:

'I stopped doing the screening altogether – any screening. We couldn't keep it up, we haven't the staff.'

However, when asked by a doctor whether the pressure of work meant they needed an extra receptionist, she replied categorically that they did not:

'We're adequately staffed, except for screening.'

And there the matter was left. The doctors were not prepared to challenge their receptionists. They might, of course, have done, if they had been more enthusiastic about the programme in the first instance.

9 Organizational Change: Teamwork

In this part of our book we have so far described how one of the three main organizational changes to take place in general practice in this country since the Second World War, namely the development of group practice, affected all the practices during our study period (see Chapter 4). We have also considered the relationships which developed between general practitioners and members of the other occupational groups who were employed by or attached to our study practices (Chapters 5–8).

Collectively, multi-occupational groupings of this latter kind have come to be called primary health care teams and to be recognized as the second major if related form of change affecting the organization of general practice in the last two decades. In this chapter, we propose to examine the collective life of the teams in the group practices both as seen through the eyes of the general practitioners themselves and as manifested in the behaviour of members of the teams towards one another in practice meetings. As in our previous chapters, we have thought it important to sketch in a brief historical account of the reasons for the development of the idea of a primary health care team and of the problems which might be thrown up in implementing it. We leave to our next chapter our description of the impact on our practices of the third major form of organizational change of the last two decades, namely the location of many general practice units in Health Centres.

THE PRIMARY HEALTH CARE TEAM

During the 1960s, it became fashionable to ascribe many of the obvious failures of the health and personal social services to meet the needs or resolve the problems of the populations they were supposed to serve to the lack of co-ordinated effort on the part of those in direct contact with the needy (Medical Services Review Committee 1962: 10). The personnel of each service were often found to be working in isolation, ignorant of the involvement of the staff of other services in related aspects of their patients' or clients' affairs. It was not uncommon to hear of situations where a family was being visited by an assortment of medical, nursing, and social work staff either unaware or resentful of each others' concerns (Hockey 1966: 21). Or there were tales of buck-passing in which the staff of one service assumed that the staff of another agency was taking care of someone, while the individual concerned received no help from any statutory body (Committee on Children and Young Persons 1960; Bell 1965).

Evidence of these kinds led to increasing demands in the 1960s from many quarters for administrative integration of the separate sectors of the National Health Service and for a unification and simplification of the personal social services for which local government was responsible (Medical Services Review Committee 1962). The advantages were alleged to be greater efficiency in the use of scarce resources and a more humane approach to those who were suffering. The structural culmination of these demands took the form, in the early 1970s, of a powerful social services department in local government and a re-organized National Health Service in which hospital services and the health services previously run by local government were brought under one statutory health authority (Local Authority Social Services Act 1970; National Health Service Reorganization Act 1973).

Neither of these administrative reorganizations affected the general practitioner service to any great extent. The general practitioners themselves had successfully resisted any suggestion that they should be directly subjected to the authority responsible for hospitals and for services such as community nursing (*BMJ* 1971: 49). They insisted upon and obtained a functionally distinct Family Practitioner Committee to manage their contracts with the National Health Service much in the same way as its predecessor, the Local Executive Council, had done. They were only formally involved in the integrated health service to the extent that one of their number was called upon to serve as a member of the newly formed district management teams (DHSS 1972c: 29).

Nevertheless, it was already becoming clear in the 1960s, that even massive changes in administrative structures would not automatically ensure that medical, nursing, and social work personnel pooled their knowledge about individuals in need and deployed their skills and other resources of cash and kind to achieve the most effective and efficient solution. If these desirable things were to happen, there had to be opportunities at the grass roots for all those actually giving medical, nursing, or social work services to individuals to confer with one another on a regular basis and take decisions jointly as to what action was warranted.

It was in this connection that, well before the statutory administrative changes of the 1970s, some medical officers of health saw the increasing number of group general practice premises that were springing up as potential natural places for bringing together doctors, health visitors, nurses, and social workers in some form of permanent relationship to serve a common clientele or body of patients; in short, they saw general practice as a base for the creation of an integrated primary health care team (Warin 1968).

These medical officers of health took it upon themselves to persuade group general practitioners in their areas to allow health visitors and other local authority health workers to work from their premises and serve their patients. They had sometimes to overcome the widespread, long-held suspicion among some general practitioners that such innocent persuasion was not part of a deep-laid conspiracy to bring them under the aegis of local government and ultimately make them public authority employees as, indeed, the medical officers themselves were (*Medical Officer* 1966: 80). To suspicious minds, planting local authority staff in their premises, under the guise of better co-operation, which general practitioners could not but favour, might be the thin edge of the wedge, especially when such staff would continue to have duties over which the general practitioners would have no control. At the very least, many general practitioners needed to be reassured that, if teamwork was to become the order of the day, it was to be clearly understood that they, and not members of any other occupational group, were the natural leaders of these primary health care teams. There were instances, however, where general practitioners had to persuade reluctant medical officers of health to attach health visitor and district nursing staff to them (*BMJ* 1966: 71).

It was not only doctors who needed to be persuaded of the advantages to them of teamwork based on general practice. Health visitors, for example, while conscious that their separation from the general practitioner service resulted in some public scepticism of their own expertise and authority in health matters, were nevertheless wary of too close an association with medical men who had not uncommonly ridiculed their work and might try to dominate them or subvert their work (Davies 1969). Midwives, too, often felt competitive with the general practitioners who, although likely to have considerably less experience than they in the delivery of babies, might nevertheless be invited by expectant mothers to be present at the home birth (Jefferys 1965: 122). For social workers, who were seeking to throw off medical domination and establish themselves firmly as independent autonomous practitioners, the teamwork concept might appeal; but they were by no means convinced that teams needed leaders in the sense of single individuals endowed with the power to determine the scope and character of the work of others. Such teamwork in hospital settings had, in their view, unnecessarily restricted their own work and hence the service to their patients (Committee on Local Authority and Allied Personal Social Services 1968: 214).

In short, the creation and smooth effective functioning of a primary health care team composed basically of doctors, nurses, health visitors, and social workers and located in group general practice settings raised particularly issues of leadership, of decision-making in clinical and organizational matters, of communication, and mutual confidence. There were also, of course, practical issues to be settled such as accommodation, privacy for work with clients, and ease of access to them.

In discussing inter-occupational relationships and roles in earlier chapters we have inevitably touched on such issues as they affected our study practices and personnel. In this chapter we propose to draw on that material and on our own observations of the interchanges between doctors and other workers in practice meetings, as well as on the doctors' own views on teamwork, to illustrate the organizational developments which occurred in the Barr and Avesbury practices during the study period.

THE TEAM - BARR STYLE

Before the move

When the study began, the Barr primary health care team consisted of its six doctors and two general practitioner trainees; two attached health visitors, a geriatric visitor, and a part-time social worker, also attached; several full and part-time employed receptionists, and a secretary. By 1976 and after the move to the Health Centre, it included an additional full-time employed practice nurse, a second old-age visitor and an attached home nurse.

At the outset, as we saw and described it in an interim report we produced, the Barr team had a clear-cut hierarchical structure based on occupational ranking and seniority within occupation. The upper stratum consisted of the general practitioner principals, the middle stratum of the attached health workers and the lowest stratum of the employed receptionist and clerical staff. We use the term stratum to imply clear distinctions in the ways in which individuals in the different occupational groups interacted with one another.

There were regular weekly meetings attended by the doctors and attached health workers, that is, by the upper and middle strata. Receptionists and clerical staff were only invited to be present when matters relating directly to their conditions of work were to be discussed. The discussions at the weekly meetings could cover the problems of caring for particular patients, organizational arrangements, or new developments in medicine. They were dominated by the doctors: the middle stratum, the attached health workers, rarely contributed, especially if organizational issues or the implications of new developments in medicine and caring were being discussed. They never chaired the weekly meetings and, according to our records of a sample of such meetings held before the move to the Health Centre, only introduced 6 per cent of the topics discussed; the remaining 94 per cent were raised by doctors.

The form of mutual address used across strata was formal if friendly. Doctors used first names when addressing each other in the meetings; so did the attached workers among themselves. The latter normally called a doctor 'doctor' without using a surname. The doctors addressed the attached workers by surname and appropriate title. The discussions themselves mainly took the form of information exchange. It was almost always doctors who asked for and gave the information. Decisions were seldom taken at the meetings, especially those with more general policy implications for the team. There was virtually no sign of overt conflict between members and little in the way of controversy. Outside the regular meetings there were few opportunities for casual contact or interchange between the different occupational groups included in the primary health care team. As far as we could judge little conferring took place except between one doctor and a geriatric visitor who worked closely together.

After the move

Four years later and after two years in the Health Centre a number of changes had taken place. There were now two regular weekly lunch-hour meetings in the practice. One of these was now open to receptionist and clerical staff. They were not merely invited to come; they were almost exhorted to. It was a disappointment to the doctors that most of them chose, most of the time, not to do so. This weekly meeting was ostensibly to consider practice policy, to exchange information, to share views, and to provide an opportunity for informal social interaction between different team members. The other regular weekly meeting was confined, in practice although not formally, to the doctors, practice nurses, and attached health workers. It was intended for the discussion of cases, especially of patients with psychological or social difficulties. It was attended by a consultant psychiatrist (see Chapter 3).

Some changes in the social climate of the practice had taken place over the years. The doctors still continued to dominate the discussions in both kinds of meetings; but there were more interjections from other health workers at the case meetings, especially encouraged by the consultant psychiatrist. The middle stratum was responsible for raising 13 per cent of the topics compared with only 6 per cent at the meetings before the move. Controversies were more likely to be voiced especially about the handling of cases, but it was most commonly the doctors who participated in such controversy. The meetings were no longer automatically chaired by the senior partner: other doctors took their turn, as did, from time to time, a nurse, health visitor, and social worker, although they appeared to be somewhat uncomfortable in this role. Doctors were now first-naming not only each other but all the other staff. They had invited all the other team members to reciprocate, but some had not felt able to do so or seemed embarrassed when they did. Outside the regular meetings there were many more opportunities for informal discussion about patients in the nursing area, the corridors and the canteen on the first floor, than there had been in the old premises.

Sharing care

The Barr doctors in 1976 believed that their practice was a team in a way and to an extent which it had not been before. They now defined a team as a multi-occupational group in which members recognized each others' skills and the right to apply them auto-nomously, not as a group of workers merely carrying out the orders of a leader. As one put it:

'We are a team in which each person is free to make his or her own contribution without interference from other members.'

They attributed the change mainly to the increased opportunities in their new premises for contact and interaction between all unit members. As a result, in the words of one of them:

'The Barr practice is now working much more as a team. It's different from the time the unit was just doctors with a few helpers.'

They were aware, however, that if team members were to be autonomous in practice as well as in theory, their special skills needed to be recognized and appreciated by patients as well as by doctors. This too, the doctors believed, was happening increasingly since their move to the Health Centre. Having modified their own views as to the value of the skills of other health workers, they had encouraged patients to accept treatment or support from them:

'Patients are more ready to be treated by health workers other than doctors, once they see them working together with doctors.'

Indeed, some patients, they told us, were electing to see the health visitor, nurse, or social worker rather than the doctor. Initially, one at least of the doctors found this difficult to accept – 'We were so used to doing everything ourselves and getting satisfaction from it' – but the advantages of teamwork were so great that they could not discourage it. Only one doctor referred to a possibly negative aspect of this so far as patients were concerned. She feared that, as the number of helpers and the involvement of each with a patient increased, the care given might be too diluted. It was all the more important, therefore, for there to be a personal doctor for each patient.

The best indication we have of the way in which the team worked in the care of patients was obtained from the weekly meetings. Patients discussed at these meetings might be known only to one member of the practice, to two, or to many of them. The decision to present the case might have been taken by one staff member only or by some or all of those known to each other to be currently involved or in contact with the individual or his family. Reasons for presenting a case varied too. A doctor, aware for the first time that his patient's difficulties could have a psychological component, might want to know whether others had information about the patient or his family which he did not have. Two workers involved with the same patient might decide to ask their colleagues for suggestions on how to deal with a diet or allergy problem. Sometimes a worker wanted to alert others to anticipated increased demands for help from a patient: 'Mary Smith's husband has left her. I think we can expect many night calls from her.' Sometimes a case was brought merely to report progress or lack of it since it was previously discussed. And sometimes it was just a cry for help: 'What am I to do next?' In short, there was at such meetings a sharing of information and opinion and a giving and receiving of support in the team as a whole.

The following extract from the researcher's notes of a case discussed at a meeting gives something of the flavour of the team interchanges:

MS BRODIE (HEALTH VISITOR)   Now that Diana [Dr Bennett] is here, I want to discuss Teresa Brien. You know, she's the young mother, whose husband is deformed. They've not been patients long, since they've only just moved into this area. She had the baby by caesarian section: the baby's fine, but the marriage is rocky. When I saw her Teresa told me that her husband is ill-treating the baby and she wants to leave him.

She's on sick leave at present but is due to go back to work. I referred her to Mary [Bancroft].

MS BANCROFT (SOCIAL WORKER)   She's a most interesting woman – from Malaysia originally. She came to London to get domestic work but met her husband within two days of arrival. It was love at first sight! He's thirteen years older than she was and has some deformity of the arms. They're very short.

DR BOURNE (GP)   Yes, I've seen him. He's a musician.

DR BARRETT (GP)   A bad musician, though. He's aspirations to be one, but he's a domestic servant.

MS BANCROFT   The relationship has been stormy. He's jealous of the baby: she's jealous of his daughter of a previous marriage, aged six. Teresa told me he ill-treats her and the baby, and she wants out of the marriage. I notified the area office (social services department), and heard from them that she contacted them the next day, and they've moved her into a bed-and-breakfast accommodation.

MS BRODIE   She came to see Diana [GP] the day after that because the baby had rolled off the bed and was bruised.

DR BELLAMY (VISITOR)   Do you think the baby really rolled off the bed?

MS BRODIE   She has to go back to work and for that she must have a signing off certificate. She also wants to get the baby into a day nursery.

DR BOURNE   She came into see me about continuing bleeding from her vagina. I never suspected any marital troubles. She didn't say anything about that.

MS BANCROFT   No, when I saw her earlier I didn't pick that up.

DR BOURNE   It seems that because her visits to us are always in emergencies that she has seen too many doctors. I suggest we should not involve more than two doctors at most and Angela [Brodie].

DR BELLAMY   I want to come back to the bruised baby. She herself and not her husband may be the injurer. After all, the baby "rolled off the bed" after she had left her husband. Are you leaving it at that?

DR BINET (TRAINEE GP)   Do you think she has a post-parturition depression? It might be that.

MS BRODIE   No, I don't think so.

MS BANCROFT   No, she doesn't strike me as flat or depressed.

DR BINET   The last time I saw her she was crying.

MS BRODIE   Well, I suppose all I can do is to maintain constant contact, along with the area social worker.

The researchers, of course, saw mainly such public demonstrations of teamwork. We were not able to examine what we imagine was the submerged part of the iceberg of co-operation that took place between members in informal encounters. We cannot say, therefore, what kinds of biases there may be in the impression we formed that teamwork did increase during the period of our study.

Structure

While there was total agreement among the Barr doctors about the value of teamwork in the delivery of care, there was some disagreement among them about how a primary care team based in general practice should be structured. The Barr doctors acknowledged that the research team's description of their practice, in its Interim Report, as hierarchical, was accurate, and most were somewhat troubled by it. They were also, since the move to the Health Centre, in much closer contact with the Avesbury group and hence more aware of the contrast between their own modes of interaction with members of other occupational groups and the more informal egalitarian style of the Avesbury doctors.

One Barr doctor, however, defended what she saw as her practice's essential character:

'Our organization is hierarchical. There is ranking in it. We are very used to it and we like it.'

In her view the ranking was reflected in the responsibility attached to different roles:

'It is the doctors who are ultimately responsible for the patients and they are the only ones who take patients on for extended years.'

She added, nevertheless, that, although the doctors generally initiated the important policy changes and made the formal decisions, they always tried to take account of the suggestions of other workers. She believed that, increasingly, ideas were originating from these other workers.

Two of the Barr doctors said they would have liked their practice to be less hierarchical and more democratic than they felt it was; but at the same time they believed they could not abrogate responsibilities which were properly theirs, because, if they did, patient care might suffer. Towards the end of the study, Dr Bourne, who was one of these two doctors, thought the practice had made some progress toward solving the dilemma. He told us:

'There is now a better balance in the organization. We are moving cautiously into a more democratic mould and this is really due to your Interim Report.'

Dr Bourne maintained that he and the other doctors had made a deliberate effort to re-distribute power and decision-making 'in the spirit of the times'. They had spread the chairmanship of their meetings to other health workers even though the others had not all taken kindly to the change. He instanced, too, the fact that the practice had recently sent a delegation consisting of a doctor, a nurse, and a health visitor to visit a Health Centre in Holland. 'A few years earlier', he said, 'this would have been unthinkable.'

The colleague who shared his views on the ideal practice structure described their practice as a 'combination of democracy and hierarchy', which, she considered, was not a bad thing:

'Complete hierarchy is absolutely out. None of us would like it. Complete democracy and nothing gets done. A blend of the two is best and that, I think, is what we have.'

She maintained that everyone was involved in decision-making, while recognizing that the doctors were more vocal than the others.

The remaining Barr practice doctors were less certain as to whether there had been any real or substantial change in the organization of their practice, and they were less satisfied with the situation than the three just quoted. They agreed that there had been a number of small changes, such as the extension of the reciprocal use of first names and a rotating chairmanship at meetings. They, too, attributed such changes to the Interim Report, the external climate, and the propinquity of the Avesbury practice. However, as they saw it, the life of the practice was still largely dominated by the doctors. It was they who at meetings 'thrashed' matters out, a process not so much of decision-making as of 'teasing-out' relevancies, and one in which the non-medical staff rarely played a decisive part. Nor could they think of any decision actually made by a non-doctor. The other workers remained far too deferential despite the attempts to encourage, even cajole, them into contributing to meeting discussions. The partners had even gone so far as to request the receptionists to attend the weekly meetings in turn, hoping in this way to draw them into the collective life of the practice. In part, they attributed the lack of basic change to personalities. The tone of their relationships with one another, they thought, had been set by Dr Bourne who tended to be somewhat formal and hence perhaps to attract staff who were more formal and correct than 'the laddies at the Avesbury practice'.

THE AVESBURY TEAM, BEFORE AND AFTER THE MOVE

We did not observe the same degree of change in the primary health care team in the Avesbury practice that we saw in the Barr group over the years of our study. Moreover, the slight change which we did see was not in the same direction as that in the Barr.

The weekly staff meetings held in the old Avesbury Road premises took place in a cramped top floor room which also served as a place where staff could make cups of coffee, eat cold lunches, and meet each other informally. Doctors, as well as the practice nurse, manager, secretary, receptionists, and attached workers helped prepare the food eaten during the lunch-hour meetings. They all wore informal clothes and addressed each other by their first names. The meetings were chaired informally by different team members. The topics discussed were more likely to include matters of general public interest and of community health than was the case at the Barr practice. Some of the visitors from overseas and elsewhere in Britain, who were often present, said they found it difficult to detect the professional identity of participants in the discussion. The team members were all likely to talk about themselves as a family: their behaviour suggested to us a group of people whose common outlook in work had spilled over into close friendships in their lives more generally.

Two years after the move to the Health Centre, the team had

expanded slightly by the addition of another geriatric visitor and a practice nurse, shared with the Barr. There had also been some staff changes. The Avesbury, like the Barr group, were holding two weekly meetings, the second to discuss cases with their attached psychiatric consultant. At this latter meeting only doctors and health workers were present, not the practice manager or receptionists.

Our measures of participation at the weekly meetings indicated that, with one exception, the non-medical workers were somewhat less likely to contribute to the discussions after the move than before, and the doctors more likely to do so. Our counts of frequency of statements of all kinds made during meetings indicated that 55 per cent came from doctors in 1972 compared with 65 per cent in 1975. The other health professionals contributed 28 per cent in 1972 but only 19 per cent in 1975. The exception was the practice manager whose involvement in the meetings increased markedly as time went on (2 per cent to 10 per cent). Towards the end of our study she was especially prominent in introducing organizational matters which required decisions.

The lesser involvement of the nurse, health visitor, and social worker contingent could have been due to the changes of personnel which occurred over the period of our study. The workers who replaced those who left were noticeably less communicative, and newcomers in any case might be expected to talk less until they felt thoroughly at home. We believe, however, that the less overt participation of the non-medical workers could have also been in part the result of a certain loosening of the close ties in the group as a whole to which a sequence of coincidental events could have contributed.

The first such event was the move to the Health Centre which, among other things, placed the non-medical attached workers on a different floor from the doctors and made casual encounters between them less likely than they had been in the old premises. This was in contrast to the experience of the Barr group who were brought into greater inter-occupational proximity as a result of the move. The move also made a canteen available where food could be purchased, thus reducing the amount of teamwork required in the Avesbury practice for the communal preparation of the cold lunches. The Health Centre also brought the attached staff closer physically to fellow non-attached workers in the Family Health

Clinic unit and made it possible for them to explore the commonality of interest and experience which binds individuals of like training. As time was not infinitive, this could have been done at the expense of other types of interaction, including inter-occupational contact.

The second event, or rather chain of events, was the gradual withdrawal of Dr Adams soon after the Health Centre move, from total involvement in the practice after he had taken on a part-time post in a professional organization, and the further expectation that he and the practice nurse who had pioneered the role twenty years earlier would soon retire altogether from the practice. As we have already suggested in Chapters 2 and 4, Dr Adams had been the leading advocate and spirit behind primary health care teamwork in his group and while he was present it thrived. As he withdrew, steps faltered and the bonds which had until then united men and women with different training and experience loosened.

Third, our own observations of the practice unit members in and out of meetings confirmed what several of the doctors had already told us in our interviews with them, namely that, for a variety of reasons which perhaps had little to do with the practice and more to do with ageing and extra-mural non-professional problems, they had less energy to devote to making the team work in and outside meetings.

At the same time, while recording that there was little in the way of development of teamwork at the Avesbury during the period of our study, and indeed noting some retreat from the integrated team achieved in the old premises in Avesbury Road, we do not mean to imply that the members of the team were any less convinced in 1976 than they had been earlier of the value, indeed the necessity, for maintaining a multi-occupational team in primary health care. Nor had they changed their view that it could most easily be achieved by minimizing the distinctions between the members of the team and by avoiding situations where possible conflicts in approach were resolved by doctor's fiat rather than by discussion. Moreover, the discussions which we recorded at the practice meetings persuaded us that, as at the Barr, sharing information among all the members of the practice group and not merely among those directly involved with a particular patient served both to support those who carried the clinical responsibility and to reassure practice members of the collective support of their colleagues.

THE RESEARCH TEAM'S ASSESSMENT

During the study period there were undoubtedly signs of increasing interchange of information and views among the members of the Barr group, in contrast to the Avesbury group which changed little. The latter had effected a style of informal interaction among team members well before it moved to the Health Centre: there was little change over time in the way it conducted practice meetings, or in the amount of participation in them of members of different occupations. The changes which did occur at the Avesbury were, if anything, to reduce the part played by the non-medically qualified members in practice deliberations, with the exception of that played by the practice manager. In the Barr practice, on the other hand, there was a slight trend to greater participation of non-medically qualified workers in the discussion at meetings, and a parallel more marked trend to a more informal style of interchange.

We were conscious, however, that the demonstration of teamwork afforded by the discussion of cases or issues at practice meetings was only one facet of the kind of teamwork envisaged by those who had been advocates of primary health care teams in the 1960s and 1970s. They had also envisaged teams as enabling shared care for patients, with two or more members of a team each helping to bring their unique knowledge or skills directly to the aid of many patients. Teamwork for some implied, in addition, the delegation of day-to-day clinical responsibility for a patient by the individual who nominally held that responsibility to another person, on the assumption that that second person had the more appropriate knowledge or skills to aid the patient and the experience to call for other help if it were required.

It was more difficult for us to judge how far these two latter facets of teamwork developed during the period of our study. The doctors agreed to indicate on their patients' records whether or not they had referred the patient to anyone else in the practice team; but the research team's checks at various times throughout the study showed that this commitment was honoured more in the breach than in the observance. If they had recorded meticulously, we could have used the sample of those records we analyzed to compare the number of internal referrals in 1972 and 1975 with some confidence that the results would tell us if there had been a distinguishable trend in the rate. As it was, the records suggest very little internal referring both before and after the move, except to the practice nurse. At the Avesbury, 17 per cent of the sample of records in 1972 showed at least one referral to the practice nurse during the year; by 1975 the figure was only 12 per cent. At the Barr, there was over a four-fold increase, from 3 per cent to 14 per cent, which was not surprising given that, in 1972, there was no permanent nursing provision, the senior receptionist standing in only infrequently in this capacity.

Another possible source of information was the interviews we conducted at home with those whose records we monitored. These tended to confirm both our view that the doctors habitually failed to record internal referrals and the considerable change in the Barr group doctors' use of their practice nurse. Forty per cent of the Avesbury sample in both 1972 and 1975 said they had had at least one contact with a practice nurse during the previous year. Only 5 per cent of the Barr group had in 1972, compared to 24 per cent in 1975. These interviews also helped to indicate, as did our third source of information – the sample of surgery attenders in 1972 and 1975 – that only a small proportion of patients had seen any of the attached practice workers, that is the health visitor, geriatric visitor, or social worker. It must be remembered, however, that our samples did not in general include those parts of the practice population – for example, the over seventy-fives and the under sixteens – who would be most likely to be referred to health visitors and geriatric visitors. It must also be remembered that the attached social workers typically saw fewer patients in a week than the general practitioners saw in a day. In other words, given that the social worker was only one person working part-time for a practice unit comprising six partners and two trainee doctors, who collectively might see close on 1,000 patients in a week, it was not surprising that our samples of those attending surgeries to see a doctor did not yield us sufficient information to show trends in the frequency of shared or delegated care.

In the absence of data to contradict the claims of both doctors and other health workers that the volume of work which was shared by two or more of them or in which the day-to-day clinical responsibility was delegated by the doctor to another member of the team had increased, we are inclined to take the claims at face value: we believe, with them, that inter-professional collaboration at the Barr practice intensified during the period of our study and at the Avesbury remained at the level which it had reached before the move to the Health Centre.

10 Organizational Change: Health Centre Practice

The idea of a Health Centre as the location for a range of curative and preventive services outside the hospital was not a new one in the 1970s. It was, for example, the major recommendation in 1920 of a Committee set up by the newly formed Ministry of Health's Consultative Council on Medical and Allied Services and chaired by Lord Dawson (Committee on the Future of Medical and Allied Services 1920: 9). The Committee proposed that general practitioner surgeries should be located in local authority buildings which would also house the latter's expanding services for maternity and child welfare, for schools and for district nursing. Although the proposals, for a variety of reasons, were not implemented, the idea of a Health Centre did not die; in a very different form it was the basis of the experiment undertaken by Drs Scott Williamson and Innes Pearse, at Peckham (Pearse and Crocker 1943: 14). Other proposals for Health Centres were made throughout the inter-war years by various bodies, including the British Medical Association (BMA 1930; 1938) and the Socialist Medical Association (SMA 1933).

It was the truncated proposals of the last-named organization which found a place in the National Health Service Act 1946. Under section 21 of that Act, local authorities were required to establish Health Centres in which they were themselves to provide a range of preventive and supportive health services while renting accommodation to general practitioners. In practice, the obligation (not the power) to establish such Centres was rescinded before the Act came into force in 1948, and in the immediate post-war years local authorities made housing and schools their first building priorities. Nor was pressure put by general practitioners on to the authorities to build Health Centres: on the contrary, the tentative proposals made by a few local authorities most commonly met with suspicion or hostility (*BMJ* 1953a: 125). As a result of all these factors, only eighteen Health Centres had been built by 1964. Although those working in the Centres were on the whole enthusiastic, those who had not found them congenial and left did not help to make the idea popular with most general practitioners (*BMJ* 1960b: 57).

In 1964, the Labour Government was returned to office for the first time since 1951. It decided to encourage local authorities to build Health Centres by making Treasury resources available to them. It did so in the belief that young doctors, in particular, might be attracted into the ailing sector of the National Health Service if they felt sure of being able to practise in well-equipped premises with supporting community-based services (Ennals 1969). Many young doctors might see renting reasonably priced surgery accommodation as an attractive and less hazardous alternative to entering into a long-term commitment with partners to purchase purpose-built or converted property (*BMJ* 1967: 90; Hall *et al.* 1975: 302). There was also the hope that general practitioners' fears of local authority control might have diminished with time and that younger doctors with no pre-National Health Service experience would not be as wary of competition from each other as many older men appeared to be, a wariness which was also thought to account in part for the reluctance to practise in a Health Centre (Irvine and Jefferys 1971). This hope seemed justified: the initial plan was for 300 local authority Health Centres by 1974; but by 1970 the target had been increased to 560 by 1976, by which time the local authorities had handed over the Health Centres to the reorganized Area Health Authorities of the National Health Service.

However, by the time section 21 of the 1946 National Health Service Act was extensively activated in the late 1960s and early 1970s, some of the reasons which the framers of that Act had had for wanting to establish Health Centres were no longer of such great moment. At the end of World War II, general practitioners were mainly lone practitioners unsupported by other kinds of health workers and lacking opportunities for any form of colleguely cover or discourse. The Health Centre then symbolized the combined ideas of the group practice and the primary health care team. By the late 1960s, as we have seen, group practices were already becoming common, and primary health care teams of a kind were developing within them, especially with the attachment of local authority staff. The moves had begun to take place without parallel Health Centre development. Health Centre practice itself was no longer so innovatory, especially when it involved doctors, as it did in the case of the Avesbury and the Barr, with long experience of working in a group with attached local authority staff.

Many of the Health Centres established in this period were in areas of new housing development. The practices moving into them were often group practices moving with re-housed populations from contracting city centres to peripheral districts. Health Centres were not established as frequently in inner city neighbourhoods, not only because populations were declining there: it was also because land values were high and local authorities reluctant to build on expensive plots if they could not guarantee that general practitioners in the area would agree to practise from them. Yet another reason was the presence of many single-handed practitioners who were often suspicious, not only of government interference with their practices, but also of each other. They continued to see each other in competitive terms (Sidel *et al.* 1972: 26).

The local authority of the London borough in which the Avesbury and Barr practices were located, however, felt confident about building a Health Centre, partly because the two groups, comprising, together, the viable number of eleven principals, had made a firm commitment to move into it and, indeed, wanted to be involved from the start in its planning. The authority also wanted to house an expanded Family Health Clinic to meet the needs of the patients of some seventy other general practitioners in the area.

We have already indicated in Chapter 2 the reasons why these two group practices wished to move into a Health Centre. For the Barr they were essentially pragmatic: the partners wanted to vacate unsatisfactory, restricted premises and were prepared to accept a tenancy with the local authority in a modern, purpose-built, well-equipped Health Centre. The Avesbury group had comparable reasons and in addition an ideological commitment to working from a building owned by the local community.

THE HEALTH CENTRE IN PRACTICE

It was clear to us and to our study doctors that some of the changes they desired would not have taken place had they remained in their old, unsatisfactory premises. For example, the expansion which took place in the personnel of their health teams and in their partnerships could not have occurred in the old premises. Nor could their educational activities. In that sense, Health Centre practice was enabling.

It could, however, be argued that these changes would have taken place if the moves had simply been to larger privately owned premises. Indeed, we are not in a position to say that any of the innovations in procedures, organization, relationships, or services provided by the groups were the direct result of practice from a local authority – subsequently Area Health Authority – owned Health Centre. We can only make the negative statement that Health Centre practice did not inhibit the developments and may well have encouraged them.

In view of the suspicions which still lurk in some general practice quarters, however, about practising in publicly owned premises, we think it useful to give an account both of the answers the general practitioners in this study gave to our direct questions about working from a Health Centre, and of our own observations of the practice units in this new setting.

PARTICIPATION IN THE PLANNING

In the first place, both practices undoubtedly saw themselves as collaborating with the local authority from the start. Indeed, a beginning of any kind was only certain after the Medical Officer of Health was able to assure his local authority that the practices wanted to move in. The tension which arises between landlord and tenant when the one party sees itself as in a bargaining and antagonistic relationship with the other did not exist. The Medical Officer of Health and the two groups saw themselves as willing and active partners in an enterprise of mutual benefit, which nevertheless required the ironing out of potential and anticipated sources of conflict.

We did not observe directly the development of the Health Centre from the first twinkle in the Medical Officer of Health's eye through the various gestational stages to the final birth and occupation of the premises; but the practices were each represented by two doctors on the planning committee and played a major role in the overall design and the finer details of the building. Their representatives as well as those of the Family Health Clinic accompanied the architects on visits to a range of other Health Centres and group practice premises.

In the retrospective accounts given to us by the doctors in the two practices it seems clear that the Avesbury was the rather more active group, and over some points of layout, which affected the overall operation of the practices once in the Health Centre, had the major voice. On occasions, they had to persuade the Barr practice of the superiority of their proposal: more frequently it was they who made the suggestions with which the Barr acquiesced.

It was the Avesbury group, for example, who proposed the common treatment centre bounded by examination cubicles which could also be entered from the consulting rooms, a proposal which at first did not meet with the Barr group's approval. The latter insisted on consulting rooms large enough to accommodate an examination couch on the grounds that patients often talked about important things while dressing and undressing. In the event, they used the examination cubicles increasingly both to save their own time and to relieve patients of what they now reassessed as possible embarrassment in having doctors obliged to wait on or for them. In retrospect, Dr Bowen believed their Health Centre to be the best he had seen, mainly due 'to Sam Adams's brilliance in designing the two-way system in the treatment area'. This opinion was shared by the Medical Officer of Health who also acknowledged the part played by Dr Adams in designing the Centre.

ADMINISTRATION – MECHANISM FOR CONSULTATION

The responsibility for the maintenance of the Centre's fabric and furnishings and for the provision of common household services such as cleaning and caretaking was initially the local authority's and it appointed a Health Centre administrator to discharge it. A married couple was taken on as caretakers and occupied a small flat on the premises. In 1974, the ownership of the Health Centre was transferred to the newly formed Area Health Authority, to some extent disturbing the relationships which had developed between the general practice occupants and their landlord (see p. 197).

The group practices and the local authority's own community-based health personnel serving the surrounding district moved into the Health Centre in May 1973. Soon after, a meeting was called of representatives of all these three units and of the local authority's health department. At this meeting a decision was taken to establish a body to be called the Link Group comprised of elected representatives of the three groups who would meet regularly to iron out any difficulties related to the use of the building, to suggest innovations to the authority, and to transmit information between the Health Centre units and the authority. It was also intended that the Link Group should encourage contact among members of all the units, by arranging social gatherings and meetings from time to time on matters of mutual professional interest.

In the event, the Link Group became a vehicle through which individual units could inform the administrator and the authority about the difficulties which they encountered, and through which remedies could be considered. It was less successful in its efforts to bring members of the separate units together on a social or professional basis.

Both the Link Group meeting minutes and the notes which our research team members made of them suggest, not surprisingly, that a number of mistakes had been made in the initial planning of the Centre. Foremost amongst them was the inadequate waiting area for mothers attending the Family Health Clinic facilities. The removal of a wall to provide more space did not wholly solve the problem. Other less serious mistakes, not necessarily involving the building, were quickly remedied; still others seemed to take a long time to iron out or were not satisfactorily resolved at all during the three years of our study.

Among the issues which were raised from time to time and seemed ultimately to be resolved, even if they took some time, were cleaning arrangements (noisy polishers used during the afternoon when patients were consulting doctors); telephones (insufficient lines and operators to deal with the volume of calls); plants (who should be responsible for watering them); cafeteria (how much part-time help should be available).

Among the hardy perennials which generated a great deal of heat but little change were the provisions for car parking both by Health Centre personnel and by Health Centre users. Another issue which created even more feeling as time went on was security, which turned out to be a multi-faceted subject. There was first of all the security of the building from the standpoint of the theft of valuable equipment or instruments or of vandalism: there was then the specific problem of thefts of psychotropic drugs used by socially deviant groups of individuals or of doctor prescription pads which the latter could use to obtain the drugs: there was also the question of the patients' records and confidentiality, since the records were stored in an open area between the reception desks and the treatment room, through which there was a continuous flow of health workers and patients.

An analysis of the discussions at these meetings of the Link Group showed that there were few signs of serious divisions of opinion between the two practices on any of the issues raised, merely an occasional sign of mutual irritation. Nor was there much evidence of conflict between the interests of the general practices on the one hand and the third unit occupying the premises – namely the authority's Family Health Services – on the other. Rather it seemed that the representatives of the two general practices, usually with the tacit rather than overt support of those representing the Family Health Services, combined to attack what they interpreted as the procrastination, short-sightedness, or sheer bloody-mindedness of the authority.

Blame for shortcomings was explicitly not attached to the first Health Centre administrator who was universally seen as 'a good guy', fighting with the rest of the Health Centre occupants against a group of nameless bureaucrats collectively known by the name of the offices in which they were located – Tristam House. A later administrator who was not as popular was more likely to be bracketed with the distant menace as partly blameworthy. When the administration was transferred from the local Health authority to the Area Health Authority in 1974, the representatives of the latter, confronted with a number of hitherto unmet demands from the Health Centre units, were able to plead unfamiliarity and preoccupation with reorganization as reasons for delays in action. Such pleas were treated with considerable scepticism, and the hostility once directed against the local authority transferred to the offending Area Health Authority officials.

In the next two years, the Link Group itself appeared, at least while we were still observing it, to have run out of steam, to feel itself relatively powerless to bring about the changes wanted by the constituent parties, to resign itself to having to accept a lower level of provision in terms of fabric maintenance, patient and staff amenities, and operational efficiency than they had originally aspired to. The half-hearted efforts to foster greater social and professional interchanges between members of the different units had mostly petered out without success. Attendances at meetings declined. The unit representatives were still mainly the same people who originally formed the Link Group, largely because they could not get others to volunteer for the job. In fact, according to some doctors, the Link Group had become something of a joke: 'a house committee for choosing colours for the re-decoration of the Centre and making decisions about curtains in consulting rooms'. They knew that these were necessary functions, but they saw them as pedestrian when what was needed was more innovatory planning, for example, the development of retirement courses for the community, involving patients in the planning.

GAINS OUTWEIGH LOSSES

At the same time, although any euphoria associated with the honeymoon period was short-lived, we did not detect any feeling after it of deep disillusionment with the Health Centre. There was irritation from time to time with the action or inaction of the authority; that was all.

Similarly, there were one or two inter-practice conflicts which caused some ill-will. One concerned smoking in the waiting areas. The Barr practice prohibited smoking in their waiting rooms; initially, the Avesbury did not. Barr patients began to make use of the Avesbury waiting area for a 'quick drag', to which the Avesbury receptionists objected. The situation was only resolved when, on the insistence of their new partner, the Avesbury practice too banned smoking in their waiting room on the grounds that it was wrong to permit it in a setting committed to health.

Another issue, one which one Avesbury doctor found 'absolutely infuriating', concerned the 'mini-waiting area' intended for
patients waiting to see a nurse. The area was also close to the
consulting rooms of two of the Barr doctors, who arranged for
patients wanting to see them to wait there. One was Dr Bourne
who explained that he got anxious about patients waiting too long
for him and so had to insist that they wait outside his room: 'It's
terribly important that they see what I am up to,' he said. So he
and his colleague continued to use the 'mini-waiting area'.

There were no clashes, however, which left the practices
regretting their move. On the contrary, the doctors in both
practice groups felt that they and their patients had either benefited from the move to the Health Centre or that most of the
fears which they had had before the move had either not materialized or been rather less disadvantageous than they had anticipated. The Barr group, for example, thought that most of their
patients had not been alienated by the modern building and busier
atmosphere which prevailed; and they were pleased that many
who had previously attended their branch surgery in a neighouring
area were willing to stay with them when they closed that surgery
down shortly after their move, a decision which they took with
some trepidation. The Barr group had also expressed some fear
initially that the Avesbury group might dominate and give the tone
to the Centre since the latter had been more vocal on many issues.
Three years afterwards, a Barr group doctor thought the danger
was reversed. With Dr Adams gone, there was little 'noise' from
the Avesbury practice. The Barr group, through its more active
role in teaching medical students, had, in his view, become the
pre-eminent one. It would be bad for the Centre, he concluded,
however, if one group became demonstrably more eminent and
popular than the other.

Avesbury doctors almost all felt some sense of loss of the team
intimacy which they had enjoyed in their old premises; but they
felt that their patients were just as happy with the Health Centre as
they had been with the Avesbury Road surgery. They also
recognized that their own sense of loss was due as much to the
gradual withdrawal of Dr Adams (see Chapter 4) and to other
non-professional difficulties which some of them were experiencing as it was to Health Centre practice as such.

On the credit side some benefits were seen as belonging to the unique properties of Health Centres and not merely to group practice and teamwork in modern, purpose-built surgery accommodation, although it was of course difficult to separate the effects of the three coincidental factors.

The four main developments in their practices which they attributed to the Health Centre as such were, first, the creation of a major nursing component in the care they were able to provide; second, a more extensive use of the community-based health-related services of the Area Health Authority on behalf of their patients; third, the ability to bring hospital-based consultant services into the primary care setting; and fourth, a much more solid and substantial contribution to the training of future general practitioners and other community-based health workers. We have already considered the third of these developments in some detail in Chapter 3 and we will not repeat it here. The fourth development, the use of the Health Centre as a demonstration and major training facility for medical and other health personnel, is reserved for special treatment in our next chapter. Before concluding this one, we want to consider briefly the impact which the expanded joint treatment area and the presence of a range of other community health services had on the practice units.

THE NURSING COMPONENT

The Avesbury doctors took much of the credit for the centrality – physical and symbolic – accorded to the treatment area in the Health Centre, an area which included examination cubicles, an open treatment room, a small laboratory, and lavatories. It was shared by the practices and, as we have already pointed out, the nurses, although employed and paid by one or other practice, treated patients from either group. The Avesbury doctors had developed this plan from their experience with the primitive makeshift arrangement in their old premises, which had persuaded them of the centrality of treatment and examination in primary health care. As one of them said:

'What we have here is an extension of what we already had in our old premises. The treatment area is the critical part of the building. It also makes this Health Centre different from all other Health Centres. Whatever diagnostic tests or investigations you want can take place in an area especially designed for that purpose, an area in which doctors and nurses work together.'

The Barr practitioners freely admitted the significance which the experience of having a treatment and examination area had had for them. One or two of them believed that sharing these facilities with the Avesbury doctors and nurses had been of very great importance to them (see Chapter 5). It had certainly facilitated the dissemination of ideas between the practice groups to an extent which was unlikely to have occurred had they been housed in separate premises.

INTRA-CENTRE REFERRALS

All the doctors were in no doubt that their knowledge of and use of the range of community health services had increased greatly as a result of their common location in the same building. Describing the range of services, one doctor marvelled: 'There are so many facilities one sometimes forgets all there is.' Those to which they most frequently referred patients were physiotherapy – which they all felt should be further expanded – chiropody, audiometry, speech therapy, dietetics, and the slimming clinic. They used the family planning clinic and the marriage guidance counsellor less frequently, as these were services which they or other members of their practice already provided.

The doctors particularly appreciated the personal contact with the clinic's senior nursing officer in charge of the authority's services, who took to attending both practices' weekly meetings. Her connections within the Area Health Authority had, in the words of a doctor: 'extended the network of available resources beyond the Centre considerably'.

The doctors felt that it was the greater opportunity for personal contact which had made them more likely to refer patients than they had previously done. It was easier in general to share the case and there was less likelihood of losing contact. One general practitioner, for instance, reported how extremely helpful it was to talk to a clinical medical officer who was looking after the school at which 'you might have a difficult customer. I always find her when I need to.'

In addition to facilitating referrals and feedback, face-to-face contact exerted a form of moral pressure which it was difficult to resist:

'Take what happens with John, the school counsellor, a side which, I must confess, I was not even aware of before meeting John. I now share quite a few cases with him and I honestly think that if I was phoned by some faceless person and asked to spend the afternoon attending a case conference, I wouldn't go; but knowing it is John, and I have to face him the next day, I go and I take others with me and the results are very rewarding.'

It was this doctor, too, who made most use of what she called the 'promotive' services of the Family Health Clinic. These were services intended to help integrate newcomers into the community: they included English language classes for immigrants, and sewing classes which she saw as having the very important latent function of introducing new mothers to one another.

At least three doctors as well as many other health workers were happy that for some patients the Centre appeared to be a 'day hospital': there were always a 'few nutty characters wandering around' and that, they said, 'was fine'. Others hoped that the Centre's 'open-door' character would make it a 'drop-in' centre for mums with small children. All agreed, however, that, to date, the Centre was 'still an illness centre with health education stuck on'.

Despite the organizational deficiencies, and notwithstanding the strength of the identities of its individual units, the doctors believed the Centre had developed an identity of its own. They all felt confident that the Centre was well known and had an excellent reputation in their part of London. A Barr doctor told us:

'The Centre has a tremendous pull, a personality or identity distinct from that of the practice, with which we do identify.'

Nevertheless, at least in the opinion of one of the Avesbury group, the Centre could not, on its own, achieve all the potential promise prophesied by those who had pioneered the idea in the first place. This would only happen when their Centre was one of a chain of comparable Health Centres, each serving between 10,000 and 30,000 people 'custom-planned to meet the needs of each area'.

THE RESEARCH TEAM'S ASSESSMENT

In this chapter we have reviewed the experience of two already experienced group practice units when they became health centre-based practices.

The pivotal place accorded the shared treatment area in the Centre and the agreement that the nurses employed by each practice should be available to treat patients of the other seem to have been the most significant factors in determining both the further development of teamwork at the Barr practice and the willingness of that practice to open itself up to outside influences. In the event, the Avesbury doctors, who had been mainly responsible for pressing the idea of a common treatment room and nursing component as well as the idea of bringing some hospital out-patient clinics and specialist advisory sessions to the Health Centre, were less able or willing to remain as innovatory after the move as they had been before. They were aware of the loss of momentum and attributed it to changes in their own personal circumstances and not in any way to the Health Centre, about which they remained utterly convinced.

In our next chapter we look at the development of the Centre as a major location for medical student training, against the background of changing ideas of medical eduation. In Chapter 16, we consider patients' reactions to the Health Centre building itself.

11   General Practitioners as Teachers

In Chapter 1, when discussing the factors which appeared in the 1960s to be putting the long-term future of general practice in this country in jeopardy, we mentioned the significance which contemporaries in the Royal College of General Practitioners and elsewhere attached to the issue of training for practice in this sector of medical services.

The issue was two-fold, involving both the preparation for general medical practice embodied in the courses for the basic medical qualification and the post-qualification preparation for those entering this branch of professional practice.

We have also pointed out elsewhere that the historical development of health services has been characterized by a series of incremental changes rather than by any substantial breaks with tradition or abrupt changes of direction. Nowhere is this more a truism than in the case of pre- and post-qualification medical education, which still, in the 1980s, bore the vestigial remains of settlements made in the mid-nineteenth century by the various bodies whose qualifications were recognized as entitling their holders to be registered with the General Medical Council. That body, established in 1858, has been responsible throughout its existence for seeing that those on its register of medical practitioners have obtained a degree or licence from an institution which it itself recognizes as fit to examine. The underlying assumption was that the registered would at least be 'safe' doctors able to treat without supervision a range of common medical conditions (Royal Commission on Medical Education 1968: 22). There have only been three modifications of any substance to the General Medical Council's functions in this respect. In 1950, registration on qualification became provisional only; full registration now follows after the satisfactory completion of a post-qualification year spent half in a medical and half in a surgical specialty, under the supervision of a consultant physician or surgeon (Medical Act 1950). The other two changes, which came after the completion of our study, dealt with registration for doctors who had obtained their qualification overseas and with vocational training for general practitioners.

Both before and after the introduction of the pre-registration requirement, which had to be discharged in hospital-based specialties, it was customary, but not obligatory, for those aspiring to a consultant post to spend several more years in a junior position in hospital, still working under the direction of a consultant. Moreover, both before and after the nationalization of the hospitals, a consultant appointment was only likely to be awarded to those who obtained the membership of the Royal College of Physicians (MRCP), the fellowship of the Royal College of Surgeons (FRCS) or equivalent specialist qualification by further advanced examination. Preparing for these examinations, which it was not uncommon for candidates to have to resit two or three times before success was achieved, usually involved taking a succession of junior hospital doctor posts where the pay was low and the workload heavy. It was well recognized before World War II that the financial sacrifice involved, if only for a limited time, was often judged too great by those with limited means and/or family-building intentions. Entry into general practice as an assistant or into an expanding salaried local government public health service, by contrast, both represented an easier financial option and could be done without sitting further arduous and highly competitive examinations.

After the war and the creation of the National Health Service, the financial sacrifice demanded of aspiring consultants diminished somewhat as the rate of remuneration of junior hospital doctors gradually increased relative to that of other doctors, including consultants; but the advent of national manpower planning and the rigorous restrictions imposed on the number of consultant posts, especially in the most sought-after specialties, intensified competition for them. Not unnaturally, therefore, general practice, in which there were fewer restrictions on entry than there had been before the war (for example, it was no longer legal to buy a retiring practitioner's goodwill) (National Health Service Act 1946, section 35') was increasingly seen by young entrants to the profession as an easier, if in other ways less attractive, option. Those who chose it were regarded by those who did not as probably incapable of mastering the esoteric knowledge of many diseases and their treatments required to succeed in, for example, the MRCP examination. Although a logical *non sequitur*, it seemed to follow that the time spent in qualifying and registering as a medical practitioner was all that was required to become a perfectly competent general practitioner, in contrast to the need for further advanced preparation for a consultant post.

Superficially, this was not an unattractive view to those responsible for securing the funding for the National Health Service. To prolong manpower training for general practice could add to the expense of the service, which was already escalating beyond expectations (Committee of Enquiry into the Cost of the National Health Service 1956: 1) and to demands for increased remuneration from general practitioners on account of the increasing comparability of their post-registration training with that of specialists (Royal Commission on Doctors' and Dentists' Remuneration 1960). Given too an effective referral system, which could act as a fail-safe device were the 'safe' doctor to prove 'unsafe', there seemed to be little need for a better or differently trained general practitioner.

Amongst those who had already become general practitioners in the 1950s and 1960s there was also some support for the existing system of entry without further demonstration of academic worth. Those who did not want change argued that basic medical education provided an adequate base and that, for the rest, only experience, not further dependent practice, could make a good general practitioner. Moreover, some felt like resisting what seemed like a growing mania, affecting many professional groups including medicine, for acquiring credentials, a trend which if unchecked might debase the value of their own primary qualification (Gerth and Mills 1948: 241; Parkin 1979: 54). If an individual did not feel equal to the challenge of becoming a general practice principal immediately after registration, he could attach himself as an assistant to an experienced man. Moreover, a national trainee scheme had been established in 1948 following a recommendation of the Spens Committee (Inter-departmental Committee on the Remuneration of General Practitioners 1946) and attracted a few hundred recruits annually during the early 1950s. The trainee was to spend one year in general practice in a supernumerary capacity with a principal approved as a trainer.

However, there were other general practitioners, prominent among whom were those who had come together to form the College of General Practitioners (later Royal), who did not share this sanguine view. They recognized that there was some truth in the criticisms of the standards of practice made by Dr Collings, a New Zealand observer, and that a case had been made out for a rigorous post-qualification period of training for those wanting to enter this branch of medicine (Collings 1950). Moreover, as long as it was possible for newly qualified doctors to become principals, so long, in their view, would general practice be held in low regard by hospital-based specialists and the general public (BMA 1950).

FROM 'SAFE' DOCTOR TO PURPOSE-SPECIFIC TRAINED DOCTOR

By the mid-1960s, opinion, at least in the College of General Practitioners, had swung firmly in favour of compulsory post-registration specialist training for general practice, although there were differences of opinion as to what the length, content and location of that training should be and whether it should involve formal examination and certification by the College (College of General Practitioners 1964; College of General Practitioners 1965: 2). The Report of the Royal Commission on Medical Education in 1968 gave a powerful boost to the advocates of a recognized period of specialist general practice training of approximately the same length as that required for recognition as a specialist and a prelude to a consultant appointment (Royal Commission on Medical Education 1968: 35). Some active opposition had to be overcome as well as the inertia of various bodies, professional and political. These had to be activated before such recommendations could be adopted and implemented. Legislative provision was eventually made to this end, closing independent contractor status in general practice to those who possessed only the minimum medical qualification (National Health Service Vocational Training Act 1976).

The advocates of a definite period of post-registration training for the general practitioner also had to agree amongst themselves what the nature of that training should be. In its turn, this depended upon greater clarification as to what general practice itself was all about, and in what respects it differed from or should embody elements of the knowledge base and skills of other specialties. It also involved reaching a sufficient degree of consensus among those who, by virtue of their elected positions in the General Medical Services Committee of the British Medical Association or the College of General Practitioners, could claim to represent the professional group at large. Such issues, as who should be responsible for the training and how judgements were to be made as to whether a trainee had reached a satisfactory standard of practice, had to be resolved. That none of these issues was solved easily or without controversy is not surprising given the underlying individualism and dislike of regulation which are characteristics of many of those doctors who choose general practice as a career.

The moves to universal compulsory training were hence piecemeal. Provision for voluntary training, as we have seen, occurred in the late 1940s and received further encouragement in the early 1960s (Ministry of Health 1964). The Government agreed to pay trainees a year's salary while they worked under the direction of recognized trainers who had to be principals with at least ten years' experience. Those wishing to become trainers had to be acceptable to a committee of their peers, drawn from the Local Medical Committee.

However, it could still be financially advantageous for the would-be entrant to take an assistantship in a practice with a view to eventual partnership, rather than become a trainee. Potential trainers too could find the former arrangement preferable because the traineeship terms, at least theoretically, involved some restriction on what the trainee could be asked to do: moreover, initially trainees could not be taken directly into partnership on completion of the training period. In practice, there were complaints from some trainees that they got little training from their putative trainer, that they were simply used as assistants to help carry a heavy workload, and that they were discouraged from attending

half-day release educational arrangements made under the auspices of the general practice advisers to the Regional Post-
graduate Medical Deans (Horder and Swift 1979). The financial
disincentives to traineeship rather than assistantship entry were
somewhat modified when, after 1966, the years spent as trainee
but not as an assistant were counted for purposes of seniority
payments (*BMJ* 1969: 60).

During the late 1960s and early 1970s, a number of three-year
training schemes were developed in various parts of the country.
These, in addition to a trainee year in a practice unit, involved a
series of senior house officer and registrar posts in hospital-based
specialties particularly relevant to general practice, such as
paediatrics, geriatrics, psychiatry, and accident and emergency
(Horder and Swift 1979). One of the features of these schemes was
a regular weekly half-day release seminar under the auspices of a
general practitioner who acted as a tutor. More and more of those
who were now viewing general practice as a career began to opt for
these three-year traineeships. These developments were encouraged by the Royal College of General Practitioners, which could
claim with some justification that more innovations had been made
in preparing individuals for its specialty than for other branches of
medicine or surgery (Freeman and Byrne 1976).

THE GROUP PRACTICES AND GENERAL PRACTITIONER TRAINING

None of the doctors in the smaller practices in our study were
general practitioner trainers and only one of them, Dr Erickson,
had had a systematic introduction which he called a training when
he became an assistant in the 1950s. Neither he nor his colleagues
had applied to become trainers. It would have been difficult in
their cramped old premises: in their new ones they had too much
to do immediately to want to take on the work involved.

By contrast, both the Avesbury and Barr practices had seen
themselves as having a training function from a very early date.
Throughout the period of our study, two doctors out of the six in
each practice were registered as trainers, and there was always at
least one trainee in post. All the Avesbury arrangements throughout that time were with *ad hoc* one-year trainees; by 1975,
however, the Barr practice had had four trainees from those

included in the three-year vocational course centred on Masters' Hospital Medical School. The Avesbury practice was expecting its first such trainee the year after the study ended.

When we asked the doctors for their principal goal in training others, most of them suggested that it was in essence a 're-orienting process', in which they had to change many attitudes to practice acquired in hospital. The aim was to loosen the bonds that tied trainees to the hospital and to a highly structured approach to medical practice and to help them tolerate the 'less well-defined, less structured, more amorphous scene of general practice'. The process had to be delicately handled so as not to be too costly in terms of emotional stress. Some of the doctors also clearly hoped that, given what they felt to be the innovatory nature of their own practices, they would be helping to provide a second generation of individuals who, in their turn, would be innovators and leaders. Beyond these general aims, the trainers claimed that they tailored their training programme to the needs of the individual trainee. This meant identifying 'gaps' in the latter's knowledge and devising programmes to fill them.

The three-year vocational training scheme in which the Barr practice co-operated brought about changes both in its training programme and in the Avesbury's:

'The trainees have become very firm about getting more teaching. They don't only want to be exposed to us, they want to see other practices. They also want to attend many outside seminars and lectures.'

Doctors at both practices felt that they had met the recent more assertive requests of trainees more than half-way. The placements were now much more oriented to training, less to service. The trainees were given a great deal of 'time off' to visit other practices and to learn more about the different areas which interested them. Commenting on these changes, a doctor concluded:

'We gain too. It rebounds on us: the trainees stimulate us with all they learn from outside.'

At the instigation of the trainees, joint seminars for trainees from both practices, generally conducted by Dr Bridges and, representing the Avesbury practice, Dr Alexander, were introduced. Both practices were committed to the principle of vocational training and, by and large, converged in terms of training objectives and programmes. They diverged, however, in the significance they accorded to the relationship between trainee and trainer and in their methods of induction into the traineeship. The differences reflected in the main the emphasis given to individual as against group responsibility in the two practices. The Barr doctors considered the relationship between trainee and trainer the crucial element in the training process: other relationships, although important, were only secondary. The Avesbury doctors, on the other hand, maintained that, although the trainee was assigned to an individual doctor, training was a function to be shared by all the doctors and by the non-medical staff. Explaining their reasoning, Dr Adair said:

'Being with us all, the trainees pick up bits they like. They are learning from many models all the time, so it enables them to select what they will do in their own practice.'

Barr practice policy was geared towards 'graduated responsibility', through a series of stages whereby the trainee was eased into the role of general practitioner. While emphasizing that each trainee's programme was a 'one-off', arrived at by the individual trainee and trainer, common to all their programmes was the requirement that the trainee spend the first few weeks simply 'sitting-in' with the trainer. After that, the trainee conducted a few consultations independently, gradually working up to a full load at any one surgery.

Induction at the Avesbury practice, in the words of both one of its doctors and a trainee, generally meant 'throwing the trainee in at the deep end'. Despite a practice decision to follow the Barr practice pattern, exigencies at the Avesbury always seemed to mean that the trainees, from the start of their placement, saw as many patients as possible on their own. In effect, having spent very little time sitting in with the principals, they were fitted into the surgery rota on almost the same basis as the 'old hands'. The research team's own enquiries certainly confirmed the differences between the two practices: during the sample weeks of the enquiry among attenders in 1972, 30 per cent of all the Avesbury patients had consultations with trainees compared with only 15 per cent of the Barr patients. In 1975, the differences between the practices decreased; the trainees at the Avesbury saw 17 per cent of the patients while those at the Barr saw 13 per cent.

Doctors at each practice emphasized different aspects of the traineeships as being of particular value to them. At the Barr practice, the relatively intense relationship between individual trainer and trainee was, as a rule, experienced by the former as highly gratifying. According to one trainer it 'added enormously' to his work satisfaction. Those who were not involved directly in training considered that they too gained: 'Our discussions with the trainees are very useful. We learn a lot – I learn a lot.' At the Avesbury practice where 'everybody takes joint responsibility to stop and talk to trainees', the advantages the doctors stressed were 'up-to-date knowledge inputs' and help with workload. Relationships with the trainees were regarded as successful if the trainee fitted in to the 'family'.

Both practices recognized that their respective styles matched some trainees better than others, and this was confirmed by the trainees. From our interviews with the eight trainees during the study period we learnt that, in general, they were satisfied with their placements. Four of them, indeed, indicated that they had not only preferred their practice's system of induction but would have had difficulty tolerating the other's: the other four, however, had some criticisms to make of the system they had experienced and saw something preferable in the other. A Barr group trainee, for example, had found their system 'infantilizing', hadn't needed 'their early kid glove treatment' and would have preferred to be left to 'get on with it' as they did at the Avesbury. An Avesbury trainee, on the other hand, would have liked a more measured induction, having nearly 'cracked' under the strain of heavy surgeries and frequent after-hours duties.

All the doctors at both practices were on the whole convinced that, despite difficulties and the occasional individual 'flop', having trainees was good for them, for the trainees and for the future status of the specialty.

BACK TO THE BEGINNING

It was also becoming clear in the 1960s to those wanting to improve the attractiveness of general practice compared to the hospital-based specialties that basing medical education exclusively in teaching hospitals was one of the main obstacles they faced. Medical students would naturally be influenced by the examples set by their clinical teachers and want to emulate them. Furthermore, in the absence of general practitioner teachers, the academic specialists and consultants could explicitly or implicitly inculcate negative images of general practice. Out-patient clinics and accident and emergency departments provided ample evidence that many of the general practitioners in the vicinity of the teaching hospitals were poor diagnosticians and managers and that they were held in low regard both by their patients and by the hospital-based staff. If medical students were to gain a more favourable impression of general practitioners and of the opportunities for good quality work in this branch of medicine, it was clear that they should have early contact with the best practitioners in the field (Royal Commission on Medical Education 1968: para. 277).

Edinburgh was the first university in Britain to establish an academic department and a professorial chair in General Practice, and to make it compulsory for medical students to do a clerkship in it. These developments took place from the middle 1950s; but, despite pressure, it was not until a decade later that comparable departments began to be established elsewhere in Great Britain.

London University itself was not notably in the forefront of these developments; many of its twelve medical schools paid little more than lip-service to the need to expose their students systematically to the clinical problems met in the general practice setting. Masters' Hospital Medical School, the school nearest to the group practices we studied, had done little throughout the 1950s and 1960s to provide opportunities for their own medical students to study outside the hospital setting. Some students managed to do so, but it was on their own initiative. There was no academic department of general practice.

Masters' did, however, ask the senior partner in the Barr practice to give an annual lecture to final year students on the opportunities within general practice, and by the time Dr Bourne had replaced Dr Barr in this capacity the climate of opinion in the medical school had begun to change. A distinguished Professor of Medicine had given his personal support to the recommendation of the Royal Commission on Medical Education in 1968 that all students should spend some time in general practice settings. He believed that the projected Health Centre, not far from the hospital itself, provided ideal conditions for this exposure and he helped to raise money to establish a library in the Centre for the use of teachers and students. Both the Barr and the Avesbury practice doctors were eager to participate in undergraduate teaching and believed that, together with the Family Health Clinic staff, they could thereby make a significant contribution to basic medical education.

THE GENERAL PRACTICE COMPONENT IN BASIC MEDICAL EDUCATION

All the doctors in our sample supported the drive for the inclusion of general practice teaching in the basic medical curriculum. They thought it essential that the aims of primary care be transmitted to students, that primary care settings be used for the purpose, and that students be exposed to work in the community as early i.ı their medical training as possible.

These views were held by the smaller practice doctors as well as by the Avesbury and Barr practice doctors, but the formers' involvement in such teaching, during the period of our study, was limited. In their old premises, they had had 'the occasional student from Masters' Hospital sitting in on a few nights a week', and they had enjoyed that. After their move, they felt they had adequate accomodation, and had offered regular student placements to another medical school, which, like Masters', was extending its curriculum to cover general practice. At the time we completed our observations they had not yet begun to take students on a regular basis.

Dr Bridges of the Barr practice was in charge of the general practice programme for all medical students at Masters' Hospital Medical School, a position which he had taken in 1973 with the support of his general practitioner colleagues. In their fourth year, students spent two weeks in an urban practice and a further two weeks in a country practice. The majority of Masters' School students came to either the Avesbury or the Barr practice when these were located in the Health Centre. In line with the longer-term aims of these practices, the Centre had become a major teaching facility for Masters' School. The School, however, left it to Dr Bridges in association with the participating general practitioners to determine how students spent their time in the practices. Dr Bridges, in turn, although providing general guidelines in the way of teaching objectives and a list of activities, left it to the practices to elaborate their own programmes. He played the most prominent part in the Barr programme.

Programmes at both practices began with a brief explanatory talk on the work of the practice, an outline of what the students were to see and do and who they were to turn to for information or guidance. In the course of the fortnight they 'sat in' on patient consultations with the doctors and accompanied the latter on their home visits. They spent time with the receptionists, practice nurses and attached health workers. They attended practice lunch-time meetings and were encouraged to participate in them. They met the Nursing Officer in charge of the Area Health Authority services at the Centre and visited the local authority social services department headquarters and other social services in the area, such as a rehabilitation centre. They were encouraged to read, using the Centre's small collection of books for the purpose.

At the end both of the first and of the second week of their placement, the pairs attached to each practice met jointly with Dr Bridges and Dr Alexander. These meetings took the form of seminars at which students could ask for information and express their views on what they had done and seen.

There were some differences in the way of dealing with students at the two practices. At the Barr practice, the doctors took turns to be responsible for the students, that is, for inducting them into the practice, supervising their activities and being available to answer questions or deal with problems. At the Avesbury practice these functions were, to a considerable extent, 'the domain of the secretariat'. While all the Avesbury doctors participated in the programmes and regarded themselves as available to the students at any time, there was no system, such as at the Barr practice, whereby students could relate to a single doctor specifically delegated to deal with their requirements.

This difference, in turn, appeared to affect the extent to which students at each practice were able 'to work on their own', something which, according to doctors at both practices, most students wanted. A Barr practice doctor put it this way:

'They all want to do more on their own. At the hospital they are always about the fourth person to see a patient, so here they very much want to be the person of first contact.'

He and his partners tried to make it possible for their students to see patients on their own, even though it involved the doctors in considerable extra work because students had to be carefully briefed beforehand and closely questioned afterwards. The students were occasionally allowed too to visit patients at home on their own. The Avesbury practice, because it had a looser relationship between the students and any one general practitioner, did not feel able to give the students this amount of autonomy in their dealings with patients.

ASSESSING THE IMPACT ON STUDENTS

In the belief that rating students' performance during the two weeks would help them see how far their own teaching objectives were being met, the doctors at both practices had agreed to assess the students' potential for general practice at the end of the fortnight, although they expressed doubt about the value of such an assessment after such a short period.

In the event, on this criterion, they rated most in the second and third categories B and C, which stood for 'good' or 'pretty good'. Both the first and last categories, A and D, comprising the 'quite exceptionals' and the 'switched-off', were used for a small minority only. Indeed, doctors from both practices suggested that exposure to general practice, as they practised it, had generally served to confirm or reinforce positive attitudes to it held by the majority and only occasionally to convert a student previously committed to a hospital specialty. As one Avesbury doctor put it:

'It's very interesting. The bulk of the students are sufficiently interested to give us the feeling that we are preaching to the converted. It's only a minority who, in a sense, haven't joined us. They are the ones already wholly committed to another specialty or who, for personality reasons, find it difficult to relate to patients as a general practitioner should.'

In so far, then, as their involvement in medical student teaching was done with a view to persuading future generations of doctors that general practice was an important branch of medicine and could be an attractive career prospect for the person who wished for intellectually challenging work, all the Barr and Avesbury doctors felt that they could record a modest success. They also believed that they had helped to minimize negative images of general practice amongst those who were likely to enter hospital specialties. Finally they held that it had helped to improve their standing with the consultants at Masters' Hospital.

At the same time, they outlined a number of shortcomings in their programmes, some of which seemed inevitable given the restricted time and resources available to them. First, ideally, for example, one practice group felt that there should be two separate general practice placement periods: the first should come in the very early stages of the course, even before the students started their pre-clinical work, and the second, as at present, in the fourth year of study. Second, given that continuity of care was one of the most important assets of general practice, they recognized that it was rarely possible in two weeks to demonstrate how a relationship could be built up over time. Again, much of their emergency work, an important component of primary medical care, occurred after hours. Because students did not 'live in' with the duty doctor they missed out on much of this work. Dr Bennett told us that from time to time she was tempted to take a student to her home to learn about the calls received at night or over weekends; but, as she said, 'it wasn't on' in London. She hoped that it would happen in the course of their country placements when they did live in with a general practitioner. Some doctors suggested that if more money was made available to the practices by Masters' Hospital Medical School, they could afford to take fewer patients and devote more time to teaching. However, this was not universally accepted as desirable: Dr Bourne, for example, thought that that might not be in the best interest of the neighbourhood they served.

Furthermore, in terms of the effect on their own day-to-day work, routine teaching was a mixed blessing. On the positive side, it kept them on their toes; working with interested, alert students was stimulating and refreshing. All the same, it was an additional strain and tended to slow down the pace of their work:

'On a busy day, with a backlog of patients building up, conflicting student and patient needs can drive anyone crackers.'

Another doctor told us: 'Whether we want to view it that way or not, it is an added burden.' Apart from anything else the presence of students could be inhibiting for doctor and patient. The doctors claimed that patient consent was always sought when they wanted a student to be present. One doctor was conscious of the need to make that consent real: 'You have to watch the patient and assess the real reaction and, if necessary, send the student out.' He estimated that students would be asked to withdraw on average from about two out of ten consultations. But not infrequently, even when the patient consented, the consultation developed differently from what it would have been had a student not been present.

THE RESEARCH TEAM'S ASSESSMENT

It was clear to us that the contribution which they were able to make to the basic medical education of Masters' School students after their move to the Health Centre was of enormous signi-ficance to both practices at the practical and symbolic levels. They had already established themselves before the moves as practices with innovatory ideas capable of attracting trainees who wanted to learn their general practice in the context of new ideas about the doctor – patient relationship or the part played by a multi-professional primary care team in helping to solve socio-medical problems. The Health Centre offered them an even greater opportunity of impressing on medical students the professional challenges involved in a career in general practice in an eviron-ment where they could co-operate with other health and social service workers.

For this reason, a close association with what many of them saw as the most influential forces determining the orientation of future generations of doctors – namely the medical school – was un-doubtedly a key element in the strategies which both of the senior partners wanted to employ to alter the shape of general practice. For the Barr practice, in particular, it was one of the major reasons for wanting to practise from a Health Centre, to which they did not have the same general ideological commitment as the Avesbury group. It was a great source of pride and satisfaction to them that Masters' Hospital Medical School, in responding to mounting pressure to expose their students to systematic teaching in a primary medical care setting, had chosen a member of their practice as lecturer and organizer and seen the Health Centre in which they worked as a major teaching site.

We end this chapter with a quotation from an interview with Dr Alexander who was then the most closely involved member of the Avesbury practice in the field of education, which conveys something of the feeling of achievement which had followed their earlier campaigns:

'If it's put to students and trainees that in 1952 general practice was virtually dead; that by 1962 it was breathing fairly regularly, and by 1972 was doing well and feeling its strength – even though its superstructure is still in the process of construction – it can all be very exciting.'

PART III

General Practitioners and Patients

12   The Boundaries of Patient Care

The extensive literature since the 1950s relating to the role of the general practitioner in contemporary society is itself an indication of the uncertainties and ambiguities surrounding that role in the recent past (Collings 1950; McWhinney 1967; Brotherston 1971). Much of this literature, whether in the form of reports from official or professionally sponsored *ad hoc* committees of enquiry or of articles or letters in professional journals, was based on the agreed premise that general practitioners either already were or were in danger of becoming little more than sorters of the medical wheat from the non-medical chaff (Curwen 1964). The wheat, the 'real' problems worthy of medical attention, it was implied, was increasingly passed to the hospital-based specialists; the chaff consisted either of problems of such a trivial nature as not to require the attention of a medically trained person at all or of matters inappropriately brought to the doctor (Horder 1977). There was agreement on all sides that, whatever the true state of affairs, it was bad for the morale of general practitioners to see themselves or be seen by others in such a light. If only to secure sufficient recruits to the service in the future it was essential to identify a more valued role for the general practitioner. The solutions which were proffered to that end fell mainly into one of two groups. The first we call the *traditional medical* solution, and the second the *holistic medicine* solution. Some, of course, saw the solution in a combination of the two approaches.

TRADITIONAL VERSUS HOLISTIC MEDICINE

The advocates of the former approach argued that general practitioners should stick to a narrowly defined medical last (Coles 1950;

Sowerby 1977). They must be skilled in the diagnosis and treatment of the major life-threatening and chronic diseases as well as of the minor acute infections likely to afflict a cross-section of patients of all ages and both sexes. They should provide every medical procedure for them except major surgical treatment or the more esoteric laboratory investigations. They should be able to reassure patients whose problems were not of this kind and either deter them from useless consultations or refer them to other qualified professional personnel, such as health visitors or social workers, who had responsibility for dealing with needs of a social or emotional kind. They should not seek to extend their role by responding to requests for help with emotional problems for which neither their training nor their conceptions of what doctoring should involve had prepared them.

In short, the traditional medicine advocates plumped for a restricted rather than a diffuse role for general practitioners. They saw dangers in general practitioners accepting tasks for which they had not been prepared and which were likely to be intrinsically and extrinsically unrewarding. They would earn respect and gratification by convincing their patients and their hospital colleagues of the breadth and depth of their knowledge of the human body in health and illness.

The advocates of holistic medicine solutions, on the other hand, argued in essence that the task of general practitioners was not to make distinctions between trivial and serious requests for help, but to treat every request as legitimate and a challenge to their diagnostic and therapeutic skills (Balint 1964). In order to do this, they had to acquire expertise in fields of knowledge which had not been adequately dealt with in basic medical education, namely in the part played by social and psychological as well as physical factors in individuals' illness experiences and in their use of services. The general practitioners' salvation, their social standing among their peers and the population at large, as well as their professional gratification, must come from the widespread acknowledgement that they too were specialists, possessors of a unique body of knowledge and skills to do with people as socially responsive animals with a complex range of reactions to emotional or physical stimuli and not as mere assembly points for a number of interrelated physical parts any one of which could go wrong (*BMJ* 1963b: 156; BMA 1970). For them, the general practitioner's services to patients consisted in accepting the inevitable diffuseness and imprecision of patients' demands for help which no other medical or non-medical professional group could or would meet and in imposing some semblance of order and meaning on them.

Within both these 'camps', variations could, of course, be observed. Among the 'traditionalists' there were some who advocated some degree of specialization based on the age or the diseases of patients while others argued for the maintenance of across-the-board generalism (McKeown 1961). Some advocated sessional hospital appointments in specialties for general practitioners; others emphasized the desirability of maintaining clinical responsibility for patients admitted to hospital for all but the most complicated medical procedures or for surgery; still others believed in increasing the 'technology' of their own surgeries, so that tests presently performed in the hospital precincts could be carried out in general practice settings (Ministry of Health 1963:47). There were also diverse views among the traditionalists on the practice of preventive medicine. Some wanted to introduce the systematic pre-symptomatic screening of adult populations for vulnerability factors such as high blood pressure; others argued against what they saw as interventionist medicine, as yet unproven and which might encourage patient dependency, if not hypochondria (Fry 1969: 161).

Amongst the holistic medicine advocates there was also diversity of opinion. There were the followers of Michael Balint, viewed by some as the founding father of latter-day holism in medicine (Norell 1973: x). Balint emphasized the need to evaluate the pertinence of 'neurotic' or psychological factors in a patient's behaviour and to operate at a 'deeper level' of analysis, so as to avoid the pitfalls of a compromised, negotiated diagnosis in which the doctor merely conspired with the patient in a process of mutual deception and left the real problems unsolved. This deeper level analysis involved interpreting rather than taking at face value the meaning and significance of the symptoms which the patient offered to the doctor. There were others, however, who, while they saw general practitioners as dealing, whether they liked it or not, with many different facets of patients' emotional and physical ills, were not followers of Balint and saw their own role as less that of interpreter as of supporter of the distressed or lonely; as responders to patients' explicit statements of their needs rather than as construers of the latent content of such needs (Thomas 1974).

In this chapter and the following two we consider the views of the doctors in our study on the character of their work for patients and their relationships with them. In the last two chapters of Part III we look at the complementary perspectives, expectations and views of the patients registered with them.

THE STUDY DOCTORS – RECRUITS TO HOLISM

Where did the doctors in our study stand on these controversial attempts to map out a role for general practitioners and establish how broad or narrow the boundaries of their concern should be? By and large, they all stood on the holistic rather than the traditional medicine side of the fence. All of them saw general practice as calling on them to provide for a diversity of human needs far greater than that for which their basic medical training had prepared them. Many admitted that this had not always been the case; their perceptions of their role had changed since they started practice. For instance, Dr Bennett of the Barr practice said she now saw nothing as inappropriate for presentation to the general practitioner, but had done so when she was younger. Then, she had not felt that she should be asked to help patients with their emotional difficulties. Dr Bridges, of the same practice, also mentioned the expanded horizons of his work. He felt he had been much influenced in accepting the expansion by the publications and activities of the Royal College of General Practitioners. Dr Osmond, a single-handed practitioner, also emphasized his initial unpreparedness for the role as he now saw it: 'I had to learn from scratch.'

Besides general intellectual acceptance by the doctors that they had inevitably to be concerned with emotional as well as physical *malaise* in their patients, there was also considerable agreement in the explanations they offered for their changing perceptions. There were differences amongst them, however, in the extent to which they welcomed the expansion of their concerns beyond the physical.

The explanation offered in one form or another by most doctors for their own changing role was the changing shape of illness in the community during the twenty or so years they had been in practice. They thought people were physically healthier than they used to be and, consequently, that doctors were dealing with less advanced, serious pathology such as the 'very, very bad cardiac condition' and the 'totally disabling bronchitis'. There were fewer cases of acute appendicitis, of severe ear infection, of duodenal ulcer, of measles, of crippling dysmenorrhea, and of acute psychiatric breakdown. Dr Cox put it this way:

> 'Twenty-five years ago, we saw a great deal of malnourishment, especially amongst children of large families and the elderly. Today, everyone is well-nourished, well-clothed and their housing has improved enormously – so the general population is physically better off.'

In the view of most of the doctors, the decline in the prevalence of serious pathology had been accompanied by an increase in psychosomatic ills and emotional distress. To quote Dr Cox again:

> 'Emotionally a lot of people are worse off, and I think the emotional thing is due to high expectations and not achieving them, striving after things which seem to be achievable, but which aren't, even with both parents working. This leads to stress and much greater anxiety than before.'

Dr Erickson, another of the smaller practice doctors, also felt that while improved housing, for instance, had brought about enormous changes in physical health, it had also generated new needs for such things as carpets and furniture, and with these needs had come hire-purchase payments and emotional problems. Likewise, Dr Amery, of the Avesbury practice, was confident that he saw less and less of what was defined in medical textbooks as disease and more and more of disordered function, almost invariably a social or emotional or even financial one:

> 'It seemed so simple thirty years ago; but not any more. Nine-tenths of those who come to us do so because they are bloody unhappy people – people so beaten down that they can no longer stand on their own feet. I try to unravel things for them to get them on their feet again – from disordered to ordered function.'

At the same time, but to varying degrees, doctors were aware that their own understanding of illness and the way in which they viewed it, and not a change in the character of illness in the community, might account for their increasing concern with the emotions. This explanation for the change in the perception of the general practitioner's role was more frequently offered by members of the Barr practice who were more likely to acknowledge the influence of Balint and social scientists on their own perceptions. For instance, Dr Balfour wondered whether emotional problems and mental illness had not always been as prevalent, and that doctors had just not understood them or had called them something else. 'We are certainly more alert to it now and so are our patients.' The present more realistic view of mental and emotional illness by doctor and patient alike, she felt, made it much easier for the doctor to be truthful, to deal with things as they really were, and not to have to pretend. Past pretence was partly the result of ignorance, partly fear of the patient's reactions. It had led to concoctions and false explanations. She was thankful such pretence was no longer necessary.

There was, however, some concern expressed by some doctors lest the balance swing to an over-concentration on psychological factors to the extent that physical pathology was overlooked. Dr Erickson had recently worked with a locum whose training was considerably more recent than his, and felt that she tended to jump to unwarranted psychological conclusions:

'For instance I saw a patient she had recently put on anti-depressants. I found a virus infection which she had missed and which most probably was responsible for the depression.'

Dr Adair of the Avesbury group also felt that doctors could be dazzled by what she termed 'the social work side' of their work to the neglect of their medical work:

'We see a mother who is tired and weary and sad and can't cope and we put it down to her life style. But this person may be anaemic.'

WHAT PATIENTS CAN LEGITIMATELY BRING TO DOCTORS

The doctors' recognition that their role inevitably involved them in whole person medicine and in a wide and diverse range of physical and emotional conditions did not of course imply that they all found the broader boundaries welcome or gratifying or that they were equally interested in all the conditions presented to them. Three of the four doctors in the smaller practices confessed that they did not like having to deal with people who came running to them for the slightest little sneeze or cough, things which would get better anyway if they waited a few days. In Dr Edmund's words, 'this is what wastes so much of our time'. All three tried, unsuccessfully they thought, to discourage patients with problems they called 'trivia' from coming to them. Four of the group practice doctors, two at the Barr and two at the Avesbury, while accepting that anything about which a patient was worried and sufficiently motivated to see a doctor was not trivial from the patient's viewpoint, nevertheless found this level of patient dependency on them either embarrassing or inimical to their view of what constituted the healthy individual. Dr Bennett, for example, was sorry that some patients regarded 'the doctor as God' with the magic to resolve all their problems, and Dr Adair suggested that young people in particular were using doctors as 'surrogate mums and dads'.

All the other group practice doctors, and one of those in the smaller practices, however, were adamant in rejecting the notion that their services were in any way being over-used or misused by patients. Indeed, one of them, Dr Bourne, was more concerned about groups of people who were *under-using* the service or not reaping as much benefit from it as they might:

'Social class V patients are not getting as good a service as they should. They don't know the value of psychotherapy. They also don't know how to use the appointments system, so hang around waiting without appointments.'

Dr Attenborough, from the Avesbury, echoed him in saying that, far from abusing the service, patients helped themselves a great deal without reference to doctors:

'One should remember that one is only the doctor and there are lots of others who are more important to the patient – friends, relatives – who support them. There is also a lot of self-medication.'

Drs Bowen, Bridges, Barrett, and Erickson, endorsing the patients' right to decide what was appropriate to bring to them, went as far as to say in one way or another that they welcomed the increasing recognition amongst patients that 'happiness' was something a doctor might do something about and brought their 'unhappiness' to the practice, either in the form of a physical pain or a frank depression. Dr Bourne thought too that it was the doctor's job to help lonely people. 'What is the answer to loneliness if no one will make themselves available to the lonely?' Dr Adams expressed a similar sentiment. Doctors had to be available to patients even when it was 'uncomfortable'. It was a doctor's job to listen to whatever people had to say:

> 'If the doctor is concerned, deeply concerned with the well-being of his patients, he must have empathy – love if you like – to relate to them as human beings. It is no longer sufficient to be concerned just with medical techniques.'

Like Dr Bourne, Dr Adams maintained that the doctor had to extend his concern to the isolated, the people without props, for whom, sometimes in some ways, the doctor – and other health and social workers – had to substitute for a husband or wife. Dr Amery endorsed this view:

> 'Medicine is all about loving and caring. If you can't do that, do something else.'

PROFESSIONAL PREFERENCES

While accepting the holistic nature of their tasks, the doctors, not unnaturally, expressed preferences for dealing with certain kinds of patients or conditions and most of them confessed to disliking or seeking to avoid others. Again, not unexpectedly, preferences were usually expressed for dealing with those conditions about which they felt themselves to be most knowledgeable and most able to achieve results.

For about half the doctors, the preference was for dealing with one or more aspects of physical disease and for the other half for treating emotional distress or psychiatric conditions; but there were a few whose preferred areas of work covered both kinds of illness. Dr Erickson's leaning was to psychiatric work. It had not always been so:

'Finding an early cancer was elating, but I have since learnt that success with it is rare. Despite an early find many such patients die. In contrast, whereas the recognition of depression used to be disheartening and made me fed-up, I now find I can, more often than not, help such patients. There are drugs to relieve their symptoms and we can talk out their underlying problems. If appropriate, I bring in other members of their family to join in the discussion and usually there is improvement within three to four weeks.'

On the whole, preferences were not practice-linked; indeed, special interests within practices appeared to complement each other to some extent. For example, Dr Erickson's preference for psychological medicine contrasted with his partner's overriding interest in somatic problems. At the Barr practice, Drs Bourne, Bowen, Barrett, and Bennett were doctors who, on the whole, found psychological problems more interesting than purely physical ones. By contrast, Dr Bridges thought that if he had any specific orientations, it was toward the physical rather than the psychological. Dr Balfour was happy to handle 'all types of problems', but considered she was better at some things – gynaecology, for instance – than at others. Three of the Avesbury doctors, Drs Adams, Alexander, and Amery, indicated that their overall orientation was predominantly psychological, but the latter two had special interests in some kinds of physical medicine; obstetrics for Dr Alexander and chest medicine for Dr Amery. Drs Attenborough and Ashton, the two youngest doctors in our sample, said they were somewhat diffident about dealing with the more complex psychological problems and felt, for that reason, that any bias they had was toward physical medicine.

EXPERTISE AND EMPATHY

During the early 1960s when general practice appeared to have reached a nadir in its professional fortunes, proposals were made by McKeown (1965) and others either to create age-band specialists in the primary care sector, what Fry called 'specialoids' (Fry 1969: 325), as appeared to be happening elsewhere in the English-speaking world, or to encourage general practitioners through association with the hospital to develop a field of particular expertise (Fry 1969: 241).

By the time that we interviewed the doctors in this study, the former proposal for age-band rather than population-inclusive clienteles had been decisively rejected by the professional bodies representing general practitioners and was no longer much of an issue until it was at least partially revived in 1976 by the Court Committee's recommendation for a general practitioner specialist in child health (DHSS 1976: 101) and as summarily dismissed again by the professional organizations. On the other hand, some encouragement had been given to the notion of developing some degree of specialist interest among general practitioners, who found that they were often welcome in the hospital for a session or two a week as clinical assistants to consultants in various specialties (DHSS 1969b: 14). Consequently, we questioned the doctors in our study not so much on their views on age-band specialization as on the scope for concentrating on problems which interested them or for avoiding those which they disliked dealing with.

The doctors generally accepted that they were in the business of providing services for all the patients on their list whatever their age or health status, and several of them talked about the value to patients of their own focus on family relationships which they thought came from treating individuals of all ages through all life stages. Yet all of them, to varying degrees, recognized that there were limits to their universalism.

Group practice doctors could to some extent avoid dealing with patients or problems which they found difficult, distasteful, or uninteresting and secure more of the work that they found pleasant or rewarding. After informal mutual negotiation among themsleves and with the other practice staff, including receptionists, patients themselves could be encouraged if necessary to consult one doctor in the practice rather than another. Patients too, by responding to the implicit and explicit clues given by doctors, might help to promote the differentiation between doctors within the same practice.

In general, doctors expressed their preferences in terms of the age or sex of the patients. Four of the six Barr practice doctors liked work with children and young persons; another was particularly concerned with the elderly and another with middle-aged women. At the Avesbury practice two doctors liked dealing with 'young mums and new babies' and two with the elderly, while the remaining two claimed to have no age or sex preference. In short, there seemed to be a degree of complementarity about the preferences in both practices, the Avesbury appearing to strike the better balance.

There also seemed to be a serendipitous complementarity in the likes and dislikes expressed by group practice doctors for particular types of patients with particular kinds of problems. For example, in the Barr practice, Dr Barrett found it particularly gratifying to deal with emergency situations – having to sort out crises and open up underlying problems – whereas Dr Bridges said he disliked 'crisis medicine'. For him, things had to be orderly and non-chaotic; whenever possible, he tried to avoid crises and to calm things down.

In the same practice, Dr Bowen found he could tolerate disturbed adolescents and drug addicts who were frankly disliked by most of his colleagues who felt incapable of helping them. Another doctor in this practice believed that a high proportion of the male homosexuals in the practice gravitated to her and she found she liked working with them. Similarly, in the Avesbury practice, Dr Amery thought he dealt with more adolescents and with more drug addicts than his partners, because on his own admission he was inclined to be more paternalistic towards them than the others were. Dr Ashton, on the other hand, said that he could feel little compassion for drug addicts and was thankful that others in the practice steered them away from him.

With the smaller practices it was rather a different matter. They did not have the internal resources to be able to spend more time with patients or on problems they felt comfortable with while steering the others in the direction of colleagues. All the same there was some complementarity in their work. One of them admitted to not liking to deal with Cypriots in general because they caused 'administrative trouble – they always have different names – each time they come they give a different name ... which makes for considerable trouble in record-keeping'. He also thought them insufficiently stoical: 'They're inclined to overstate their illness. They never have a pain; they always have a terrible pain. Anything they have is very bad, very sick.' Fortunately perhaps for the Cypriots, another of the smaller practice doctors singled them out as the group he particularly liked to treat. He found them 'warmer, more friendly, less remote' than the average patient.

Serendipitous complementarity, however, could not prevent doctors from having to deal from time to time with patients whom they disliked for one reason or another. These were patients, not unnaturally, who tried the doctors' patience, brought into question their competence, or raised their antipathies. They included for one or other doctor 'rich, parasitic, self-inflated patients'; 'hysterical manipulative women'; 'opinionated, fussy, rigid people'; 'all those locked into *folie de deux* relationships – mothers and daughters, husbands and wives, mutually and symbiotically dependent on each other's neurosis'; 'those with disease concepts so foreign to me that I don't know what they are saying or wanting'; 'those whose behaviour is so embarrassingly at variance with everything that medicine stands for'.

THE LIMITS OF TOLERANCE

All the doctors recognized that their tolerance was not infinite. The difficulty, if not impossibility, of escaping from their patients' demands provides the probable explanation for the greater circumspection employed by the smaller practice doctors in the selection of their patients in the first place. They put off would-be patients by allowing their receptionists to say that they had a full list. All the small practice doctors indicated that they were reluctant to take on patients who were going to mean trouble. They instanced drug addicts, squatters, dosshouse inmates and alcoholics who were also lay-abouts – 'people generally beyond rehabilitation in its widest sense'. One of the doctors did not want to take on older people because he thought they were particularly likely to make heavy and unreasonable demands on him. It was all he could do, he felt, to keep pace with the needs of patients who had aged with the practice.

It was clear that doctors at both group practices felt under great compunction to accept and continue to keep anyone who chose to register with them. They disliked having to label any patient as unacceptable. It was only Dr Adams of the Avesbury practice, however, who argued that the distinction between the acceptable or unacceptable patient was the inevitable consequence of the method of providing primary health care through registration with independent contractors. He thought that, if doctors were simply attached to Health Centres which had an overall responsibility for the health of the local population, no person requiring help would be without it.

While not discouraging or preventing would-be patients registering with them, the group practice doctors acknowledged taking the initiative in removing patients from their lists. They did so very infrequently and generally only after discussion at a staff meeting. Dr Bennett at the Barr practice had excluded three patients from the list in the recent past. Two were psychotic and followed her wherever she went – to her home, on her calls to patients, night and day. The third was an unpleasant psychopath who 'kept abusing us' and causing scenes in the waiting room:

> 'If patients break the rules we must take action. It's not so much if they break the rules with us, but with the whole group. We can tolerate a lot of unpleasantness; but when we see it's a hopeless situation and getting worse ...'

Throughout the study period we had no first-hand knowledge of any removals at the Barr practice. We were present, however, at several meetings at which the removal of a Mr Casey was discussed. The following are relevant excerpts from our minutes and illustrate the kinds of situation and the reluctance of the group to rid themselves of a difficult patient:

DR BOURNE   Michael Casey came in yesterday evening – drunk. I gave him ten minutes, but after that as I was already late for another appointment, I told him he would have to go. I told him this, I admit, just at the point he was telling me he had been in hospital and the ward sister had chucked him out. On hearing the consultation had to terminate he broke a chair, and wrote 'shit' outside my door. Then he went to the ladies' lavatory and did the same. What do I do? Do I (a) throw him off the list, or (b) give him a warning that if he ever does it again, which he will, I will throw him off?

DR BARRETT   He frightened various members of staff.

DR BRIDGES   Get rid of him – he provokes rejection.

TRAINEE GP   I am afraid of him and he is not helpable.

DR BOWEN   Putting him off the list means forbidding him to come to the Centre. The Centre is a community facility, you can't keep anyone out.

DR BOURNE   You can: the hospital threw him out.

DR BRIDGES   I threw someone else off. Then I'm tougher than
   you. You must decide: we will back you up.
DR BOURNE   Then he must have a warning that if he is rude to
   anyone at all – he's out.

Two weeks' later, Dr Bourne reported that Mr Casey had come
in to repay money he had once borrowed from him and he had
given him the final warning – 'so far so good'. Three years later,
Michael Casey, still Dr Bourne's patient, died of cancer. Dr
Bourne, whom he had named as his executor, was the only
mourner at his graveside.

Our minutes of the Avesbury meetings provide only two instances of the removal of patients from their lists. The first was
Daphne Butt:

MS AUDEN (HEALTH VISITOR)   There is the question of Daphne
   Butt remaining on the list after her abusive telephone call to
   Barbara [Almont] two weeks ago.
MS ALMONT (HEALTH VISITOR)   Phillipa [Dr Attenborough]
   has had to 'section'* her three times already and she has been
   very threatening. She said she wanted a doctor and then said
   she'd murder Phillipa if she came. She has already done Peter
   Allan [area social worker] in.
DR ATTENBOROUGH   The problem is how to get her off the list
   without her taking vengeance. And all her kids would have to
   come off too.
DR ASHTON   Why is she so angry?
MS ALMONT   I'm not sure, but I think she is mad enough to
   carry out her threats.
DR ALEXANDER   I don't think you are quite doing her justice,
   Barbara, because you were deeply offended by her last call.
MS ALMONT   Yes, she rang up saying she had a sick child, but
   not to send Dr Ashton, that fucking comedian, round. At the
   time, I was very annoyed; I'm a lot calmer now.
DR ADAIR   But we must also remember that other foul-
   mouthed lady we had who eventually calmed down. It was
   just her way of expressing herself. [To Ms Almont] Do you
   feel this is for real?

* The Mental Health Act 1959, sections 25 and 26, allow a social worker
to secure an emergency admission to a psychiatric hospital.

MS ALMONT   Yes, and also because of what she did to Peter Allan.

MS AUDEN   Is she going to come off then?

DR ATTENBOROUGH   Well we're not doing her any good.

DR ADAIR   She is your patient, Phillipa, the final decision must be yours.

DR ATTENBOROUGH   Yes, she comes off.

But it fell to Dr Adair to do the deed. She gave us the following account of her interview with Mrs Butt:

'I had her into my consulting room and told her that however upset she was, whatever she felt, we simply couldn't keep her – it was impossible – and that she must find someone else. She cried, but eventually accepted it and said "Could the children stay?" I said "no" but whenever they stayed with their granny, she could bring them up to see us. In effect, it means the children stay with us, because it is always the granny who brings them up anyway.'

The second Avesbury patient to be removed was Maria Polski who, according to Dr Amery, made a lot of demands, most of which he had to refuse. She was also in regular treatment at a homeopathic hospital on which she made similar demands. She rejected the advice of both and tried to play one off against the other. He accepted that many patients used alternative care for different things, but she involved both simultaneously for the same condition. He had told her it was 'not on', and that she had better commit herself to homeopathy for the time being.

The smaller practice doctors were no more likely than the group doctors to remove patients from their lists. Hostility to the doctor or rudeness to the receptionist were for them usually the last straws:

'I will not keep a patient on my list when – either because of his hostility to me or mine to him – I have lost confidence in his capacity to get on with me or I feel that the patient has lost confidence in me.'

PREVENTIVE MEDICINE?

In most of the reports on the future of general practice in the 1960s and early 1970s, stress was laid on the need for general practitioners to become seriously involved in preventive medicine and the promotion of health (Ministry of Health 1963: 39; RCGP 1972: 57). It was widely claimed that the separation of curative and preventive medicine at the community level, with the former function being performed by general practitioners and the latter by local health authority-employed doctors and health visitors, meant that many opportunities for promoting healthy behaviour at times when patients were likely to be susceptible to advice were missed. It was further pointed out that the separation of the curative and preventive functions had arisen in the specific social and economic climate of the nineteenth century and had been perpetuated by pre-National Health Service inter- and intra-professional rivalries (Honigsbaum 1979: 180). While the vestiges of these rivalries remained and were given room for expression, if not reinforced, by the administrative divisions within the National Health Service, there were now opportunities in group practice and in Health Centres for ending the sharp divisions and for drawing general practitioners into many of the tasks of preventive medicine.

Calls for the ending of the division of curative and preventive tasks in the primary health care field and for an expanded role for the general practitioner in preventive medicine found ready acceptance among all the doctors in our sample. 'It's like the family and religion – good in principle,' said Dr Bourne, epitomizing the sentiments of them all. He went on to claim that:

'The direction of general practice is toward prevention. It is important that doctors orientate themselves and their work towards health, not only disease. Although there are limitations, it should be the goal.'

In all the practices we studied there was some evidence to show that consideration had been given to ways in which the traditional work of the doctors themselves should be extended to include activities which could properly be called preventive. Such activities could roughly be categorized under three headings: immunization of well populations, screening of a-symptomatic populations for risk factors or for early signs of preventable disease, and health education.

There was virtually no disagreement among the doctors about the value of childhood immunization against a number of major infectious diseases; but, in the main, it was the attached health visitors who encouraged it and employed practice nurses who performed it and not the doctors themselves. However, during the study a television programme dealing with alleged fatal and brain-damaging effects of whooping cough vaccine was screened. 'All rather horrific', according to a health visitor attached to the Barr practice who reported to a practice meeting that many patients had been disturbed by it. She estimated that, as a result of the programme, 30 per cent of those who should have been immunized had not been. Her own faith in the procedure had been shaken and she asked for guidance from the doctors. After reviewing the available evidence a practice policy of recommending immunization was agreed, but not without some doubts being expressed by some doctors worried by the pronouncements of the anti-vaccine lobby (*BMJ* 1974: 81).

The wisdom of routine monitoring or screening of a-symptomatic populations was also challenged by some doctors while whole-heartedly supported by others. None questioned the desirability of regular check-ups for infants and toddlers and each practice made arrangements for this to be done at special weekly clinic sessions where a doctor was available. They believed, however, that much of this work rightly devolved on the health visitor, their own role being at least partly token, to reassure mothers about their children's normality since they rarely found much pathology.

The controversies arose on the questions of the screening of adult patients. A majority, nine doctors in all, took what could be called the middle ground: they believed that general practice should be the locus for the detection of risk factors, provided something could be done about them. They usually instanced blood pressure testing of all adult patients attending the surgery for whatever reason as a means of detecting hypertension.

Two doctors were enthusiastic believers in screening in the form of general health check-ups as a means of extending the doctor's traditional role of only responding to illness by 'dishing out pills'. As Dr Balfour put it:

'Of course we have to treat heart disease, but we would do so much better to give advice before they deteriorate to that extent.'

This doctor was an advocate in particular of regular screening of elderly patients in the practice, feeling that it was possible thereby to prevent a good deal of the more serious morbidity and handicaps of old age. Her enthusiasm was admired but hardly shared by all the other doctors. She herself recognized that 'interventionist' medicine was:

'Still an act of faith. We do not know how much good it can do.'

She acknowledged too that it could mean more, not less, interference in people's lives.

Five of the doctors we considered were on the whole 'anti-screeners', in that they had serious reservations about any move to provide routine tests for their adult patient populations. Two of the five emphasized what economists would term the opportunity costs of screening; in other words, they saw it as giving them less time to do other work which they considered more valuable. As one of them said:

'We haven't time to solicit trade by asking healthy people to come and see us.'

and the other agreed:

'It's all a question of resources. If you have screening clinics you can't do other things, which is mostly seeing patients when they are ill.'

Others of the five were mostly worried that screening procedures would create unnecessary anxieties or that well patients would be precipitated into semi-invalidism. One suggested that it was more important for doctors to be alert to all the implications of manifest symptoms rather than concern themselves with latent conditions which might not develop.

During our study, the degree of commitment to screening of the doctors in the two group practices was put to the test. On the initiative of Dr Balfour of the Barr practice, the two groups had all agreed to implement a screening programme whereby patients in selected age groups attending the Hearth Centre for a consultation with any doctor would be invited by the receptionist to see a nurse for blood pressure and weight tests and for investigation of their smoking habits. The object of the programme was to systematize the detection, monitoring, and surveillance of hypertension, obesity, and excessive smoking. It only seriously got under way, however, at the Barr practice where the doctors had no difficulty in obtaining their receptionists' co-operation as well as that of the nurses, who were also committed to the scheme. At the Avesbury practice, the doctors were lukewarm and took no steps to persuade the receptionists and nurses to carry the programme through. In the event, as we have shown in Chapter 8, it was the receptionists who brought the scheme to a premature end by failing to steer patients in the direction of the nurses.

Health education too was something which, almost unanimously, the doctors felt they, as well as other attached and employed health workers, ought to do. They saw health visitors as having the opportunity for health education on a group as well as on a one-to-one basis. They saw their own part as essentially related to the consultation; but there was little evidence in their tape-recorded consultations with patients that the doctors seriously engaged those of their patients who might be at risk from smoking, drinking, or eating too much in any discussion of their habits in these respects. Listening to a sample of tape-recorded consultations, members of the research team identified doctor-initiated discussions of such issues in only 12 per cent of the sample. Nor were the consultations notable for any deliberate attempts to help people 'to help themselves – to regain confidence and independence', the avowed objective of meaningful education according to at least two of the doctors. The evidence, indeed, confirmed what one doctor admitted:

'We are still in the diagnosis and treatment business with a bit of health education stuck on. It's unrealistic to see our work any other way, though prevention, despite its limitations, should be our aim.'

While, therefore, the doctors appeared to be making little use of the consultation as a vehicle for health education, they supported and took some part in initiating the ample displays of health educational posters and leaflets in the public parts of the Health Centre.

THE RESEARCH TEAM'S ASSESSMENT

In our view, all the doctors in our study, sometime before their moves to the Health Centre or shared group premises, had accepted the view that general practice involved them, whether they liked it or not, with a much wider and more varied range of ills than their medical education had prepared them for.

Intellectual acceptance of wide boundaries and of the need to develop skills which were not conceived of, let alone taught, in the medical school curriculum did not automatically lead to emotional acceptance of an holistic approach to patients. For some, preference, expertise and empathy remained firmly embedded in the treatment of patients with frank physical disease uncomplicated by psychological disorder. For others, practice in the primary care setting allowed or encouraged a greater concentration on the psychological component of patients' distress.

The doctors also varied in the extent to which they felt morally obliged to meet all the demands which patients made upon them. Some believed that they must respond non-judgementally to the needs which patients demonstrated, however difficult it was to meet them. Others did not feel the same moral imperative. They could and did avoid some kinds of call for help on the grounds either that their own area of competence did not enable them to help or that the request was in some way illegitimate.

Finally, the doctors, and especially those in the group practices, were aware of the suggestions that they should move from the responsive, demand-oriented illness treatment service which they had traditionally provided into the prevention of illness and the promotion of health. The moves actually taken involved the non-medically qualified staff of their units. There were few signs that they themselves were dealing with much more than the alleviation of the pain and distress which patients brought to them. Indeed, some of them expressed ambivalence about the wisdom of taking on a role which, in creating greater health consciousness, might paradoxically have the effect of diminishing self-reliance.

In our next chapter we examine in more detail the ways in which this group of doctors thought about the traditional medical tasks of diagnosis and treatment and in the following one their views about their relationships with patients. In our final chapter we return to consider some of the dilemmas which breaking new ground can create for the general practitioner.

13　Clinical Tasks

The practice of medicine, at its most basic, has been said to consist of making a diagnosis and in the light of that diagnosis instituting appropriate treatment (Passmore and Robson 1974: 1.3). Generations of medical students have learned that their first duty is to arrive at a diagnosis, if only in a tentative fashion, by taking a history of the patient's symptoms (obtained by asking a series of specific questions) and by looking systematically for physical signs. The object of both the history taking and the physical examination is essentially to exclude possible alternative diagnoses by their systematic elimination, and the method itself is seen as the very embodiment of the principles of scientific discovery and hypothesis testing. The diagnosis reached will then determine prognosis and prescription.

This clinical procedure is the quintessence of what it has become fashionable to call 'the medical model' (Noack and Muller 1980: 39) on the assumption that the primary task of medicine is to detect and treat organic disorders. Only when investigations have shown no physical lesions which could explain the patient's distress are functional or psychological explanations sought.

In the 1950s and early 1960s, the appropriateness of slavish adherence to this way of processing patients in the general practice setting began to be questioned (Ministry of Health 1954; 1963: 8). Michael Balint, and the general practitioners who were attracted by his ideas, had begun to feel that mental distress due to many complex social and psychological factors was a very frequent causal element in the somatic symptoms which patients presented to their general practitioners (Balint 1964: 24). To regard psychological factors as merely residual explanations for somatic ills was to adopt a crude, mechanistic approach, when every illness had essentially a multi-causal origin and multi-faceted consequences.

Balint argued that it was therefore necessary in the clinical encounter not only to ask questions but to 'listen at the deeper level' and to take account of 'the patient's characteristic utterances and emotional behaviour' (Balint 1964: 17). The purpose of that encounter should be, not so much to reach and attach a diagnostic label, as to understand the significance of the complaint to the patient. The approach did not require general practitioners to throw away all they had learned in the course of becoming doctors: it did require them to modify the focus and content of their customary dialogues with patients, to listen more and to question less.

Balint, indeed, challenged the classical conception of medical practice, which regarded diagnosis and treatment as two separate processes, the second invariably dependent upon and following the first. His notions blurred the distinctions between the two processes. In particular, in his scheme of things, listening was a vital ingredient of both diagnosis and therapy. Through listening, the diagnostic process could itself become therapeutic; equally, through listening, the therapeutic process retained a perpetual investigative if not diagnostic function (Balint 1964: 121).

Our treatment of this theme cannot be exhaustive. Although we had long interviews with the doctors, we could not hope to cover every aspect of their clinical work. We have, therefore, selected for exposition and comment a few topics which seemed to us to have contemporary significance. These touch on the applications of the holistic view of the general practitioner's clinical tasks to the process of diagnosis, on the use of the extending range of investigative procedures as an aid to diagnosis, and on the use of various treatment options.

APPROACHES TO DIAGNOSIS

Despite the fact that almost all the doctors in our sample veered towards whole person medicine, at least four amongst them were emphatic that, in reaching an explanation for the patient's distress, priority had to be given to physical factors. For example, Dr Erickson, who defined himself as a 'generalist in the widest term', and who, on balance, found dealing with psychological problems more gratifying than treating physical disease, nevertheless always sought to exclude a physical cause before looking for psychological ones. 'In this respect,' he explained, 'I am still a member of the old school.'

By contrast, Dr Attenborough, although claiming that she was not skilled in treating psychological disorders, maintained that she seldom thought in terms of a diagnosis 'unless by diagnosis is meant writing down the situation as you see it'. Dr Bridges said he followed the Royal College of General Practitioners' precepts and 'formulated patient presentations in terms of problems with many facets rather than as a hospital-type diagnosis'. He liked to think that by doing so he did not over-estimate any one aspect, 'emotional, physical, social or psychological'. The other doctors too tried to be aware of all the factors which could account for a patient's condition or contribute to it, 'to find out what was wrong, whatever the nature of the problem'. Several of them admitted, however, that there were times when they took what Dr Bowen described as 'the surface view'. By that he meant that he did not consider all possible explanations, either because he was too pressed for time or not in the mood to open up complex emotional or social situations. It was then, that is, when he felt guilty of superficiality, that he was grateful for the framework for continuity which primary care arrangements in this country gave – 'a next time' and a second chance to do better.

INVESTIGATIVE PROCEDURES – CLINICAL IATROGENESIS

During the 1950s and 1960s, scientific progress within medicine led to an expanding array of investigative procedures designed to increase the certainty of the diagnostic function. The advances largely took place in hospital-based laboratories or radiological departments with a research as well as a service function, and initially access to their facilities was generally confined to hospital-based consultants. By the 1970s when our study took place, however, most general practitioners were aware that they had the right to direct access to most hospital-based pathological laboratory facilities, even if some of them chose not to exercise it. Moreover, technical improvements meant that some of the simpler procedures could be carried out in any reasonably well-equipped room in a Health Centre or group practice centre.

As we showed in Chapter 2, all the doctors interviewed had

welcomed the opportunity to utilize hospital facilities for investigation without having to refer their patients to an out-patient department. The Health Centre doctors also welcomed the facility which the new premises offered to take blood and urine samples from their patients for dispatch to the local hospital laboratories. In Dr Adam's words: 'It makes it mechanically easier to do the right thing.'

We wanted to know, however, whether any of them felt that the very existence of an expanded range of diagnostic facilities might encourage over-utilization, as a result either of pressure from patients or of anxiety on their own part not to commit sins of omission (Scheff 1966: 105; Rubsamen 1979: 442). We had in mind the belief, expressed by critics of modern medicine in general and American medicine in particular, that the demand for investigative procedures always tended to expand to meet the supply and could also lead to an increase in costs without any corresponding benefit in the form of reduced morbidity (Powell 1966; Bunker and Wennberg 1973). There was the further proposition too that investigative procedures created an unhealthy dependency upon medicine, what Illich in 1975 called clinical iatrogenesis (Illich 1975: 39).

We found that most of the doctors we interviewed were conscious of the dangers of such unintended consequences of investigative fervour. They agreed, in Dr Erickson's words, that there was such a thing as doctor-induced pathology. Some went quite far with this contention, one suggesting that 50 per cent of the patients seen by a doctor would get better anyway, 25 per cent would actually benefit from the consultation, and 25 per cent would be worse off:

'Mainly because of unnecessary drugs or being sent for unnecessary investigations or being given ridiculous advice.'

Several claimed that they protected patients from the interventionist actions of specialists. Dr Bennett, for example, claimed that she and her Barr colleagues were 'cagey' about referring patients to a hospital where they were 'likely to end up being operated on'. Dr Adams, too, thought that investigations could be overdone: 'to impress the hospitals without doing anything really useful.' Others mentioned their opposition to 'executive-type check-ups' and reliance on 'clever machines' which were no substitute for clinical judgement.

Some of the Health Centre doctors claimed that their concern with the iatrogenic effect of their own 'weaponry' predated the publication of *Medical Nemesis* (Illich 1975). Nevertheless they thought Illich had done a good turn to doctors and patients alike, even if he had somewhat overdone it. Current public concern with iatrogenics might be exaggerated – 'an over-reaction' – but it had lead to a re-examination of investigative and prescribing patterns. They recognized that there was always some danger attached to the application of medical knowledge. A single-handed practitioner said he often felt he would like to return to an era in which medicine was relatively harmless, but that he was locked into a system in which risks had to be taken: while recognizing 'a negative in the balance of our usefulness, if you like', most believed, as he did, in the enormous benefits medical science offered the population. Their scepticism had not led them to abandon the investigative tools they had acquired or to which they now had routine access:

'Society without medical science would, by definition, be a different society. It's like a four-wheeled vehicle which does a lot of harm; but on balance we benefit from it.'

TREATMENT OPTIONS

We discussed with the doctors the range of treatment options open to them in general, not specific, terms. We were not concerned with their views of the relative efficacy of one or other pharmaceutical product or dietary regime in the management of one or other condition, but rather with their attitudes to three controversial issues which had surfaced in the late 1960s and early 1970s. The first concerned the phenomenal increase in the prescribing of pharmaceutical products; the second, the practice of repeat prescribing; the third, the purposive use of the doctor's charismatic authority, rather than active chemical substances, to effect beneficial changes in patients.

Chemotherapy – psychotropic drugs

It was not only the appropriateness of the widespread and increasing use of investigative procedures for diagnostic purposes which began to be questioned during the 1970s. The substantial increase in the range and use of pharmaceutical products for treatment purposes had also begun to be a cause of public and professional concern (Mapes 1980: 33). And since these products reached the public predominantly through general practitioners, it was their behaviour which was coming under scrutiny. Much of the increase in the consumption of pharmaceutical products was due to the development and prescribing of drugs for the control of conception, heart disease, infections, neurological disorders, allergies, and inflammatory conditions. Most of the drugs concerned had beneficial effects in preventing unwanted pregnancies, prolonging life, reducing pain and discomfort, or decreasing handicaps. But many of them, it was later discovered, had undesirable or dangerous side-effects, which might outweigh the benefits (Melville and Mapes 1980: 121; Teeling-Smith 1980: 7).

In the same period, there had also been a substantial increase in prescriptions for psychotropic drugs, an increase which led to a growing concern about the use of these drugs (Office of Health Economics 1975). The concern was of two kinds – safety and cost. First there was evidence that barbiturates and amphetamines, extensively prescribed in the 1950s and 1960s, were pharmacologically addictive in that they induced effects such as impaired alertness and physical distress on withdrawal, comparable to those produced by illicit narcotics such as heroin (*BMJ* 1954b: 1534; *Lancet* 1954: 75.) Moreover, it was becoming clear that legally prescribed barbiturates and amphetamines were becoming available to young people through theft or personal contact. Some were using them, not for therapeutic purposes, but to obtain a kind of intoxicated euphoria frowned upon as immoral by the majority of the population (Laurie 1967: 75).

As awareness of the ill-effects of the major psychotropic drugs became known, general practitioners, the major agents for the distribution of these drugs, began to be wary of them and to restrict their prescribing. The pharmaceutical companies, however, had developed another class of psychotropic drugs which came to be called minor tranquillizers and hypnotics as well as anti-depressants, all of which appeared to be free of addictive and other untoward side-effects. These claims were endorsed by at least some academic clinical pharmacologists (Trounce 1970: 103). These drugs, moreover, seemed particularly effective in treating anxiety states and mild depressions, that is, the kind of conditions which general practitioners recognized lay behind a substantial proportion of the conditions with which their patients presented.

The DHSS, while apparently accepting that the drugs in this group were not addictive, a view which was not shared by all medical opinion (Lader 1981: 13), was obviously anxious to contain costs and hence sought to persuade general practitioners to resist demands from patients for such drugs as well as the blandishments of the interested drug companies (Parish 1971: 61). In society at large, there was a more general questioning of the efficacy and the social implications of extensive drug use in which such moral issues as the creation of psychological if not pharmacological dependence on chemical substances were raised (Illich 1975: 31–60).

The response of the doctors in this study to our questions about their use of drugs showed that they were all aware of the current debates surrounding prescribing, of the dilemmas which they daily faced in this regard, of the pressures which they were under to prescribe, of the fallibility or precariousness of the stances which they themselves had adopted, and of the need from time to time to re-evaluate and re-examine their assumptions and procedures, and their consequences.

Where barbiturates were concerned there was unanimity. They had all ceased to prescribe them for anyone who had not already become an *habitué* and for whom withdrawal could bring great distress. According to their own accounts, however, they differed somewhat in the amount of effort they made to help the habituated to withdraw.

There were still greater divisions of opinion and practice among them on the prescribing of minor tranquillizers and hypnotics. Eleven of the sixteen doctors reckoned they were high prescribers of drugs, including psychotropic drugs and inert placebos,* as well as those with effects on specific parts of the body. Of these eleven, seven were prepared to defend their practices on grounds either of pragmatism or effectiveness. One, for example, thought he had a higher than average proportion of 'marginally, not grossly, inadequate' patients on his list and that this accounted for his high

---

* *Dorland's Medical Dictionary* (1965) defines placebo as 'An inactive substance or preparation, formerly given to please or gratify a patient, now also used in controlled studies to determine the efficacy of medicinal substances.'

prescribing rate. A single-handed doctor thought that prescribing levels were a function of the resources available to the general practitioner: where he was on his own the resources tended to be minimal. He claimed that his own tranquillizer prescribing had diminished when his patients had had access within the premises to a marriage guidance counsellor, and that a dietician in the group practice premises had reduced his prescriptions for slimming tablets. 'She earns her keep in the reduction in prescribing costs,' he said. A Barr group practice doctor thought some of his patients were better *on* than *off* drugs and another in the same practice felt that his rather lavish prescribing meant that many depressed and anxious patients were able to cope in a way which they otherwise could not. An Avesbury doctor, who at first said he felt somewhat guilty at yielding to pressures from patients, on reflection added:

'Patients are living in an increasingly hostile world and sedative drugs may be the only way to keep them in one piece. It's a relatively small price to pay to give them tranquillity and help them to live in peace with their families.'

Other doctors who expressed a sense of guilt tended to blame themselves for yielding to patient pressures. 'It's a sort of self-defence situation,' said one. 'If you are not going to prescribe you have to take time to say why,' said another. Yet another who thought his patients manipulated him blamed himself: 'I often attempt to stone-wall, but end up prescribing.' The theme of patient pressure was, indeed, a common one as instanced by Dr Bennett's statement:

'I'm afraid I still tend to over-prescribe although I am very conscious of it. I find it hard not to accede to patient requests. I feel very happy if I manage not to prescribe, just to give advice and not pills. But there is an awful amount of pressure – the magic is in the pill and it's hard to eradicate – although I feel drugs won't help as much as the patient's own attempts to get to grips with his problems.'

Repeat prescribing

The second controversial treatment issue we explored with the doctors was repeat prescribing. Although repeat prescribing does occur during the course of a consultation (according to our taped consultation 42 per cent of the prescriptions given during consultation were 'repeats' not new ones), the term is now commonly understood to mean the giving of a prescription to a patient who has not been seen by the doctor.

To some extent, therefore, the repeat prescription can be viewed as an alternative to the consultation, one, it might provocatively be suggested, likely to be favoured by doctors working within a system based on capitation rather than fee-for-service payments. In Britain, at any rate, the 'repeat prescription' outside the consultation appears to have been an established procedure in voluntary hospital out-patient departments, people's dispensaries and panel practices before 1946 and to have been carried over into the National Health Service. Dunnell and Cartwright (1972: 41) found that in 1969 nearly three-quarters of prescribed medicine taken by a national sample of adults in the two weeks prior to an interview had been obtained by repeat prescription.

Towards the end of the 1960s it became commonplace to suggest that the way in which some doctors managed patients requiring or demanding continued drugs could be both a reason for the escalating cost of drugs to the National Health Service and intrinsically undesirable (Committee of Enquiry into the Relationship of the Pharmaceutical Industry with the National Health Service 1967). It was argued that patients were often able to obtain drugs without due consideration by their general practitioner as to their appropriateness. This, it was held, was likely to occur when a patient came to the surgery or telephoned to obtain a prescription, and when the script was written out by the receptionist who took it to the doctor for signature without the patient's case notes, possibly in a batch of similar scripts for other patients (Parish 1971: 71). Evidence that this was by no means an unusual way of dealing with patients' requests for continuing drugs stung such bodies as the Royal College of General Practitioners into seeking to improve the ways of managing such situations, so that their members would not be vulnerable to attacks of irresponsibility. In particular, general practitioners were admonished not to give patients repeat prescriptions for long periods without insisting on a further consultation and assessment of the need, it being recognized that a consultation was not always necessary as a prelude to a prescription (BMA/DHSS 1978).

At the same time, Balint and his associates, notably Marinker, developed the theory that the repeat prescription differed qualitatively from the 'normal' consultation (Balint *et al.* 1970). Marinker argued that, whereas the consultation normally progressed through history taking, examination, and investigation to diagnosis and rational treatment, the repeat prescriptions was 'a hybrid' of treatment and diagnosis. Moreover, it was not only a form of treating and describing a condition; it also constituted a truce or peace settlement between a patient and a doctor who had jointly failed to negotiate an illness acceptable to both. Marinker further argued that the reason for the failure could, in the main, be traced to the patient's personality. The typical repeat prescription patient had both greater dependency needs than the average patient and greater difficulty in maintaining intimate relations, that is, relations in which he could be dependent. For patients such as these, the remote but sustained link with their doctor afforded by the repeat prescription was a preferred treatment. He described the procedure as:

'A mechanism for containing the doctor-patient relationship within tolerable bounds for the patient, a way of preventing any intimacy or examination of private areas of the patient's life.'
(Marinker 1972: 251)

In general, the doctors in our sample who were familiar with the work of the Balint group appeared to be well acquainted with such views on repeat prescriptions and several referred spontaneously to them. These doctors tended to see repeat prescribing, as they did other forms of treatment, as of the order of either substantive or symbolic medicine, or of both. In contrast, the doctors who were less familiar with Balint's work discussed prescribing mainly in terms of substantive medicine. We are not suggesting that the difference was attributable only to the influence of Balint's work, but rather to the likelihood that the doctors who exposed themselves to his teachings were, in any event, more sympathetic to ideas such as those developed by him than were doctors who did not.

All the doctors viewed repeat prescribing as a valuable and necessary procedure for patients with long-term physical conditions, which they felt could only be controlled pharmacologically. Diabetes, epilepsy, congestive cardiac failure, hypertension, schizophrenia, and hyper- or hypo-active thyroids were the conditions most frequently referred to, conditions which, in Dr Adair's words, 'probably meant medication for life'.

In discussing repeat prescribing some doctors distinguished between 'life saving' drugs and the drugs with somewhat doubtful chemo-therapeutic properties, that is, bordering on the realm of placebo. Dr Adair said she was quite happy to prescribe 'the cough bottles for the chronic bronchitics and the pints of whitewash for the tummy sufferers' provided patients were checked at intervals appropriate to their condition. Dr Bridges placed the placebos firmly in the context of the doctor-patient repeat prescription relationship as defined by Balint and his followers:

> 'Certain personalities need them, and they need them only as a means of contact with the doctor; the actual drug is irrelevant.'

Dr Bridges added that the doctor too was sometimes pleased to have only this limited form of contact. Dr Bennett elaborated the theme agreeing that one of the main functions of the repeat prescription was 'as defined by Balint'; it suited the patient who needed something but did not want to analyze his problem, the patient who kept the doctor at a distance. But she thought the doctor had to guard against using such interpretations facilely: 'sometimes I ask one of these patients to come and see me and the patient is surprised and pleased'.

The doctors who accepted the main gist of Balint's ideas usually accepted also the symbolic interpretations of the relational significance of the repeat prescription. Others denied it. For example, a single-handed practitioner would not accept that there was a distancing element in the process; and a group practice doctor felt his relations with all his patients, whether or not receiving continuing chemotherapy, were relatively close.

Whether or not they accepted the Balint concept of the repeat prescription, the doctors stressed the need for regular monitoring of patients on repeat dosages, while admitting that, for the most part, they had not really achieved this goal. For example, one doctor thought she maintained proper surveillance over 'women on the pill', but was less happy about her scrutiny of requests for other kinds of drugs. Another hoped he picked up the bulk of the patients who might be, as it were, 'vicariously prescribing for themselves', but could not be certain that this was so. Others acknowledged that there were patients whom they failed to recall because they did not know what else to offer them or would rather not see them; but most considered that there were instances in which it was wise to let well alone a patient 'stabilized' by repeat prescribing.

Long-term prescribing of the minor psychotropic drugs, not unexpectedly, was controversial. As in the discussion of chemotherapy in general, several doctors, while admitting that they prescribed tranquillizers on a long-term basis, expressed qualms about it. For instance, Dr Bowen said:

> 'I'm in favour of repeat prescriptions for some physical conditions, but am less happy about chronic repeat tranquillizers. If however, this is the only way of enabling some patients to function – and where intervention means trouble – I let them go.'

An Avesbury doctor would have liked to reduce patient dependence on these drugs. She told us of a patient who 'was started' on diazepans in hospital:

> 'He ticks over, does odd jobs here and there. We have an on-going relationship and I feel he could manage without drugs. Perhaps putting my foot down is what is needed therapeutically, but I have neither the courage nor the conviction to do it. It is always easier to give than not to give.'

Dr Ashton too saw long-term tranquillizer use as possibly the only solution for some patients:

> 'Life is slutty and one of the most difficult jobs in general practice is to decide the best way to actually reduce misery.'

Doctor as drug – listening as therapy

Most of the doctors recognized a connection between the level of their prescribing of chemical substances and their use of the only other form of therapy open to them, namely, the use of themselves as therapeutic agents. Nearly all of them, either explicitly or implicitly, indicated that if they had more time to spend with each patient they would be able to reduce the volume of prescribing. Only one doctor suggested that high levels of prescribing, especially of anti-depressant drugs – 'they work' – should not necessarily be seen as compensation for the shortage of the only other form of effective therapy, which involved the doctor's time and attention. His consultations and prescribing confirmed that he practised what he preached: he had longer consultations than his colleagues *and* a higher prescribing rate.

We were interested in our interviews with the doctors to see how familiar they were with the ideas of Michael Balint and the extent to which they felt these ideas had influenced their own practices with respect to psychotherapy. We discovered that it was the group practice doctors, and most particularly those from the Barr practice, who were best acquainted with Balint's concepts and arguments and most likely to feel that he, and the seminars his work had generated, had influenced the way in which they thought about their role in patient care. Among the concepts which had caught their imagination, since it appeared to account for much in their own experience with patients, was that of 'doctor as drug' (Balint 1964: 1, 4).

From our talks with doctors it was clear, however, that the insight which the concept had given them was variously interpreted and applied. It could, it seemed, like so many summary propositions, become something of a convenient catch-all phrase, concealing a variety of meanings which, if not actually contradictory, gave different emphases to different facets of the umbrella term. For some, the concept implied that the doctor, because of the patient's view of his potency, was, whether he chose it or not, inevitably a part of the therapeutic process, a drug:

> 'When the patient has come to you because he believes in you – has invested you with the power to help him – then you probably are the person to do so.'

For others, the use of self as drug was an elective rather than an intrinsic unavoidable function. As one doctor put it, if the patient was prepared to work with him, 'it was a good thing', but, he added:

> 'To be a therapeutic agent, you have, like any other drug, to suit the person being treated. You don't want any side-effects.'

And at least one doctor saw dangers for both doctors and patients in accepting the implications of the term 'doctor as drug':

'Patients may see me in a quite unreal light – as a god-like figure – and one must be careful not to believe it oneself.'

Most of the doctors who accepted the validity and usefulness of the term, were prepared to accept that, as with many drugs, there was always the risk of addiction and long-term dependence, which was not good for patients, let alone for doctors. One doctor outlined the tactics he employed to try to avoid such consequences, by contracting with patients to see them for longer consultations, on a 'six sessions' basis:

'If you can't get anywhere in six sessions, you are unlikely to do so in eleven, twenty or seventy-six sessions. The idea in using the limited contract is to work within a framework which explicitly pushes people back into living and so prevents them becoming chronically dependent on me or on anything – on magic, or diet, or drugs, or yoga – but rather provides them with a frame of reference within which to face up to their own difficulties, to accept themselves as they are and to go back to their life.'

Setting the limit in advance, this doctor argued, protected the patient from feelings of rejection when the treatment ended. There were times, however, when he confessed to being faced with transference difficulties and the need for help in dealing with them. The help was forthcoming from the psychiatrist attached to their practice. For another doctor, awareness of the dynamics of the doctor–patient relationship had not made it easier to avoid or solve the problem of patient addiction. 'Unfortunately', she said, 'the old umbilical cord is too strong.' Although she tried to keep the 'dosage' down and wean her patients from dependence on her and towards coping on their own, there were still too many who required repeated reassurance from her.

For this doctor, and for others who accepted that as doctors they were potentially powerful drugs, some patient dependence seemed inevitable. Some patients, they maintained, needed only short-term intensive support. One, who was gratified by his patients' trust in him rather than 'chary' of it, thought a positive response to 'a cry for help' often made a patient aware of the true nature of his needs and that this awareness was a first step towards cure and independence. Another suggested that the 'drug', when effective, was likely to increase patient autonomy and decrease dependence on the doctor or anyone else. Another argued that it was part of the doctor's job to respond to a patient's need to be dependent. If the doctor was able to cure the patient of this need, that was excellent, but not always possible. He returned to the theme of lonely people and his belief that it was the doctor's duty to succour them, if they had no one else to be dependent on. He added:

'In any event, as a profession we purvey dependence. In theory, we believe in self-care, but don't know how to teach it.'

The differences found among the doctors on the meaning of the concept 'doctor as drug' were replicated when they were asked to describe their techniques for dealing with patients in whom they diagnosed anxiety or depression, with or without physical manifestations such as rashes, asthma, and so on. They all believed that these symptoms required 'talk'; but as they enlarged on their ways of providing help it was clear that 'talk' too had different meanings. Some emphasized the initiative they took in giving advice to patients: it was *they* who did the talking. Others suggested that their technique consisted in listening, in encouraging *the patient* to talk. It is important not to exaggerate the differences in techniques, but there did appear to be a tendency for those who, in response to our questioning, detailed the content of their own talk to be wary of interpretive, psychoanalytical theories, and for those who emphasized listening to believe in such theories and to seek to work on that basis in so far as the conditions of general practice allowed.

An example of the former was a Barr practice doctor who said he tried not to get too involved in the psychotherapeutic role. If 'long, uphill talk' was needed, he referred the patient to their social worker or psychiatrist. Another of his colleagues also disclaimed using interpretive therapy: he merely tried 'to pick up truths and link them back' for the patient. He frequently told a patient 'You'll be better in a week or two,' and, more often than not, because *he* said so, he reckoned that the patient's condition improved. Another single-handed doctor also laid great store by telling patients how long their condition was likely to last. Shaping expectations in this way, in his view, lessened patient anxieties, gave them something to look forward to and protected him from early return visits. 'It's a bit of a con trick', he admitted, 'but it works well with eczema and rashes.' An Avesbury doctor declared himself inclined to take patients' problems at face value and to give them 'pep talks', rather than 'probing grandfather's incestuous relations with step-aunt'. Another from the same practice talked about the importance of the directions given at the end of the consultation:

> 'The directional business from powerful people – Mummy and Daddy figures – like when you say: "Now you go home and gargle with salt water" or "Buy some Radox and put it in your bath." Being clean – how much it helps.'

By contrast, five doctors felt that they had been much influenced by psychoanalytical theories and normally adopted one of its cardinal techniques – listening. One of them, however, recognized that his own methods were eclectic:

> 'Counselling, support, admonition, disciplining, let alone psychotherapy are all built into my day.'

THE RESEARCH TEAM'S ASSESSMENT

The strong impression we formed in our explorations of the elements of their clinical work with the study doctors was of individuals who had abandoned any dogmas they might once have possessed and adopted a pragmatically based eclecticism.

Their espousal of holistic medicine tenets had alerted them to the need to explore dimensions of patient experience which went far beyond the areas considered relevant in the more narrowly conceived medical model. They were also alive to the twin criticisms which were currently being made of modern medicine, that it was at one and the same time too ready to institute elaborate hospital-based investigation and too prone to treat patients symptomatically with powerful drugs which could have untoward side-effects or socio-psychological consequences. They recognized the real danger that their practices might result in various kinds of iatrogenic illness.

In the last resort, however, and for reasons of expediency as much as on grounds of principle, some continued to give tacit priority in their diagnostic procedures to investigations which would exclude treatable 'organic' causes of pain or discomfort before socio-psychological factors were considered.

Most of them were uneasy at the extent to which minor tranquillizers had become the only remedy they offered to anxious and unhappy people. They believed that such drugs could only be palliatives, helping individuals to cope with the difficulties of their everyday lives. They also recognized the potential significance of their own behaviour in their encounters with patients as a factor in the capacity of the latter to overcome emotional obstacles to health. They were reluctant, however, to make what they considered were moral judgements concerning the undesirability of dependency about people whose lives they felt were empty or stressful. We turn in the next chapter to a fuller discussion of the doctors' views on the nature of their relationships with patients.

14 Relationships with Patients

We have so far looked at the boundaries which the doctors set themselves in their central concern with patients and at their views on the appropriate use of the range of investigative procedures and therapies available to them. We now want to examine their views on the nature of their relationships with patients.

It is probably true to say that most doctors throughout history have recognized that success with patients depended upon more than clinical acumen or diagnostic skills. Indeed, if the autobiographical or hagiographical writings of many medical men in the past few centuries were to be examined, they would probably indicate that success was attributed to the doctor's personality and the impression he made on his patients as much as to his technical abilities or his knowledge (Swift 1982).

Nevertheless, until relatively recently, very little serious attention was paid by medical writers to the nature of the relationship which was formed between doctor and patient and the part it played in the therapeutic effectiveness of their encounters. It was probably taken for granted, however, that a satisfactory relationship must necessarily be one between an authoritative doctor and an obedient patient. While George Bernard Shaw (1906) and other sceptics were willing to challenge the medical profession's claims to superior knowledge and hence to authority in their relationships with patients, the majority of the population was not. The term 'doctor's orders' came to symbolize the power with which the doctor's role was generally endowed, just as the word 'patient' symbolized passivity (Jewson 1976).

It fell to the American sociologist, Talcott Parsons, in the 1950s, to argue that public acceptance of the reciprocal relationship of an authoritative doctor with a compliant patient fulfilled several necessary social functions: in his view, it enabled society to deal effectively with sickness in its midst by ensuring that the sick went to technically competent experts and felt obliged to take their advice in order to get well; it protected the sick who needed authoritative legitimation to be relieved of some of their normal social obligations in order to concentrate on getting well; it permitted examination of parts of the body in a manner which in normal circumstances would not be socially acceptable (Parsons 1951: 428). Some members of the medical profession may have been delighted if not a little surprised to have a justification of their authority from such an unexpected quarter.

It was in the 1950s and 1960s, however, that writers began to point out that this ideal relationship of justifiable trust leading to patient compliance with the doctor's orders was not always achieved. Much of the blame for failure was laid at the door of the doctors and in particular at their lack of skills in communication (Davis and Eichhorn 1963); but Freidson, another American sociologist, as well as others, argued that the tidy, mutually rewarding, reciprocal relationship of the Parsons model might be more myth than reality: the relationship could embody conflict as much as consensus (Freidson 1970). Balint too suggested that the motivations of both patients and doctors in their encounters were much more complex than Parsons's simple, reciprocal ideal model suggested and required a much deeper form of psychodynamic analysis (Balint 1964).

In our interviews with doctors we did not ask them to consider all these controversial views on the doctor-patient relationship head on or at any depth; but we did ask them to talk generally about their views on the nature of the relationship and the factors which increased or diminished its effectiveness. What follows is a distillation of the stances they adopted on the question of the balance of authority and egalitarianism in the doctor–patient relationship, as well as on the problems of handling actual or potential conflict in that relationship, including their own emotional reactions.

AUTHORITY IN THE DOCTOR-PATIENT RELATIONSHIP

When asked to describe the relationship between doctor and patient that they would regard as ideal nearly all of the doctors used epithets suggestive of an egalitarian relationship rather than one based on a dominant and a subordinate participant. 'Natural', 'friendly', 'informal', 'honest', 'open', 'frank', 'rational' were the adjectives which they used as they responded initially to our questions. One or two added a qualification to the effect that a degree of distance must be maintained beyond that of really equal friends, for example:

'No one should be allowed to feel the need for you, the doctor, as a person.'

and

'For therapeutic reasons there must always be some distance between doctor and patient: the relationship must be retained as a professional one.'

Only one, Dr Edmunds, from a smaller practice, favoured a relationship in which the patient was encouraged to see the doctor as a powerful figure. In his view, it was patient recognition of this power which enabled the relationship to be therapeutic. Without it the consultation would be ineffective:

'If patients are not going to take the doctor's advice and do as he says, well, what's the point of coming to see him in the first place?'

How far did the doctors feel that their relationships with most patients approximated to the egalitarian ideal, tempered with professional distancing, that they painted for us? Most believed that they did; but they differed first as to whether the relationships had become progressively more egalitarian over time, and second, if they thought there had been such a change, as to what it might be due.

Of the four smaller practice doctors, Dr Erickson and Dr Osmond felt that there had been little change in the character of the relationship over the time they had been in practice, maintaining that it had never been other than a mainly egalitarian one:

'I wasn't put on a pedestal by my patients twenty years ago and I'm not so now.'

Dr Erickson nevertheless thought that deference went with age, that is, that older people were more likely to accept a doctor's edict as binding on them. The other two thought there had been a change towards a less authoritarian relationship; but while Dr Cox welcomed it: 'the doctor hasn't the same magic and that suits me'; Dr Edmunds regretted it, feeling that: 'over the years, the doctor-patient relationship has deteriorated'.

The Barr practice doctors felt that their relationships with most patients had become more egalitarian over time, and, in the main, they welcomed it. They differed among themselves, however, in their views as to what the change was due. Some saw it as predominantly a change wrought by patients. One of these said:

'Because patients know so much more now, we have to spend more time with them.'

Others in the practice talked about the role of the media and 'the general social climate' in altering the character of the doctor-patient relationship. Three of them, on the other hand, emphasized the conscious efforts that they, as doctors, had made to render relationships less authoritarian:

'One tries to face patients with the truth of one's limitations, to create an honest relationship. It matters to yourself. If you're not pretending to be something you're not, you can handle patients' problems so much better.'

There were admissions as well from two doctors in the practice that many, if not most, of their relationships with patients remained unequal ones, sometimes because the patient was unwilling to make it an equal one and sometimes because they made it difficult for the patient. Dr Bowen, for example, instanced the case of a barrister, a distinguished QC, who still relished being told what to do despite his own attempts to share decision-making about treatment. At the same time, he recognized a tendency in himself on occasion to be 'abrupt, laconic, cold' and to shut patients up, while at other times he was able to 'be more civil' and 'to let the patients talk'. Dr Barrett also thought that, although less prone than formerly to make a god of him, patients still took their lead from him. It was he who still determined the tone and direction of the consultation, that is, exercised the real authority, albeit his style was now more informal, thus giving the appearance of greater patient participation in the decision-making. It was Dr Barrett, too, who attributed his own change of style as well as that of his Barr colleagues to the influence of the Avesbury practice which had rubbed off on them after their common move to the Health Centre.

As we have shown in Chapter 2, Avesbury ideology was in principle egalitarian. The practice goal was to 'eliminate hierarchies', including those between doctor and patient. Dr Adair told us: 'We positively detached the badges of office, the white coats, the stethoscopes.' And Dr Alexander described for us the steps he personally took to reduce social distances on joining the practice:

'I wanted to be accepted as one of them. So I shed my pins tripes and went to the pubs frequented by our patients and it worked. Within a few months patients had a different attitude to me, many calling me by my first name.'

Nevertheless, all the Avesbury doctors recognized that their relationships with patients, while manifestly friendly and informal, were unequal in many ways. Dr Alexander, for example, despite trying hard to become just another member of the community to which his patients belonged, admitted later that only 10 per cent of his patients were prepared to challenge his advice, even though he saw this as a great advance on the previous position. Dr Attenborough, too, felt she had to be selective in moving to egalitarianism since it could be unsettling for some patients. Dr Adair, while as ideologically committed as the rest to goals of equality, was also prepared to admit that inequality seemed to be built into the doctor–patient relationship:

'We can't deny that we are and will always be in a managerial and directive position.'

And Dr Amery, who acknowledged that in any case his natural style tended towards the paternalistic, wondered whether a strong-minded doctor was not sometimes more effective therapeutically than one more open to patient manipulation.

COMPLIANCE

Authority in the conduct of doctor–patient encounters is only one aspect, if an important one, of authority in the relationship in general. Another aspect is that of compliance. If compliance is defined as the extent to which doctors' advice, whether to do with drug taking or behaviour modification regimens, is adhered to. Compliance could, of course, legitimately be seen as involving the doctor in meeting the patient's requests for help; but, while we discuss this aspect of compliance in Chapter 15, we are here considering it from the standpoint of the doctor.

Among the doctors in this study, only one seemed to feel that patients always or nearly always followed his advice. Among the remaining doctors, there was a general awareness that many patients did not follow their advice, although differences of opinion were expressed as to how widespread such non-compliance was, whether or not it was growing, whether it was or was not a bad thing, and what it signified. One Barr group practice doctor, who felt that non-compliance was common, had always been so, and that it was not necessarily a bad thing, put it thus:

'I think patients have always disregarded the doctor's advice. We didn't use to realize that, but assumed they were doing what we told them. Now we know that about half of it won't be carried out, and that's not a bad thing actually.'

These sentiments were matched by those of an Avesbury doctor who estimated that 'about half the patients poured the stuff down the drain anyway'. He felt that, except for certain life threatening conditions, such conduct was not important. A single-handed doctor confessed to ignorance on the extent of the problem which he knew to exist: 'We still don't know how many prescriptions end up in the gutter,' was how he put it. An explanation for this non-compliance phenomenon was offered by a Barr doctor who thought that patients consulted primarily for reassurance. Once they had that 'they hardly bothered with anything else' the doctor might say or prescribe. On the other hand, in her view, chronically ill patients or those with clearly established pathology were more likely than their forebears to respond to a doctor's advice and adhere to his prescribed treatments, because the modern doctor had more effective remedies to hand than had his predecessor.

What was perhaps surprising about the doctors' views on non-compliance was the extent to which they were prepared to accept, condone, and justify it. Only two of them, one a single-handed practitioner, the other from the Barr group, thought that the failure of patients to follow the doctor's advice indicated an unacceptable or undesirable rejection of that advice. When it was patent that a patient had done so, both of them felt that the right course was to show the patient their displeasure in no uncertain terms and the need to comply.

Two principles appeared to underlie the tolerance of the rest of the doctors for non-compliance by their patients: first, respect for and desire to extend patient autonomy, and second, awareness of the fallibility or tentative nature of their own judgements. These were well expressed by one of the Avesbury doctors:

'My attitude is fundamentally one of agreement and support of the patient. I've always felt my function is purely advisory. When a patient comes to me with a problem, I give him my view of it, and very often it can only be a matter of opinion. Often I will offer him more than one – others as well as mine – and leave it to him to choose. It has to be his decision. Frequently I will agree with the patient's view of treatment.'

In the view of most doctors, however, acceptance of the patient's right to non-compliance did not exempt them from persevering with attempts in some circumstances to get patients to comply with a prescribed treatment. Most instanced the need for patients to finish the full course of antibiotic treatment and others mentioned patients on anti-convulsion drugs or on lithium. An Avesbury doctor argued that, in such attempts, doctor perseverance was an important prerequisite to patient perseverance. It was the doctor's responsibility to make all the implications of non-compliance with a regimen clear to the patient. Sometimes, when she thought she had done so, it later emerged that she had not and that the patient had retained or received a false conception of his illness and its treatment.

A stratagem used by several doctors to increase compliance was a form of surveillance. Dr Cox told us that he checked the adherence of some hypertensive patients to his prescribed regimen by counting the number of tablets they had left:

'If the answer's right, that's fine. If not, it's important they know I know. In this way I have changed a lot of people from loose to precise tablet taking. If they are elderly and liable to forget, I get their children or someone else involved.'

ANY DOCTOR? ONE DOCTOR? CONTINUITY AND PERSONAL
DOCTORING

It has long been customary for general practitioners, as well as for
those anxious to defend the national system for providing access to
all forms of health service through the general practitioner, to
claim that continuity of care is highly desirable. By continuity in
primary care is meant care from the same doctor through different
episodes of ill-health (RCGP 1972: 21).

The exclusive relationship of a patient with one doctor is a
dictum which early achieved sacred cow status. A cynic might
suggest that this was a not surprising defensive tactic on the part of
professional men at a time when they faced fierce competition
from their peers (Titmuss 1958: 172; Freidson 1975: 45). However,
even after intra-professional competition diminished in the 1950s
and 1960s, resistance by many doctors to group practice or to
partnership of more than two or three was often predicated on the
grounds that such arrangements might jeopardize or violate the
intimacy of the personal doctor–patient relationship. This last was
taken for granted as a good thing (Fox, T.F. 1960), not only by the
resisters to group practice but by those who in increasing numbers
chose to form large partnerships or enter already established
group practices. These last sought by a series of devices to
discourage patients from 'shopping around' casually among the
partners, or using immediate availability as the main criterion for
their choice. Most patients too according to a survey in the 1960s
set store by personal doctoring and continuity of care; however,
the substantial size of the minority of patients interviewed who did
not, cannot have provided great comfort to those who argued for
patient loyalty to a single general practitioner (Cartwright 1967:
149). We consider the views of patients in this study in our next
chapter.

Not surprisingly, when asked to give their views on continuity of
care and personal doctoring, the smaller practice doctors did not
see difficulties in achieving these objectives, which they took for
granted as desirable. In the two-man practice, a patient might
choose occasionally to 'see the other chap to check on the first
one'; but the doctors believed this was rare and felt they could
safely leave it to the patients to maintain a high level of continuity,
even queueing to see the doctor with whom they were registered

when the other one might be more quickly available.

The Barr group practice doctors, too, with no exceptions, extolled the virtues of continuity of care by a single doctor. One of them suggested that any problem presented by a patient was related to a past problem and would probably be related to the next. Another emphasized the need to establish an atmosphere of trust, which could only be done over time. One or two conceded that it could sometimes be a good idea to get someone new to look at the problems and that some patients could benefit from seeing more than one doctor. There was, however, no doubt about practice policy as a whole on this issue. It was explicitly to establish and maintain patient allegiance to individual doctors. Except in emergencies, the receptionists encouraged patients to see their own doctor even if it meant a slightly longer delay.

At the Avesbury practice, things were different. The ostensible professed policy of the practice, as expressed by Dr Adams in his account of the origins and objectives of the group, was to emphasize teamwork, not personal doctoring. Patients were to be encouraged to see all members of the group, including those without medical qualifications, as potential counsellors. Indeed, if anything, patient allegiance to a specific doctor was to be discouraged as an undesirable proof of patient dependency on an individual. The 'group' should be the corporate 'family doctor'.

In fact, only one of the six doctors in the practice adhered to this view when we interviewed them again in 1975. That doctor still maintained that efforts to encourage loyalty to individual doctors fostered dependency in the patient and smacked of an ego trip for the doctor. With a reference to the horse and buggy doctor cf a popular radio and TV soap opera programme of the 1970s she claimed:

'Either you have a group practice or you have six doctors each with his or her own list, and it's back to Dr Cameron.'

The essence of group practice to this doctor was the capacity to avoid the danger of a doctor knowing the patient too well and:

'not seeing what was under his nose. If one doctor doesn't see it, another doctor will.'

All the other doctors in the Avesbury practice, including Dr Adams himself, had changed their minds about the desirability of encouraging patient allegiance or had never fully accepted the policy. Dr Adams said he had now come to the conclusion that care by a succession of doctors could not take the place of continuity. A second doctor thought that medical work was more interesting if you knew your patients. Another member of the group made a similar admission:

'Yes, I try to keep as many patients who I know to be mine and about whom I have unique knowledge which no one else in the group has. It seems a pity and foolish for them to be seen by someone else. Also it makes for more work.'

In short, there seemed to be a general consensus, first, that while patients had every right to elect to see more than one doctor, this could be a manipulative device (for example, to obtain more drugs); and second, that if patients spread themselves around or were spread by the doctors themselves around the practice, that was bad medicine. Fortunately, it seemed to them, this did not occur frequently. Most patients deliberately opted for a personal doctor, a doctor they regarded as their 'own' and who, except in emergencies, they would always elect to see. Nevertheless, in contrast to the Barr practice, it was still policy at the Avesbury to leave the choice of the doctor to be seen to the patient, at least at the start of any new episode. Significantly, the Avesbury receptionists asked patients: 'Who would you like to see?' At the Barr, the receptionists' first question was: 'Who is your doctor?'

THE CONCEPT OF AVAILABILITY

A closely linked but analytically separable issue is that of the availability of the patient's personal doctor for consultation and treatment. Clearly, the more available he or she is the greater the likelihood of maintaining continuity of care and personal doctoring.

Under the provisions of the National Health Service Act 1946, the general practitioner principals who signed a contract to provide unrestricted services to patients who registered with them had to make themselves or a competent substitute available for medical advice throughout the twenty-four hours of every day in every year. They were also obliged to visit their registered patients in their own homes in circumstances in which the latter could not reasonably be expected to come to the doctor's surgery.

By any standard, these appeared harsh terms for the general practitioners, but ones which, during the events leading up to the Act, their negotiators were prepared to accept in order to preserve what was for them the cardinal principle, the general practitioner's status of independent contractor (Stevens 1966: 67; Forsyth 1966: 14; Honigsbaum 1979: 284). Not surprisingly, therefore, consideration of how general practitioners could best meet these obligations has been a live and controversial issue ever since. The question has been how to reduce the totality of personal commitment required in ways acceptable to the executive arm of the National Health Service through whom the contract is made. It has also been apparent that the obligation to provide services at all times and in patients' homes as well as in the surgery is closely linked to the more global issue, the survival and viability of a primary care sector based on a general practitioner service still financed largely by payments from central government funds for each patient registered.

There were, in fact, several questions which were likely to tax general practitioners at the time of our study. The first was how far the problems involved in managing personal availability were factors in the doctors' choice of the size of practice to join. The second was the lengths to which doctors were prepared to go to reduce their personal availability to patients who wished to consult them and not a substitute. The third was the extent to which they felt it was desirable or possible to reduce patients' expectations of their personal availability.

For Dr Osmond, the additional costs of single-handed practice, in terms of both the physical energy and the finance required to obtain substitute relief, had clearly not been sufficient to prevent him quitting a partnership for solo practice. Nevertheless, he recognized that, while increasing his availability to his patients by being single-handed, he could not escape the need to provide cover for himself at some times of the day, week or year:

'I think continuity is desirable, which means the same doctor must be available at all times, day and night. But it's just not compatible with modern life and with the other demands on a doctor's time. So although it's ideal, it's not practical.'

For the other smaller practice doctors, the formation of a partnership or the decision to share practice premises with other doctors was undoubtedly taken with a view to managing the availability problem, among others, at less personal cost to themselves in time or money. So too were the decisions taken by the group practice doctors to work in such organizations (see Chapter 4).

The specific arrangements whereby the doctors made themselves available to patients were undoubtedly related to practice size; that is, the smaller practices had similar arrangements, but these differed in a number of ways from those of the group practices. In the first instance, the former conducted fewer surgeries weekly than the group practices, since they held morning and evening surgeries only, whereas the latter had afternoon surgeries as well. They also closed on Thursday evenings and, unlike the group practices, relied on commercial services to give them coverage from 11 p.m. at night to 8 a.m. in the morning.

These differences suggest that, at least marginally, the doctors in the smaller practices were less available for rapid consultation by their patients than those in the group practices. Against this, however, it must be said that, except during their vacations or bouts of illness and for one evening weekly, the smaller practice doctors were personally available to their patients twice a day without appointment. By contrast, the group practice doctors operated a rota which allowed everybody at least the equivalent of one full day's surgery off every week and could also provide cover for doctors with study leave or other professional engagements. Moreover, both group practices operated an appointments system which could mean that a patient who wished to see a particular doctor could not do so for several days. Hence any one doctor was less available to those patients who wanted a consultation with him or her only than were the smaller practice doctors. Moreover, a patient was less likely to see his own doctor than was the patient registered with a smaller practice who, except after 11 p.m., was likely to have a one in two chance of so doing.

None of the smaller practice doctors thought that their availability constituted any sort of problem for their patients, and they all attributed it to their walk in and queue system which they all said they would not change to an appointments system. They were not altogether happy, however, with the need to use a commercial agency for night calls. One doctor told us that ideally he would do them too, but found that, at his time of life, after doing a day's work, he was no longer able to handle them. None of the smaller practice doctors were in the first flush of youth and they all chose to accommodate to their workload in this way rather than by reducing their availability during normal surgery hours.

They also had a deliberate policy of discouraging home visits on grounds both of the time involved for them and the inferior conditions for examining patients in the home. Dr Erickson said he had virtually eliminated home visiting for children by telling mothers:

'There will be no delay in the waiting room. The child with a temperature will go into the examination room right away and be seen in a few minutes.'

His home visiting was now mainly confined to the over-eighties.

In contrast to the smaller practices, all the group practice doctors considered an appointments system essential. They also considered it essential that one of their number be available to answer requests for night and weekend calls. Dr Adams described the reasons for this policy thus:

'The fact that patients are not seeing a complete stranger in the middle of the night but a doctor who works here, knows the patients who are particularly vulnerable, either physically or psychiatrically, has access to their records and is likely to respond in the same way as the patient's doctor and will in any case talk to that doctor in the morning is very important.'

There was, however, a difference between the Avesbury and Barr doctors in their general attitudes to individual availability and in their assessments of their achievement in this regard. Most of the Avesbury doctors thought it was important for patients to be able to see a doctor on the day of request and, by that standard, they felt they were providing a reasonable degree of accessibility. As one of them said:

'Our availability may not be good enough, but it is infinitely superior to that of most practices in Britain.'

This seemingly complacent remark was echoed by others, one of whom went on to claim that, if a patient could not wait to see a doctor at the end of a surgery session, he or she could always see a nurse.

Two Avesbury doctors, however, who set more store on personal doctoring were less satisfied with their arrangements. One of these recognized that it had become less easy in recent years for patients who wanted to see him to do so within a reasonable period of time, partly because of the increase in his extra-mural activities and partly because his caseload had increased. He added:

'I suppose we are all getting older and some of my colleagues feel more tired and hard-pressed and less able – or willing – to carry the load they formerly carried.'

There was consensus amongst the Avesbury doctors, however, regarding home visits. Like the smaller practice doctors, they tried to educate patients not to demand what they, the doctors, had come to consider inappropriate visits. Telephone requests were vetted and, if at all possible, patients encouraged to come to the surgery – 'in most cases you find they can come in', or the consultation might be conducted over the phone. In general, the doctors felt these educational efforts had been successful and there was now 'considerably less stone-walling for a visit or else' than there had been.

In contrast to the Avesbury, all the Barr doctors felt that ideally each should be available at all times to his or her patients and all but one were critical of their own level of availability. The one exception thought it was not too difficult for his patients to get an appointment with him, mainly because he had fewer outside commitments than his partners. The others accepted that they had become less available over the years, to the point that the situation was no longer entirely satisfactory. There was now just not enough doctor time in the practice as a whole to meet patient demand, mainly because their other interests – teaching, research, committee work for professional bodies, and so on – had made inroads into surgery time. They were aware, too, that their system favoured the chronically ill, who made appointments well in advance, over patients who became ill suddenly, especially if, as not infrequently happened, the duty doctor was absent on an emergency call. They had tried various procedures, but none could, in fact, compensate for the shortage of doctor time. Yet, as one doctor explained, none of them were prepared to give up their other commitments or thought the others should do so. They saw these commitments as of value to the community, to the practice as a whole, and to themselves individually. Another doctor concluded:

'We really don't know how to improve our availability, and unfortunately our confusion goes through to the receptionists.'

Their concern about their levels of availability in the surgery did not apply to their home visiting provision. Although Dr Bridges thought it might be desirable to have a 'back-up' doctor available to the doctor on night or week-end duty, they agreed they rarely experienced difficulties in meeting home visit requests. Moreover, in contrast to the doctors at the other practices, they maintained that it was not their business to discourage home visits. If a home visit was what the patient wanted, the patient should have it. Furthermore, most of the doctors at this practice considered a home visit a valuable opportunity to learn more about the patient, his home and his background, and useful for the practice of family medicine:

'One goes to see one member of the family and the others, without being aware of it, open up.'

Nevertheless, despite their conscious efforts not to discourage home visits, the Barr practice doctors, like those at the other practices, reported a diminution in demand. The Barr doctors thought this diminution was because more patients than formerly had telephones and could phone for advice without requiring a visit. Patients were also more mobile and might not want to wait at home if they felt a visit to the surgery would expedite a consultation. The change was not regretted:

'It's a relief. Home visits are time-consuming and exhausting; and while it's of value to see the patient's home at least once – it adds to your knowledge and you understand the problems better – continuous visits rarely add more.'

COPING WITH UNCERTAINTY – MANAGING THEIR EMOTIONS

By its very nature, medical practice, especially in the primary care sector, involves uncertainty at many different levels. General practitioners are daily confronted by patients with complaints which may be either trivial, self-terminating and capable of self-treatment, or the harbingers of illness, perhaps irreversible, involving great pain, discomfort, and long-term disability, or premature death. With experience, they may come to be more certain as to how potentially threatening the conditions are; but that certainty can never be absolute and there must consequently be some continuing uncertainty on the part of all doctors about the diagnoses they reach (F. Davis 1960; Mechanic 1968: 23).

At another level there is also uncertainty about the efficacy of the different forms of intervention available and their potential to harm as well as to help the patient. Doctors must also face the uncertainty of not knowing enough about every patient in the round to predict the outcome of their treatment in the individual case. Consequently, they cannot know precisely how much or little to tell individuals about their conditions or expect from them in the way of behaviour change. To these clinical uncertainties must be added those which afflict all adult members of a society to a greater or lesser degree as part of the business of living in a complex industrial society.

Renee Fox, an American sociologist, writing at the end of the 1950s, suggested that both the general ambience of the medical school and its formal curriculum helped prepare doctors for their life tasks, which would include the management of uncertainty (Fox, R. 1957). It is of course questionable whether such implicit, latent functions of a medical school do adequately prepare their neophytes for this inherent aspect of their future work (RCGP 1972: 19; Balint 1973: 2; Armstrong 1980: 81). What does not seem to be in question is the role which uncertainty at many levels continued to play in the anxieties which the doctors in our sample, to varying degrees, acknowledged.

When asked whether their work, and if so what parts of it, made them anxious, virtually all the doctors recognized that while anxiety was inherent in the work, the level rose when they felt uncertain about the significance of a patient's symptoms or how best to deal with them. They assumed, however, that if they were unable to control their anxiety, it would be an indication of their ultimate unfitness for the job. A few pointed out that, like people in other demanding occupations, there were times when pressure built up and, particularly if it coincided with strains in areas of their lives other than the strictly professional ones, their capacity to contain anxiety could be impaired.

It was perhaps not surprising that among this sample of self-conscious, analytically-minded doctors some of them should also have mentioned changes in their own lives and the process of ageing in particular as pertinent to the issue of coping with professional work with patients. One Avesbury doctor, for example, confessed that night duties had recently become too much for her:

'I reckon thirty-two years is enough. It's not a matter of principle, it's personal. I have never been able to settle at night when I'm on duty. I walk around like a cat on hot bricks, almost glad when a call comes. The others don't suffer this way; they just go to sleep or out to dinner and do a visit when necessary. I could never do it that way.'

Another Avesbury doctor also attributed his desire to lessen his workload to ageing:

'As you get older, you tend to feel that someone younger should worry about some of the things that have to be done for our patients.'

Along with anxiety, the emotion which many doctors found they had to manage was the hostility they felt for some of their patients, a problem which we have touched upon in Chapter 12. Managing it involved a variety of tactics, from avoidance, which was easier in the group practice setting, through concealment, to confrontation. Two of the younger group practice doctors, for example, told us frankly that they let their hostility be known to others in the practice in the hope that one or more of them would be willing to take on the patients in question. Another emphasized the value of the group practice setting for him in this regard:

'I can only cope with some patients by complaining loudly about them behind their backs.'

A smaller practice doctor, with less room to manoeuvre, tended to send patients he disliked to hospital for investigation, care, or an opinion, sooner than he would otherwise have done. Two other doctors, one from the Avesbury and the other from the Barr practice, tried to deal with their own hostility by concealment:

'I over-correct. I become extraordinarily charming and never avoid seeing them.'

A group practice doctor, however, claimed that he found it best to confront aggression with aggression: 'be hostile back'. This response could fail, but usually he thought it worked because behind his spontaneity was 'a sort of insight' and interest in the peculiarities of people's lives, which hostile patients could appreciate.

PATIENTS AS SOURCES OF FRUSTRATION AND REWARD

John Berger, in a book entitled *A Fortunate Man* (1967), drew a picture of a rural general practitioner whose life of dedicated service to his patients seemed to have brought him fulfilment and contentment of an enviably high order. Much of this, it was implied, was due to the nature of the relationships which develop between a family practitioner and his patients in a rural setting of great natural beauty which gave to all those living and working there a sense of timelessness, tranquillity and security.

Autobiographical accounts by many general practitioners, however, suggest that, although it may help, it does not need an idyllic village scene and bucolic country folk to set the scene for a satisfying sense of purpose and achievement (Hale and Roberts 1974). The relationships which are generated from the patients' need for advice and support from a knowledgeable and sympathetic human being and the doctor's reciprocal need to respond clearly occur in less salubrious surroundings (Robertson 1970: 15).

And so it was with the general practitioners in this study. The district in which most of their patients lived could not be called beautiful; many of their patients were transients rather than old-established inhabitants; their home visits often involved them in the discomfort of traffic jams and parking difficulties; yet all this did not prevent all but one of them from seeing themselves as relatively fortunate people with the privilege of a working life which, although not without frustrations and difficulties, enabled them to feel that they were helping others.

Their frustrations arose mainly from three sets of causes: their own limitations or inadequacies; their patients' limitations or inadequacies; and a miscellany of factors which they saw as outside their own control or that of their patients, such as the ill-deployment of resources at national, district, or area level, insufficient time to see patients, or having to deal with patients other than one's own. Frustrations, moreover, were usually the result of the interaction of factors of more than one kind. For Dr Adair, it was her own limitations coupled with the conditions in which she sometimes had to work:

'I only feel frustrated when I feel I'm being driven. I can't bear to be driven any more. But it's me – I get tired.'

Others located their frustrations in themselves and in the patients:

'It's when you can't help – when the patient can't be helped.'

Generally speaking, the doctors in the smaller practices were more likely than the group practitioners to see patient behaviour as a source of frustration:

'People I can't really help, who can't learn to handle themselves.'

'The people who don't get better – no matter what you do.'

'The patient for whom – whatever you do – it's not good enough.'

What were the rewards? Trying to be analytical, we felt we could discern three kinds of rewards in the words which the doctors used to express their satisfactions with their work.

There were, first and foremost, the rewards of visible or measureable achievement in terms of improvements in the health of their patients:

'Seeing people get better. Things don't hurt any more or their emotional or social problems are sorted out and they lead happier lives. There are huge rewards in general practice.'

Such rewards were mentioned by all the doctors.

A second kind of reward, mentioned by more than half the doctors, was the relational one, including the pleasure derived from patients' expressions of gratitude:

'Knowing patients, liking them, and feeling they trust me. Often, on return from holiday, I feel how nice that they know I will help them. It is rewarding.'

'As gratifying as seeing a patient recover is the knowledge that he knows he can turn to you in a moment of trouble, and that together you can try to work through his trouble.'

'It's when you treat a condition and the patient is delighted and says 'thank you'.'

The third kind of reward lay in the satisfaction derived from successful problem solving. Four doctors talked about this aspect of their work with patients not as the only reward but as a major one:

'It's the intellectual challenge – the jigsaw element of fitting pieces together, being the detective.'

'It's the relationship you build up and it's making uncomfortable people feel comfortable. But it is also the interesting mathematical-type problems – the tying together of symptoms.'

'It's making the correct diagnosis in both physical and emotional terms and because of that, being able to lighten the patient's burden somewhat and a new relationship occurs which makes all the difference to one's acceptability in future relationships with them.'

We cannot, however, do better than end this chapter with the confession made by at least three of our doctors when discussing the nature of their relationships with patients, and summed up in the words of one of them:

'Doctors need patients. Perhaps today, I need them more than they need me.'

15   Patients and their Doctors

Both the initiators of the study, the DHSS, and the general practitioners who agreed to participate in it wanted the research team to study patients' attitudes and behaviour as well as those of doctors and other health workers.

In this chapter we concentrate on patients' attitudes to their doctors and to medicine. We explore, in particular, their views on how wide the boundaries of general practice medicine should be, what they looked for in their general practitioners and in their consultations with them, and what they wanted their relationships with their general practitioners to be. We also consider how far patients felt these expectations or desires were met by their own practitioners. Where possible, and this was not always so, we see whether reported behaviours confirmed the attitudes expressed. Again, where possible, we compare patients' attitudes in 1975 with those expressed in 1972, in order to see whether there were any significant changes during the period of our study. In the following chapter, we switch from concentration on the doctor to consideration of patients' views about the organization of their general practice units more generally, including such matters as the appointments system, waiting time, the availability of the doctor, and relationships with practice personnel other than doctors. In both chapters, we draw attention to differences where they existed in the preferences and experiences of patients registered with the different practice units.

The views expressed came from two samples of patients, neither of them fully representative of the entire population registered with the study practices (see Chapter 1). One sample consisted of individuals interviewed in their own homes, whom we here call 'home interviewees'; the other consisted of those consulting a

—

general practitioner during four sample weeks, whom we call 'attenders'. Both these samples also reported some of their experiences of general practitioner services. In addition, we have utilized from time to time the evidence we obtained from recording a sample of doctor–patient consultations in 1975.

MATTERS FOR THE DOCTOR

In Chapter 12, we described the doctors we studied as holists rather than traditionalists where the boundaries of the medical role were concerned. By that we meant that they drew no hard and fast distinctions between the pain and distress which could be attributed to the malfunctioning of the human body and that which appeared to have no such organic origin. They also considered it their duty to deal with it all whatever its cause and its manifestation. However, they differed among themselves on the extent to which they felt primacy should be given to the task of excluding physical causes of illness before dealing with its possible psychological causes or manifestations: there were differences among them too in what they felt it was appropriate and legitimate for patients to bring to them.

While we did not explore patients' views on such issues directly, a number of the questions we did ask bore upon them and allowed us at least to get a feel of what patients' views on the boundaries of the general practitioner's role should be.

One forced-choice question to home interviewees, for example, was whether they thought it 'very important', 'important', or 'not important' to be able to discuss 'problems which were not strictly medical as well as medical problems with a doctor'. In 1972, two-thirds chose 'very important' or 'important' as their response: by 1975, this proportion had increased to three-quarters (see *Table* 7) suggesting that expectations of the general practitioner, at least as someone interested in patients as people, increased over the period.

On the other hand, very few patients saw the doctor as the most appropriate person to deal with such difficulties as marital problems, domestic arrangements for handicapped people, or social readjustment after mental illness. We reached this conclusion by analyzing the home interviewees' responses in 1975 to questions as to whether they felt professional help of any kind, and if so, of

Table 7   *Percentage distribution of home interviewees in each study year viewing opportunity to discuss non-medical problems with their/a doctor as 'very important', 'important', and 'not important'*

	1972	1975
	%	%
very important	28	33
important	39	42
not important	32	22
unknown	1	3
total N = 100%	(503)	(509)

which kind, was needed in nine kinds of hypothetical difficulty people can experience (Brooks 1973) (see *Table 8*). Several features of the response were interesting: for example, the home interviewees were more self-reliant and less likely to feel professional help of any kind was required than we had expected. What is relevant to the issue of the expectations which the population had of its general practitioners, however, is that the latter were still seen as the most likely source of competent help in the more somatic manifestations of ill-health. Where social implications were paramount, the doctor was only one professional among others who was seen as an appropriate agency.

Although there were no marked differences in the responses of patients of different practices to the broad question of the importance of being able to discuss non-medical problems with their doctor, there were differences in their answers to the questions of the kind of help needed for each of the nine difficulties 'people can experience'. The differences were in part accounted for by differences in the age, sex, and social class composition of patients in our sample registered with the different practices. In general, older patients and working-class patients were less likely than younger patients or middle-class ones to suggest 'outside help', as defined. We drew this conclusion from comparing responses by age and social class to the need for outside help. We found, for example, that 93 per cent of the sixteen to twenty-four year-olds advocated outside help in at least four of the hypothetical difficulties presented to them, compared to only 76 per cent of those aged sixty-five and over. Similarly, 89 per cent of those in social classes I

Table 8   *Percentage of home interviewees who (a) think 'outside help needed'* with nine hypothetical difficulties, and if so, (b) from a doctor*

difficulty	(a) external help needed N = (509)	(b) doctor nominated as appropriate external help	
	%	%	(N = 100%)
a woman of 35 with loss of appetite for a week or longer	76	99	(388)
the mother of a girl of 10 who wets her bed nearly every night	81	83	(412)
a boy of 15 with a boil on his neck	66	79	(334)
the parents of a teenager who have just found out he is taking drugs	72	76	(369)
a young mother of a baby of 6 months refusing to go on solid food	76	46	(385)
the wife of a man who appears to be habitually drinking too much	47	43	(276)
a married woman of 35 who has just returned from a mental hospital and is having difficultly adjusting to family and social life	80	35	(408)
a woman of 75 with long-standing arthritis, living alone and becoming unable to manage housework	93	14	(479)
a married couple who quarrel so much they are beginning to think seriously of a divorce	45	14	(278)

* 'Outside help' defined as help *other than* from family, friends or neighbours.

and II would seek professional help in at least four of the difficulties, compared to 83 per cent of those in social classes III, IV and V. Since there were more younger and more higher social class patients in our samples of group practice interviewees (see Chapter 2), it was not surprising that group practice patients, and especially those at the Avesbury, were overall more likely than those of the smaller practices to suggest outside help. We also found that, when outside help was thought necessary, those in higher social class groups were rather more likely than those in lower social class groups to suggest other professional sources of help as well as the doctor. For example, 40 per cent of the middle-class home interviewees (social classes I and II) would think a nurse appropriate to deal with a boil on an adolescent's neck, as compared with only 18 per cent of those in social classes IV and V, who were much more likely to say they thought the doctor should deal with it.

Our home interviewees were responding in such questions to what were essentially hypothetical difficulties, most of which they personally were not likely to be encountering at the time; but we had some evidence from the attenders' enquiry and from our taped consultations that most patients presented their doctors with physical symptoms (see *Table 9*). In a sizeable minority of consultations, however, such matters as their personal relationships or their social circumstances at home or work were discussed.

Before drawing conclusions from these findings, it must be pointed out that there were difficulties in classifying the patients' reasons for wishing to consult, some of which were expressed in very vague terms. The records the doctors themselves made of the attenders' consultations (see *Table 9*) suggested 'emotional symptoms only' rather more than did our own codification of the reasons given by the same patients immediately before the consultation.

The discrepancy could have arisen for any one of a number of reasons: for example, the attenders concerned might have wished to conceal from us their real reason for consulting; they may have

Table 9   *Percentage giving different reasons for consulting the doctor derived from (a) tape-recorded consultations, 1975; (b) attenders' own statements; and (c) doctors' accounts of the attenders' reasons in 1975*

reasons	(a) tapes	(b) attenders' statements	(c) doctors' recording
	%	%	%
physical symptoms only	59	61	74
emotional symptoms only	7	4	8
both or ill-defined	34	35	18
Total N = 100%	(215)	(917)	(865)

changed their minds about what to raise when in the consultation; the doctors, on the basis of prior knowledge of the patients, may have discounted the latter's desire to present emotional distress as bodily symptoms. If we had had to rely on this source of evidence alone, given the difficulty of codifying, we would have hesitated to draw any conclusion at all; but because our data came from more than one source, each of which told approximately the same kind of tale, we felt fairly confident in making a further assertion. It was that the doctor, while still seen as the appropriate professional person to approach with somatic symptoms, is also consulted by a large minority of patients about states of mind and body which are difficult for patients and their doctors to describe as only physical or only psychological in origin and in manifestation.

Women were only slightly but consistently more likely than men to consult for emotional or ill-defined symptoms. So were those in their middle ages, those under twenty-five and over sixty-four more commonly consulting about physical conditions only. These differences however were not reflected in practice differences; there were virtually no differences in this regard among the attenders of the five practices.

TRIVIAL COMPLAINTS

Following evidence that many general practitioners during the 1960s felt that patients brought too many trivial, self-terminating complaints to them (Cartwright 1967: 44), we asked the doctors in our study how far they felt this was true. As we indicated in Chapter 12, all the Avesbury and Barr practice doctors as well as Dr Erickson rejected the notion that any of the complaints patients brought to them could be labelled trivial, on the grounds that whatever worried patients could not be trivial for them. On the other hand, they wanted to encourage patients' independence in health matters and hence to wean patients from excessive dependence on them.

If we had asked patients whether they took trivial complaints to their doctors, we could rightly have expected to obtain denials. We did, however, think it worth-while, as another kind of indicator of their views on the doctor's role, to ask home interviewees whether, overall, they felt general practitioners were asked to deal with too many trivial complaints or whether people in general were too reluctant to consult about minor ailments. Not everyone (8 per cent) was prepared to answer the question; but amongst those who did and who did not say that both statements were true (11 per cent), six times as many felt patients generally were more prone to consult about trivia than felt there was too much reluctance to consult, and this ratio did not differ significantly according to practices. In short, it seemed that patients were more prone than the doctors in our study to take a moral stance and to suggest that there was a good deal of unnecessary consulting.

EXPECTATIONS OF THE CONSULTATION AND THEIR SATISFACTION

In Chapter 12, we discussed the views which the doctors in our study had expressed about some of the more controversial issues concerning the most central of their professional tasks. We did not ask our samples of patients the same kinds of questions. As a result, we cannot say what they felt about the appropriateness or otherwise of doctors seeking to exclude possible physical causes of distress before looking for psychological or relational causes; of the ready prescribing of minor tranquillizers and sleeping pills; of the system of repeat prescribing; or of the doctors' use of listening as a therapeutic as well as an investigative device.

Nevertheless, patient responses to some of the questions which we did put to them and our analysis of their behaviour in the taped consultations helped us to obtain a picture, if a somewhat blurred one, of their expectations of their general practitioners when they consulted, and of the extent to which these expectations were met and they went away satisfied.

The attenders were asked before they consulted the doctor what problem had brought them to see a doctor on that specific occasion; and as we have already indicated most of them mentioned symptoms which we and their doctors characterized as purely physical in origin or manifestation. They were then asked, with a series of prompting questions (*Table 10*, col. 1) to which they could answer 'yes' or 'no', what they wanted the doctor to do for them in the consultation. Column 2 shows the proportions giving positive and negative answers to each of these prompts, in descending order of positive responses in 1972. Column 3 shows

Table 10   *Percentage of adult attenders wanting and not wanting the
doctor to do specific things during the consultation in 1972 and
whether or not they got them (N = 837)*

(1) *wanted doctor to*	(2) *yes* *no*		(3) *percentage of those wanting who got it*	(4) *percentage of those not wanting who got it*
	%	%	%	%
give a prescription	54	46	87	48
give advice	51	49	81	50
explain symptoms and conditions	45	55	72	35
put mind at rest	42	58	86	49
give a check-up or examination	31	69	57	19
give a certificate	18	82	84	9
give some treatment (e.g. injection, bandaging, ear syringe)	12	88	28	3

the proportion of those who wanted each item who obtained it,
and column 4 the proportion of those who did not say they wanted
each item who nevertheless received it.

The figures in column 3 of the table suggest that over four-fifths
of those who consulted their doctor because they wanted a
prescription, reassurance, a certificate, or advice were likely to
have obtained them. It was interesting to note, however, first, that
only just over half the sizeable minority (31 per cent) of attenders
who wanted a check-up or examination had had one: and second,
that comparatively few (12 per cent) wanted the doctor to treat
them physically in some way, and that of these, less than a third
received any such treatment. Those who wanted explanations
were more likely to obtain them than those who wanted to be
physically examined; nevertheless, over a quarter of the former
(28 per cent) did not feel that they had been offered the explanation they sought.

It is also clear (column 4) that about half those who did not go to
get a prescription, advice or reassurance nevertheless obtained or
felt they had obtained these things from their doctors. A not
insignificant minority (35 per cent) of those who had not expected

explanations in fact obtained them, and nearly one in five of those not expecting a check-up or examination received one.

We repeated this analysis for the 1975 attenders but have not reproduced the results in a full table here because there was little significant change in the overall pattern of wants and their fulfilment from that found in 1972. For example, 57 per cent of the patients wanted a prescription compared to 54 per cent in 1972 and 89 per cent of these were successful as compared to 87 per cent. At the other extreme, 10 per cent wanted treatment and 27 per cent of these obtained it, compared with the 12 per cent wanting it, 28 per cent of whom obtained it, in 1972.

Nevertheless there were some small changes from 1972 to 1975 (*Table 11*). These changes suggested that, in the three years between our two surveys, patient expectations had risen. At the same time, their chances of being examined had increased, but their chances of obtaining advice or reassurance from the doctors had diminished. We were aware of the difficulty of interpreting trends of this kind and, particularly, of the danger of assuming too readily that diminished response to patient demand indicated deteriorated patient care. For example, patients who do not get the reassurance sought are perhaps better served than if they received reassurance based on deception or half-truths. In short, the doctor's purpose might not necessarily be to reassure in every instance; failure to reassure on demand cannot be taken as an unequivocal measure of the quality of the doctor's care in the consultation.

We did not either need to be reminded of the difficulty of interpreting the data drawn from responses to standardized ques-

Table 11   *Percentage of adult attenders wanting and obtaining advice, reassurance, and examinations in 1972 and 1975 (N in 1972 = 837; N in 1975 = 891)*

service	% wanting it		% of those wanting who obtained it	
	1972	1975	1972	1975
advice	51	55	81	71
reassurance	42	48	86	81
examination	31	38	57	68

tionnaires on patient expectations of their doctors and the extent to which they believed them to be met. It is possible that, in both study years, reassurance may have been essayed by the doctor but misinterpreted or rejected by patients. Yet again, patients who indicated in their responses to our questionnaire that they wanted reassurance may not have made it clear or explicit in the consultation itself. That this last may, indeed, have been the case in many instances emerged from our sample of taped consultations in 1975 (*Table 12*). The proportions of patients making what we, as researchers, were prepared to accept as verbal requests for the services listed in that table were considerably less than the proportions of attenders we had interviewed only a few months earlier who told us they wanted them.

Table 12   *Percentage of patients in taped consultations who asked and did not ask for specific things and who were offered them (N = 216)*

(1)	(2)		(3)	(4)
service	asking	not asking	of those asking who were given	of those not asking who were given
	%	%	%	%
prescription	25	75	96	51
advice	19	81	100	42
information/explanation	16	84	100	32
reassurance	14	86	99	16
certificate	10	90	100	11
treatment	1	99	100	0

To take only two examples, 57 per cent of our 1975 attenders told us they wanted a prescription, but only 25 per cent of the patients in our recorded consultations actually asked the doctors concerned for one. The desire for explanation provides the second example. A half (49 per cent) of our 1975 attenders said that they wanted explanation; but, according to our reckoning, only 16 per cent, or slightly more than one in six, of the consulters asked for it explicitly.

What possible explanations can there be for the discrepancies between the expressed expectations of attenders and the recorded behaviours of patients in the consultation? One possible explanation is a bias in the sample of consultations we recorded. For example, we know that 72 per cent of the attenders obtained prescriptions compared with only 62 per cent of the patients in the taped consultations, which indicates a possible bias in the consultations.

It is unlikely, however, that any such bias was great enough to account for such substantial differences and we need to examine other explanations. A second one is that the researchers' definition of what constitutes a request for an explanation differed substantially from that of patients as a body. A third possibility is that patients do not succeed, for whatever reason, in asking the doctors for the items they want, once they are in the consulting room.

What conclusions is it legitimate to draw from these data? It seems clear that the doctors in our study complied with most of the explicit requests for information, advice, explanation, reassurance, prescriptions, and certificates which they received and that they met many of the expectations before they were actually voiced (see *Tables 10* and *12*). It is also clear that they gave such services to many patients who had not formed prior expectations of receiving them. In short, in their consultations they not only complied with overt patient demands; they also took the initiative in providing services which patients had not themselves recognized as needed or wanted.

There were, however, some exceptions to these conclusions. The doctors in our study were expected by only a minority of patients to examine them, and they met these expectations in less than 60 per cent of these cases; and they only examined less than one in five of those who had not expected an examination. Much smaller proportions of patients (12 per cent in 1972 and 10 per cent in 1975) saw the doctor as likely to give them simple physical treatments, and, in the event, most of those who did were disappointed.

In general, where the consultation itself was concerned, we found that the great majority of the attenders in both 1972 and 1975 gave positive responses to three of our questions. The first asked whether they felt they had been able to tell the doctor all they wanted to about their health or other problems. In 1972, 95 per cent said 'yes' to this question and in 1975, 93 per cent. The second question asked whether they felt the doctor had answered all their questions and told them all they wanted to know. The percentages replying positively to this question were almost the same, 95 per cent in 1972 and 94 per cent in 1975. The third asked them whether they felt the doctor was hurried or unhurried, and, despite the fact that many of the consultations were five minutes or less in length, the same high levels of attenders described the doctor as unhurried (94 per cent in 1972 and 90 per cent in 1975).

We were mindful, of course, that attenders had had little time to reflect before answering our questions, that they were still on what they probably regarded as doctors' territory, and that these facts might account for the high level of positive responses to these questions. It was for this reason that we put comparable questions to our home interviewees about the usual surgery consultations they had had with their doctor. In this instance, the answers were not related to a specific occasion. They tended, however, to confirm the picture we had obtained from the attenders. Over 90 per cent of the home interviewees in both 1972 and 1975 said that they felt able to tell the doctor all they wanted to when they consulted, and that he or she answered all their questions.

Much of any remaining scepticism we felt about these high levels of positive response to questions about the doctors' willingness to let them give a full account of their symptoms or problems and to give them as much explanation as they asked for was dispelled by the analysis we made of the taped consultations. We looked specifically for evidence of attempts by doctors in these consultations to cut patients short in their descriptions of symptoms or troubles, to avoid answering their questions, or to terminate the consultation abruptly. We found some evidence of all of these, but the incidents were so infrequent that we gained a good deal of confidence in the authenticity of the attenders' and home interviewees' answers.

PRACTICE DIFFERENCES IN EXPECTATIONS OF THE
CONSULTATION AND IN SERVICES GIVEN IN IT

The analysis, so far, of patients' expectations of the consultation was of the entire sample of attenders, which included more than twice as many group practice attenders as smaller practice attenders in 1972, and three to every two smaller practice attenders in 1975. When we looked at the figures for each of the practices, however, we found that neither expectations nor their fulfilment varied greatly between practices. The smaller practices' attenders consistently, in both 1972 and 1975, were more likely than the larger practice attenders to want prescriptions and certificates and to receive them from their doctors. The former included rather more older people who were more likely to expect prescriptions. Although we did not know the social class of attenders, we believe that there were rather more working-class men among the male attenders at the smaller than at the larger practices, which could account for the greater need for certificates.

Nor was there much difference in the proportions of each practice's attenders who had had their expectations met. The Avesbury patients in both 1972 and 1975 were more likely to say that they had not had the check-up or examination they expected than were those attending the Barr or Erickson practices. The Cox practice attenders in 1972 had resembled the Barr and Erickson practices; but, for some reason which could possibly be connected with the retirement of one of the partners in 1974, they were even more likely than the Avesbury attenders in 1975 to claim that their expectations had not been met (*Table 13*).

Table 13 *Percentage of attenders expecting an examination at each practice in 1972 and 1975 who did not obtain one*

	1972		1975	
	%	(N = 100%)	%	(N = 100%)
Avesbury	56	(65)	39	(97)
Barr	37	(95)	22	(124)
Cox	38	(42)	57	(28)
Erickson	43	(49)	32	(57)
Osmond	–		24	(25)

The absence of any other substantial or consistent differences between the practices' attenders is itself worthy of note. It suggests that the practices in this study were seeing patients who, in total, had comparable expectations of the consultation. What variation there was could be accounted for by differences in the age and sex of attenders and, we suspect, in their social class.

OVERALL SATISFACTION WITH THE CONSULTATIONS

One of our final questions to the attenders was how they felt about the visit as a whole. This again was a forced-choice question to which they were given five possible responses. Between 1972 and 1975, there was an increase in the proportion who were less than satisfied. This occurred at three of the four practices where attenders were interviewed in both years (*Table 14*). Among all the attenders in 1975, about the same proportions gave each of the two best options 'very satisfied' (45 per cent) and 'satisfied' (44 per cent). To compile *Table 14* we combined these two categories and have shown only the percentage in the sample as a whole and in each practice which gave any of the other three optional answers, that is, 'mixed feelings', 'rather dissatisfied' and 'dissatisfied'. In passing, however, we noted that the 'satisfied' group practice attenders were considerably less likely than the smaller practice attenders to say that they were 'very satisfied'; they chose much more commonly the 'satisfied' answer. The tendency for rather more of the group practice patients to express some criticism or dissatisfaction with their visit was thus accompanied by a tendency of the satisfied to put their satisfaction in less eulogistic terms.

Table 14   *Percentage of attenders expressing mixed feelings or dissatisfaction with their consultation by practice in 1972 and 1975*

practice	1972		1975	
	%	(N = 100%)	%	(N = 100%)
Avesbury	11	(273)	15	(267)
Barr	7	(306)	16	(280)
Cox and Charlton[1]	7	(134)	6	(85)
Erickson and Edmunds[2]	4	(140)	8	(190)
Osmond[3]	–		6	(112)
All attenders	8	(853)	12	(934)

[1] Dr Charlton had retired by 1975.
[2] Dr Erickson had been joined by Dr Edmunds in 1975.
[3] Dr Osmond's attenders were only interviewed in 1975.

There were, as far as we were able to ascertain, several contributory reasons for the greater degree of mixed feelings and dissatisfaction among group practice attenders. First, for example, in both years younger attenders, and especially younger women, were noticeably more likely to express themselves in this way than were older men and women; and since there were more of the former attenders in the group practices this could account in part for the practice differences. Second, those who were not seeing their own doctor, or who had no doctor they considered their own, were more likely than those seeing their own doctor to express some dissatisfaction; this too was more likely to occur at the group practices. Third, those who would have liked to consult earlier and blamed the practice rather than external factors for the inability to do so were also more likely to express dissatisfaction, and such attenders were also more likely to be found among the group practices. *Table 15* shows how these three characteristics of 'less than wholly satisfied' attenders were distributed among the different practices, together with the practices' less than wholly satisfied percentage rate.

Table 15   *Percentage of attenders with each of three characteristics (col. 1) who were not wholly satisfied (col. 2) and percentage of such attenders at each practice (cols 3–7) and in total (col. 8) in 1975*

(1) attenders' characteristics	(2) percentage not wholly satisfied		(3) Avesbury	(4) Barr	(5) Cox	(6) Erickson	(7) Osmond	(8) all practices
	%	(N = 100%)	(N = 267) %	(N = 280) %	(N = 85) %	(N = 190) %	(N = 112) %	(N = 934) %
aged 15–34	18	(463)	56	56	31	44	47	50
not seeing own doctor	18	(302)	55	39	4	29	8	37
wanted to consult earlier and blames practice	22	(87)	46	64	26	7	13	37
not wholly satisfied	12	(934)	16	14	6	8	7	12

QUALITIES IN A DOCTOR

Besides asking home interviewees what kinds of condition their general practitioners should be able to deal with and recording the attenders' reasons for consulting, we also asked the home interviewees to name the qualities which they considered made a good doctor. From the spontaneous answers to this question it seemed that it was interpersonal skills and the capacity to empathize which were valued. Most referred to a readiness or ability to listen, kindness, sympathy, patience, and understanding. For example, one patient defined a good doctor as 'someone who listens to you, doesn't just give you a prescription and push you out'. Another said: 'He puts you at your ease, he doesn't make a fool of you'; and, in the same vein, a third described the perfect doctor as someone who 'treats patients as human beings and as intelligent people and doesn't patronize or bully them'. Many too emphasized the capacity to reassure:

'A good doctor is someone who doesn't shrug off patients' worries even if they are unfounded – these are illnesses in themselves – but puts their minds at rest.'

In all, over four-fifths of patients in these samples emphasized interpersonal skills or qualities. In contrast, only two-fifths referred spontaneously to qualities generally associated with technical skill and knowledge, such as efficiency, competence, thoroughness, and these proportions did not differ appreciably among the home interviewees of the different practices or from 1972 to 1975. At the same time, the spontaneous stress on interpersonal qualities cannot necessarily be taken to mean that most patients did not value technical skills in a doctor. It was probable that, in general, patients took professional competence for granted, assuming that, as qualified people, doctors were technically proficient, and that they, as lay people, could not describe the technical skills needed for the role, whereas they could specify humane or social standards. Indeed, when we analyzed the answers to a subsequent question, in which we had tried to force them into saying whether cleverness and knowledge in a doctor were more or less important than kindness and understanding, over a half in 1972 and a third in 1975 were not prepared to make a judgement. Significantly, of those who were willing, about twice as many opted for cleverness and knowledge as for kindness and understanding (see *Table 16*).

However, as the table also indicates, there were some differences in the frequency with which home interviewees at each practice responded to this question. These practice differences were not associated, as were some others, with size of practice.

Table 16   *Percentage of home interviewees who rated cleverness or kindness as most important in a doctor in 1975 by practice*

quality	Practice					
	Avesbury	*Barr*	*Cox*	*Erickson*	*Osmond*	*All*
	%	%	%	%	%	%
cleverness	74	54	76	72	59	68
kindness	26	46	24	28	41	32
N = 100%	(80)	(65)	(41)	(115)	(22)	(323)

The Avesbury patients resembled two of the smaller practices, while the Barr practice patients were more like the Osmond patients. The response to this question, on the other hand, did not appear to differ significantly, as we had thought it might, according to either the age or social class of the respondents. There was a tendency, which we had expected because it fitted with a common sex stereotyping, for women to be rather more inclined than men to choose kindness rather than cleverness when they were pressed into a choice. In 1975, of the women home interviewees, 24 per cent in a forced choice chose kindness and understanding compared with only 16 per cent of the men.

FEELINGS ABOUT RELATIONSHIPS WITH GENERAL PRACTITIONERS

In Chapter 14, we discussed doctors' views of what their ideal relationship with their patients should be and what it was. Most of them, it will be remembered, believed that they should encourage an egalitarian relationship, in which friendliness, tempered by some distancing to prevent the growth of too much dependency, was cultivated. We also considered doctors' views of the importance for patients of a personal doctor.

Once again, the information we obtained from patients does not allow us to say exactly how they would have reacted to the views expressed by the doctors. We did, however, ask them some questions about the kind of relationship which they wanted with their general practitioner and how far they felt they had such a relationship. First, in response to a forced-choice question, home interviewees in all the practices in both 1972 and 1975 overwhelmingly opted for a relationship with their general practitioner which was friendly as well as business-like. Only one in seven (14 per cent) in 1972 and one in six (17 per cent) in 1975 said they would prefer one which was business-like only. We also asked them whether their present relationship was business-like only or friendly as well. About a quarter at each practice felt it was the former. Virtually all those who wanted a business-like relationship felt they had it, but many of them felt it was also friendly. A small minority of those who wanted the relationship to be friendly as well as business-like, however, did not feel it was (9 per cent in 1972 and 10 per cent in 1975), a percentage which did not differ significantly from practice to practice.

A PERSONAL DOCTOR?

In trying to establish how important having a personal doctor was, we obtained some information from both attenders and home interviewees which threw light on their attitudes. In the first instance, for example, we found that among the group practice attenders in 1972 and 1975, 14 per cent and 11 per cent respectively claimed that they did not have a doctor whom they regarded as their own. There were rather more of such patients at the Avesbury than at the Barr, which, given the philosophies of the practices, we had expected to find. These findings had some degree of correspondence with those from the home interviews, where the proportion who either said they had no single doctor they regarded as their own or that they regarded more than one of the practice's doctors as a personal doctor was very similar. Once again, there were relatively more of both at the Avesbury than at the Barr.

We went on to ask the attenders at the Avesbury and the Barr if it mattered or not to them whether they saw a particular doctor on that occasion, and we gave them a choice of three answers. In 1972, as *Table 17* indicates, the two practices' attenders differed considerably in their response in the predicted way. In 1975, the differences, although still present, had narrowed appreciably.

Not unexpectedly, the older the attenders the more likely were they to say that it mattered a lot whom they saw, and the least likely to say it did not matter at all. In 1972, 66 per cent of patients

Table 17   *Percentage of Avesbury and Barr attenders who said it mattered
'a lot,' 'not much', or 'not at all' which doctor they saw, 1972
and 1975*

	1972		1975	
how much it mattered	*Avesbury*	*Barr*	*Avesbury*	*Barr*
	%	%	%	%
a lot	30	47	37	43
not much	16	20	14	13
not at all	54	33	49	44
N = 100%	(276)	(306)	(270)	(286)

over forty-five said it mattered a lot compared to 37 per cent of
those under forty-five. In 1975, the age difference remained but
had narrowed somewhat: the proportions were 48 per cent and 33
per cent respectively. It was not surprising either to find that
women were more prone than men to say it mattered a lot: 44 per
cent of them did compared to 33 per cent of the men in 1972, and
there were comparable differences in 1975.

We asked the home interviewees from all the practices how
important it was to have a doctor whom they could consider their
own and again gave them a choice of three answers. Not surprisingly, those registered with the smaller practices, with very few
exceptions, said it was either 'very important' or 'important'.
Those registered with the group practices were considerably less
likely to say it was 'very important'; but it was only a minority (13
per cent at the Avesbury and 16 per cent at the Barr in 1975) who
said it was 'not at all important'. Again, a minority of patients in
both practices in 1975 who thought it important to have a personal
doctor did not feel they had one (16 per cent at the Avesbury
and 10 per cent at the Barr). So did 10 per cent of the home
interviewees in the Erickson practice after he was joined by Dr
Edmunds.

The differences between the group and smaller practice home
interviewees about personal doctoring were also to some extent a
result of their different age and social class backgrounds. The
older the home interviewees the more likely they were to regard a
personal doctor as very important: for example, in 1975, 42 per
cent of the under twenty-fives thought so but as many as 67 per

cent of the over sixties; and the smaller practices had more older patients. Working-class patients, that is, social classes III (manual), IV and V, too, were more likely to think it very important; 64 per cent did compared to 50 per cent of the upper middle class (social class I); and the former were more common among the smaller practices' home interviewees. These structural differences were not sufficient in themselves to account for the great differences in attitudes to personal doctoring. It could be that the individuals who chose to register with a single-handed practice did so precisely because they felt it would ensure personal doctoring. On the other hand, we may simply be registering the attitudes which have been formed by the experience itself of being with a small practice, where there was at most a choice of two doctors, or of being with a large practice group, where it was possible, at least theoretically, to see five or six. In fact, in 1975, 60 per cent of group practice patients who had had at least one contact with a doctor during a twelve-month period had seen only one doctor, and a further 30 per cent only two. It was only a minority of consulters, amounting to just about one in ten, which had had contacts with as many as three.

COMPLIANCE AND DEPENDENCY

The study doctors, as we have shown in Chapter 14, almost all maintained that ideally patients should feel free to reject the advice they offered and should not become dependent on them. None of the questions we asked patients were designed directly to see how far they felt they should be or were dependent on doctors; but we did ask the home interviewees a number of questions about some issues which could be said to reflect their views on the authority of the doctor and their faith in medicine.

First, for example, we asked them whether they were the kind of person who always followed the doctor's advice and did what he suggested when they were ill. In 1975, 67 per cent answered this positively, without reservation, and a further 17 per cent said they would, but with some qualification. Only 16 per cent said they would do what suited them if they thought 'doctor's orders' did not. The proportion of patients who would not comply 'if it did not suit them' had not changed since 1972.

The home interviewees from the smaller practices were rather more likely to follow the doctor unquestioningly than those from the group practices (72 per cent in the smaller practices said they would do so compared with 61 per cent in the group practices). This difference was largely attributable to the age and social class differences of the two groups, since those who would suit themselves were more likely to be young and upper middle class. In 1975, 21 per cent of younger patients (under forty-five) and a similar percentage of those in social classes I and II said that they would do what suited them, compared to only 12 per cent of patients over forty-five and 11 per cent in social classes IV and V.

We also asked more specifically about taking the full course of pills prescribed by the doctor or stopping them when they still had some left if they felt better. In this instance over a quarter (26 per cent) in 1975 said they would not complete the course, the implication being that they did not accept the doctor's advice. We are not sure, however, that all the home interviewees were responding to what we had in mind when we asked the question, which was to see whether whole courses of antibiotics were followed or whether they stopped on the disappearance of the symptoms. Some may have had in mind such things as taking prescribed analgesics or other drugs which could have been prescribed to take 'as required'. Those who responded negatively to the question which asked them whether they always followed their doctor's advice were by no means the same group as those who said they would stop taking pills when they were better. For example, 58 per cent of those who said they did not always follow the doctor's advice when ill said they would continue to take a full course of pills even if they felt better, while 23 per cent of those who said they always followed the doctor's advice when ill would stop taking a full course of prescribed pills if they felt better. This suggests that non-compliance has more than one dimension. Our own questions were perhaps not subtle enough to distinguish the various ingredients which blend the different mixtures of compliance and non-compliance.

A time trend could be discerned in responses to the question, 'In general, would you say that with the medical knowledge doctors now have they can help people a lot, or do you feel they can't really do very much?' In 1972, 95 per cent gave a positive reply while in 1975 the proportion had fallen to 86 per cent. This is consistent with the trend to a more sceptical or critical stance among patients to which we have already pointed and on which we comment in our concluding chapter.

REPEAT PRESCRIPTIONS

In Chapter 13 we discussed doctors' views on the controversial issues surrounding repeat prescribing and pointed to their general awareness of the problems of habituation to which it might give rise, as well as of its value to them as a potential time saver.

We did not question home interviewees in like manner, but a series of questions which we put to them in 1975 touched peripherally on some of the issues. For example, we discovered that as many as a third (34 per cent) of the home interviewees were then having one or more drugs by repeat prescriptions, which they had obtained without seeing the doctor. It must be remembered, however, that the sample of home interviewees was biased towards those with chronic somatic conditions: had it been a truly random sample of patients the percentage would have been a good deal smaller.

We also asked those currently receiving repeat prescriptions two further questions: for how long had they been receiving them, and how long ago it was since they had consulted their doctor about the condition for which they were receiving the prescription. The distribution of answers is shown in *Table 18*. They suggest that the

Table 18   *Percentage of home interviewees on repeat prescription, according to the length of time (a) since first given it and (b) since consulting the doctor about the condition for which the drug was prescribed. (N = 164)*

length of time	(a) since first prescribed	(b) since consulted doctor about condition
	%	%
5 years or more	39	6
1–5 years	43	14
6 months to 1 year	6	13
3–6 months	6	13
1–3 months	4	23
Less than 1 month	3	30

majority of those on repeat prescriptions in 1975 had been receiving them for a long time (82 per cent had been on them for over a year). However, over half the patients had had a consultation with their doctor about the condition involved within three months: a fifth (20 per cent) had not had one within the year.

THE RESEARCH TEAM'S ASSESSMENT

What conclusions can be drawn from this broad review of patients' opinions about their general practitioners and the services they obtained from them?

One of our first conclusions was that patients, to a greater extent than the doctors themselves, saw the latter as there to advise them on illnesses which have a physical rather than an emotional manifestation. Moreover, they appeared to think that the doctors too frequently had to deal with trivial complaints from patients. They presented themselves, on the contrary, as essentially stoical and unlikely to seek medical advice except in potentially serious illness.

A second conclusion that we drew from our interviews with attenders and our taped records of consultations was that when they visited their doctors they generally wanted explanations and advice and generally expected to be given a prescription. In the consultation itself, however, they were less likely to make explicit requests than could have been anticipated from the statements they made to the researchers prior to the consultation. It was also clear that only a small minority of those visiting the doctor in his surgery expected to have a physical examination and even fewer received one.

In general, patients were satisfied with the consultations they had with doctors, but they were less likely to be satisfied if the doctors had not met their expectations. We were, however, conscious that the instruments we used to elicit expectations and satisfactions (that is, the standard questionnaires) were crude ones and should not be made to carry too much in the way of interpretation. We felt it was possible to say, however, that patients' speech, as listened to in the tapes, was consistent with the view that what they often wanted was an opportunity to present the problem in all its complexity to the doctor, in the expectation that he or she would have the knowledge, skill, and sympathy to show them how to deal with it.

A third conclusion which we reached was that throughout the period of our study the desire for a personal doctor was shared by a majority of patients, even in the larger practices. Choice of doctors in those practices did not primarily mean indifference as to which doctor was seen, but rather a search among the available doctors for the person most likely to show sympathy, understanding and knowledge of the problem.

Yet another conclusion was that many patients did exercise their independent judgements about how to take the drugs which their doctors had prescribed. Their replies to our questions on this subject supported the doctors' belief that their opinions were more likely to be challenged, especially by the young and the middle class, than they had once been.

16 Patients and the Practices

We devoted the whole of Chapter 15 to patients' views about their general practitioners, to what they wanted from them when they consulted and, more generally, to the character of the relationship they would have liked to have with them. We did this because it seemed to us that from the patients' standpoint, in both formal legal terms and in reality, the general practitioner was the key individual in the general practice setting. Furthermore, the central, core activity of general practice, its *raison d'être*, was the consultation between doctor and patient. Other services, including those offered by other individuals in the setting, had grown up around it. For example, while seventy-seven out of every hundred of our home interviewees in 1975 had had a consultation with a doctor in the preceding twelve months, only 15 had seen a practice nurse, and even fewer the practice health visitor or social worker.

Nevertheless, the doctor did not exist in a vacuum. Patients' opinions of how far their self-defined needs were met were undoubtedly influenced by the physical setting in which the doctors' services were offered. They were also influenced by the administrative arrangements made by the practice units to regulate patient access to the doctors and other staff, to issue repeat prescriptions and to communicate with hospitals and other referral agencies. They were even more strongly affected perhaps by the general ambience or atmosphere of the practice. This would have been created by the human beings who together with the general practitioners constitute the practice unit. These individuals included the receptionists who mediated the patients' access to the doctor and who could be perceived by patients as efficient or inefficient, friendly or hostile, helpful or obstructive, as facilitating approaches to the doctor or as impeding them (see Chapter 8). They also included, especially in the larger group practices, a corps of nurses, health visitors, geriatric visitors, and social workers, who usually undertook direct services for patients at the request of the general practitioner or provided a complementary counselling service at their own volition (see Chapters 5, 6, and 8). In so far as patients came into contact with these staff they would have contributed directly to the views they formed about the service. Indeed, the very presence of staff other than doctors, even if patients had no direct experience of using their services, may well have influenced patients' perceptions of what the general practitioner had to offer them.

In this chapter, therefore, we present data from our interviews with attenders and home interviewees which throw light on their attitudes to the buildings in which the practices were situated, on the practices' methods of making the doctors' services available to them in the surgery and at home, and on their opinions on the optimum size of a practice unit. We finish by discussing their satisfaction with the service as a whole.

THE BUILDING: REACTIONS TO THE HEALTH CENTRE

Before their move in 1972, some of the doctors in both group practices had expressed the fear that their patients might find the Health Centre building a somewhat less friendly and more formidable place than the premises to which they had become accustomed (see Chapters 2 and 10). We therefore asked the home interviewees in 1975 whether they found the Health Centre a friendly place and, if they had known the old premises, which of the two they preferred. The attenders were also asked this latter question.

In quantitative terms, the responses we obtained from both the home interviewees and the attenders from the two group practices were broadly similar. A substantial majority of the home interviewees in 1975 (70 per cent of the Barr and 75 per cent of the Avesbury) was prepared to categorize the Health Centre as a friendly place. The minority in both practices was, however, sizeable. When they were asked whether they preferred the old or the new premises, however, an even bigger majority favoured the Health Centre over the older premises (79 per cent of the

Avesbury home interviewees and 91 per cent of the Barr's). This majority gave as its major reasons for preferring the Health Centre its greater spaciousness, its cleanliness, and its range of clinical facilities. The minority who preferred the older premises usually referred to its friendlier, less formal atmosphere. The views expressed by the home interviewees were, in broad outline, confirmed by the attenders. Only 11 per cent at both practices who had known the old said they preferred it.

To have expected unanimity among patients would have been unrealistic. The degree of consensus reached could, in the circumstances, be interpreted as an endorsement from the general body of patients of the practices' decisions to move to another building. Indeed, many of those interviewed in 1972 before the move had had many criticisms and complaints to make about the physical properties of the practices' premises. At best they were seen as old-fashioned and overcrowded. After the move there was a notable absence of criticisms of the Health Centre building as such. For example, Avesbury home interviewees made an average of 1.6 criticisms each of the old Avesbury Road premises in 1972, compared with 0.2 criticisms of the Health Centre in 1975. The Barr home interviewees were less likely to make criticisms of their old premises (only 1.0 criticisms each) but even this was reduced to 0.2 per person after the move to the Health Centre. In particular, well over 90 per cent of the home interviewees of both practices said they were happy with the consulting rooms, the examination cubicles and the treatment area.

Nevertheless, there was one aspect of the layout of the building which did evoke a considerable amount of criticism, albeit criticism which might not have been voiced at all if we had not asked a specific supplementary question about receptionists. We first asked the home interviewees whether they were at ease with the receptionists at the desk in the Health Centre and only 4 per cent of the Avesbury and 9 per cent of the Barr said they were not. However, when we went on to ask them whether they felt they had enough privacy to tell the receptionist all they wanted to, a majority at both practices (64 per cent at the Avesbury and 72 per cent at the Barr) said they had not. The contrast between the first and second response is a salutary reminder of the fact that the way in which questions are formulated elicits, possibly even constructs, particular kinds of patient response.

VIEWS OF THE SMALLER PRACTICE PATIENTS ON THEIR DOCTORS' PREMISES

The smaller practices moved from their old to their new premises only during 1975. The Cox practice was the first to do so in June that year, by which time we had already completed all but twenty-three of our home interviews with that practice's patients. The Erickson and Osmond practices did not move until several months later, that is, after we had completed our interviews with their patients. Hence we only have the opinions of twenty patients about the relative merits of the two premises. This small group divided sixteen to two in favour of the new premises, another two not being willing to voice an opinion.

In 1972, however, the home interviewees of the Cox practice had voiced an average of 1.2 criticisms of their practice's premises and the Erickson home interviewees 0.6. In both instances, the main criticism was of cramped waiting rooms. In 1975, when Dr Erickson had been joined by Dr Edmunds but before the move was made, the volume of criticism had mounted, no fewer than 1.3 criticisms being made per patient. The sense of crowding, of too little space, had understandably grown with the advent of another doctor and the patients which he brought with him. Not surprisingly, perhaps, a substantial minority (28 per cent) of the home interviewees were not prepared to call it a friendly place in 1975.

GETTING TO SEE THE DOCTOR IN THE SURGERY

Most of the general practitioners who, in the early days of the National Health Service, contracted to provide full services for patients registered with them adopted the arrangements common among their predecessors, the panel doctors, to make themselves available. In short, they indicated on the plate outside the surgery that they would be present for about two hours in the morning and again in the evening to see patients on a first come first seen basis. After morning surgery they would make home visits to patients who requested them. The advantage of the system from their viewpoint was that it was administratively simple and cheap. A receptionist/secretary or a wife performing similar functions could cope relatively easily with the requests from an average practice enrolment for home visits and with the correspondence with hospitals, the Local Executive Councils and so on. Patients who had experienced the panel system were accustomed to the queueing system, recognizing that it might involve them in long waits to see the doctor, a wait which they often attempted to shorten, not always successfully, by arriving at the surgery as or before it was due to open. Middle-class patients used to seeing a doctor privately by appointment may well have seen a long surgery wait as the price they had to pay for the undoubted benefit of a free service to which they had not been accustomed.

It was in the 1960s that the lay press and many general practitioners began to recognize that the open queueing system could involve long waits for patients, that it discouraged doctors from giving their whole attention to the patient when he or she eventually reached the consulting room, and that it could have disadvantages for the practitioner (*BMJ* 1963d: 959; Cartwright and Marshall 1965). Little by little, originally on an experimental and partial basis, general practitioners, and especially those in group practices, began to institute appointments systems. By the early 1970s, most group practices used them, while most single-handed practices and many two-man partnerships retained the open surgery, first come first served system. In 1964, Cartwright (1967) found that patient opinion was divided: a majority of patients in the practices which had appointments schemes liked them; on the other hand, a majority of those in practices without them approved the system they had. Thirteen years later, Cartwright and Anderson (1981) obtained very similar results in a repetition of the earlier study. Meanwhile in the professional press, some analysts, including practitioners who had at one time enthusiastically adopted an appointments system, were aware that such systems might discourage patients most in need of their services from consulting at all (Lloyd 1974). There was a growing awareness too that the appointment system might have greater advantages for doctors, by reducing the pressure on them to see all comers, than for patients.

As we have already pointed out (Chapter 8) both the Avesbury and the Barr practices had appointments systems in 1972, while the two smaller practices did not. The two group practices made some detailed changes in the way in which they dealt with patients who did not or could not make appointments during the period of the study but retained their systems in essence. So too did the smaller practices after their move to new premises.

We asked the home interviewees in both 1972 and 1975 whether they were satisfied with the appointments system or the queueing system used at their practice. In both years, a majority in every practice expressed satisfaction with what they had, but the size of the majority in the Erickson practice was considerably greater than in the other practices. At the same time, the move of the group practices to the Health Centre marginally increased the proportions satisfied with the system whereas the small change in the Erickson practice was in the opposite direction (see *Table 19*).

Table 19 *Percentage of home interviewees in 1972 and 1975 satisfied, dissatisfied or with mixed feelings or indifference to their practice's use or non-use of an appointment system*

| | Avesbury | | Barr | | Cox | | Erickson | | Osmond |
	'72	'75	'72	'75	'72	'75	'72	'75	'75
	%	%	%	%	%	%	%	%	%
satisfied	61	68	52	59	62	63	90	83	86
indifferent or									
mixed	25	21	29	31	21	26	6	12	11
dissatisfied	14	11	19	10	17	11	4	5	3
N = 100%	(146)	(118)	(127)	(108)	(89)	(71)	(107)	(171)	(35)

From comments made in the interviews and from evidence obtained from attenders in the two years it seems that the question we put was not really sensitive enough in itself for us to distinguish whether it was the existence or not of an appointments system which was the object of satisfaction, or the way in which it appeared to work out for individuals when they wanted to consult. However, we did ask those who expressed mixed feelings or dissatisfaction for their reasons. Only a few of those in the smaller practices who did make adverse comments suggested an appointments system as an alternative: it seems they were often reacting to an unusual long wait in the recent past. There was, however, a wide variety of complaints from the group practice patients. Some alleged that they still had to wait for a long time despite the system; others that they had difficulty in making the appointment in the first instance, that they had to come to the Centre to do so, that they often had to wait for many days to see the doctor of their choice. One patient alleged that 'You could die in the time that elapsed before your appointment!'

The attenders were not asked what they thought of their practice's system in general; but they were asked a series of questions intended to elicit both their experience in respect of the consultation they had then come for and their feelings about it. For example, they were asked how long before the consultation they had decided to come or to make an appointment; whether they would have preferred an earlier visit and, if so, whether it was they or the practice which had been responsible for the delay. We also recorded the amount of time they had to wait before seeing the doctor from the time of their arrival on the premises, in the case of the smaller practices, and from the time of their appointment, in the case of the group practices. After they had seen the doctor we asked them to say whether they felt the wait they had was reasonable or too long.

There was a gradation in both 1972 and 1975 in the proportion of attenders at each practice who had made the decision to consult only in the last forty-eight hours, from the 51 per cent of the Barr attenders to the 71 per cent Erickson and Edmunds attenders. It was true that the patients without appointments systems were all at the higher end of the gradation in terms of consulting soon after taking the decision to do so; but there was little difference in the middle range between the Avesbury with 59 per cent and the Cox attenders in 1975 with 61 per cent. Clearly there were factors other than the existence or not of an appointments system which helped to determine how quickly the decision was consummated.

A better gauge of the extent to which practice procedures for seeing patients themselves contributed to delay in the consultation came from combining the answers to two further questions. These asked whether they would have wanted an early consultation and, if so, whether the practice arrangements or other unrelated factors were responsible for their failure to come earlier. There was little difference in the proportion in each practice who would have liked to have consulted earlier than they did (in both years between 20 and 30 per cent said they would); but, as *Table 20* indicates, there was a great difference between the practices with and without appointments systems in the extent to which the practice arrange-

Table 20 *Percentage of attenders in each practice wanting an earlier consultation who blamed the practice arrangements for the delay in 1972 and 1975*

practice	1972		1975	
	%	N = 100%	%	N = 100%
Barr	43	(88)	61	(82)
Avesbury	42	(66)	45	(60)
Erickson	17	(41)	2	(41)
Cox	14	(28)	19	(27)
Osmond	–	–	13	(30)

ments were held to be responsible for the delay. The practices with appointments systems, and especially the Barr, were much more commonly held by their attenders to have frustrated an earlier contact.

The chief reason generally given for the introduction of an appointments system is that is saves patients' time in the waiting room before seeing the doctor. As *Table 21* shows, however, the existence of appointment systems at the Barr and the Avesbury did not eliminate what we considered fairly long waits for many patients. We considered a wait of fifteen minutes or less from the time of the appointment to the time the patient was seen by the

Table 21 *Percentage of attenders in each practice waiting less than 15 minutes and more than 30 minutes from time of appointment or of arrival to seeing the doctor in 1972 and 1975, ordered from shortest to longest wait in 1975*

	practice								
	Avesbury		Barr		Erickson		Osmond	Cox	
time waited	'72	'75	'72	'75	'72	'75	'75	'72	'75
	%	%	%	%	%	%	%	%	%
up to 15 mins	30	40	32	37	44	30	22	27	4
15–30 mins	37	36	38	31	32	39	28	31	11
30+ mins	33	24	30	32	24	31	50	42	85
N = 100%	(258)	(256)	(218)	(180)	(138)	(201)	(118)	(135)	(97)

doctor as reasonable; but in both 1972 and 1975 this was achieved by less than half the patients. In 1972, the Erickson patients with no appointments system were just as likely to have as short a wait, although by 1975 the proportion waiting for less than fifteen minutes had fallen there. In the Cox practice, a considerably greater proportion of attenders had to wait more than fifteen minutes before seeing the doctor, especially in 1975. Indeed nearly nine in every ten had to wait more than half an hour.

If patients at all the practices had put the same value on being able to consult the doctor of their choice within a day and on not having to wait more than a few minutes after reaching the surgery, we would have expected complaints about delays in getting to see the doctor to be greater among the large group practices' patients, and complaints about the time spent in the waiting room to be greatest at the Cox practice. As we have already seen (*Table 20*) our first expectation was met. More of the Barr and Avesbury practices' patients than of the smaller practices' patients complained of practice-induced delays in getting to see the doctor. The second prediction, however, was not fully borne out. Those attending the Barr and Avesbury practices, whatever the length of wait, were more likely to complain that it was too long than were the equivalent patients in the Erickson and Osmond practices (see *Table 22*). In short, it appears that patients of practices without appointments systems were rather more willing than their counterparts at those with appointments systems to countenance a long wait, except where an inordinate percentage (85 per cent), as at the Cox practice, were waiting over thirty minutes.

Table 22   *Percentage of attenders waiting more and less than 30 minutes at each practice in 1975 who complained that it was too long*

practice	waited less than 30 mins		waited more than 30 mins	
	%	(N = 100%)	%	(N = 100%)
Barr	8	(122)	43	(56)
Avesbury	7	(191)	36	(61)
Cox	(2)*	(15)*	38	(72)
Osmond	3	(58)	12	(58)
Erickson	2	(134)	23	(61)

* Numbers too small to percentage.

ASKING FOR A HOME VISIT OR AN EMERGENCY CALL AT
NIGHT

We noted earlier that all the doctors, in line with their colleagues
nationally, believed they had made fewer home visits than had
been customary in the 1950s and 1960s. While they had acknowledged the value to the doctor of knowing something about the
home circumstances of their patients, they argued that it was now
easier for most patients to reach the surgery without difficulty and
that they could be of greater use to the patient when they had the
equipment and facilities of the surgery around them than in the
patient's home. At the same time, they had recognized the
possibility of some special pleading on their own behalf since home
visits could be tiring and time-consuming (see Chapter 14).

We were mindful, too, that some patients' associations and
Community Health Councils were aware of situations in which
doctors had refused to make home visits when patients needed
emergency advice or treatment or where to come to the surgery
was likely to involve them in considerable hardship or risk. It had
also been suggested that patients were becoming more diffident
about asking for a home visit for fear of a rebuff (Simpson 1979).

In an effort to discover whether or not patients were increasingly diffident about requesting a home visit, we asked the home
interviewees in 1972 and again in 1975 whether they felt they could
ask for a home visit. In both years, only a small minority felt they
could not, and it had only increased from 5 per cent in 1972 to 8
per cent in 1975. The practice differences in the extent of change
were not noticeable, except in the case of the Erickson practice
where initially only 1 per cent had expressed any reluctance
compared with 8 per cent in 1975. We concluded that patient
diffidence was not a major factor in these practices in controlling
demand for home visits.

We also found, as we had expected, that it was only a minority
who had had a home visit from a general practitioner during the
twelve months prior to the home interview. Indeed, the percentages (21 per cent in 1972 and 19 per cent in 1975) were
comparable to those found by Cartwright and Anderson in 1977
(1981: 41) in their national study (19 per cent). Another small
number, 2 per cent only, had requested a home visit and had
instead talked to a doctor over the telephone or been advised to
come to the surgery.

When, however, we questioned the home interviewees about their practices' arrangements for emergency cover at night and over week-ends, we were somewhat surprised to learn that about half in each study year claimed not to know what these were. The Avesbury patients appeared to be the best informed, the Barr patients among the least. In fact, it was a small minority of home interviewees who had had a night call at all during either year. The group practice patients were more likely to have had one; but there was some reduction in the proportions at the Avesbury (from 12 to 7 per cent) while the Barr percentage remained constant at 10 per cent.

PRACTICE EFFICIENCY AND SIZE

We asked home interviewees two questions which could be said to tap their views on the efficiency of the practice with which they were registered. The first, directed to all the home interviewees, was simply whether they thought the practice was well run. The second, addressed only to those who were then receiving repeat prescriptions, asked them whether they were happy with the arrangements made by the practice for them to obtain these. In both years there was virtually unanimous support for the view that the practices were well run. Only the Cox home interviewees differed; 10 per cent of them were critical in both years. Similarly, less than 10 per cent of those receiving repeat prescriptions at any of the practices voiced any dissatisfaction with the way the system was administered. At the smaller practices, most home interviewees said they came in personally to ask for them and waited until they were obtained. Some sent proxies. It was rather more common for patients at the large practices to telephone ahead and to collect them later. The difference reflected social class differences in the composition of the home interviewee samples.

Finally, we invited home interviewees to comment on the size of the practice to which they belonged. We asked them whether they were satisfied with its present size or whether they would prefer it to have more doctors (in the case of the small practices) or fewer (in the case of the group practices).

Most of the group practice home interviewees in 1972 and 1975 were happy with the size of their practices. Only 13 per cent at the Avesbury and 11 per cent at the Barr in 1972 would have preferred a single-handed doctor and by 1975 these proportions had fallen respectively to 4 and 7 per cent. In 1972, the Erickson home interviewees were also satisfied, with the exception of 13 per cent who thought it would be better if he were in a group or partnership. That was roughly the same as the proportion of group practice interviewees who would have preferred their doctor to be single-handed. By 1975, when the practice had become a two-man partnership, only 74 per cent expressed a preference for that size of practice or were indifferent. Of the remainder, 14 per cent would have preferred it to revert to a single-handed practice and 12 per cent to expand to a group practice.

The Charlton-Cox home interviewees in 1972 were less wedded to their practitioners' practice size than the Erickson patients had been in that year. Over a quarter of them (26 per cent) thought a group practice would be preferable and 4 per cent opted for a single-handed doctor. By 1975, Dr Charlton had retired and Dr Cox had decided to soldier on alone. His decision, however, appeared to meet with the approval of only a minority (29 per cent) of the home interviewees. Six per cent did not express an opinion; but the remaining 65 per cent would have preferred either a group practice or a partnership arrangement.

PATIENT SATISFACTION WITH THE SERVICE AS A WHOLE

What conclusions can we draw about the extent to which such features of the practices' organization as their premises, their arrangements for patients to consult, the time patients had to wait on the premises before seeing the doctor, their out-of-normal hours provision and method of dealing with requests for home visits or repeat prescriptions, rather than the quality of the relationship which patients felt they had with their general practitioners in or out of their consultations, helped to form opinions of the value of the service as a whole?

We attempted to reach a conclusion, if a somewhat crude one, by relating a measure of expressed satisfaction with the service as a whole, derived from answers given by home interviewees, to the number of criticisms or negative statements they made about various specific aspects of the practice's organization, such as those we have dealt with in this chapter. In order to do so we used a statistical measure, Eta, which in this case has been employed to indicate the strength of the associations between criticisms or negative comments and the overall measure of satisfaction with the service. The higher the value of Eta, i.e. the nearer to 1.0 and the further from 0.0, the closer the association of that particular component of the practice with the level of overall satisfaction expressed. *Table 23* shows the association of opinions on seven components of the general practice service, three of them doctor-centred and four practice-centred, with the overall measure of satisfaction with the service as a whole.

Table 23   *The association of levels of criticisms of various components of the general practitioner service with satisfaction with it in general, based on home interviews in 1972 and 1975*

	Eta value	
	1972	*1975*
doctor-centred components		
1 doctor's affective skills	0.517	0.417
2 doctor's persona	0.473	0.357
3 doctor's technical skills	0.395	0.328
practice-centred components		
4 practice efficiency	0.369	0.154
5 doctor's availability	0.343	0.304
6 premises	0.324	0.123
7 receptionist service	0.204	0.199

Two features of *Table 23* require comment. In the first place it is clear that the specific variables we included collectively in one or other of the *doctor-centred* components contributed more to the level of satisfaction expressed with the service as a whole than did the variables we included in any of the *practice-centred* components. This was true in both 1972 and 1975.

In the second place, the Eta values in 1975 were all lower than they were in 1972, especially in the case of the practice-centred components. This reflected a reduction in the number of specific criticisms of various components of the service in 1975 and yet a lower level of general satisfaction expressed in that year compared with 1972.

On several occasions throughout this book we have commented on a long-term tendency, recognized by the doctors too, for patients as a body to become more assertive, to have higher expectations of the services and to be more critical. *Table 24* contains two measures of satisfaction for each of the four practices we studied from the outset for both 1972 and 1975, the percentage 'very satisfied' and the percentage 'not wholly satisfied'. The measures, based on a forced-choice answer to a single question, are inevitably crude; but since they were put to all the home interviewees in 1972 and 1975 it is possible to argue that substantial differences within a year among practices imply either differences in perceptions of the service or differences in the language used to express similar perceptions. Changes over time within each practice unit imply either a change in the composition of the home interviewees or a change in perceptions between 1972 and 1975.

Table 24   *Percentage of home interviewees in each practice who expressed themselves very satisfied, satisfied, and not altogether satisfied with the general practitioner service in 1972 and in 1975*

measure of satisfaction with unit's service	practices							
	Erickson		Barr		Cox		Avesbury	
	'72	'75	'72	'75	'72	'75	'72	'75
very satisfied	84	66	69	54	64	60	59	48
satisfied	15	27	24	39	28	30	28	40
not wholly satisfied	1	7	7	7	8	10	13	12
N = 100%	(118)	(172)	(132)	(111)	(102)	(71)	(151)	(119)

For the reasons just listed it is not possible to interpret the figures in *Table 24* unequivocally. However, some things are clear. First, in 1972, many more of the home interviewees of the Erickson practice, then single-handed, on both the positive measure of 'very satisfied' and the negative one of 'not wholly satisfied' appeared to think more highly of their general practitioner service than was the case elsewhere. The differences among the other three practices were not so great; the two-man partnership, again on both measures, lay between the two large practice groups. It was not possible to infer, therefore, that size of practice in itself had much to do with the general level of satisfaction.

In 1975, after Dr Erickson had been joined by Dr Edmunds, the

Erickson home interviewees were still the most likely to express themselves as *very* satisfied; but their lead on this measure had been cut. All the other practices also experienced a fall in the percentage saying they were *very* satisfied; but the fall was not as great as at the Erickson. They did not, however, experience a change of any note in the percentage who were not wholly satisfied.

If the answers to a single question by the home interviewees had been the only indicator of patients' views of their general practitioner's service we would have had little confidence that it could be taken seriously as a measure of real opinion. However, this indicator provided roughly the same gradations in the percentages for each practices in both years as did the answers to the parallel question we asked the attenders, namely how satisfied were they with the consultation they had just had (see Chapter 15). In short, the congruence of the two indicators from different samples of patients suggests a degree of validity for the results.

THE INFLUENCE OF DEMOGRAPHIC CHARACTERISTICS ON PATIENT'S SATISFACTION WITH THEIR PRACTICE

It remains for us to consider how far the demographic make-up of each practice's home interviewee sample (that is, its age, sex, and social class characteristics) might account for the practices' differences in the expressed levels of satisfaction.

As illustrated in *Tables 25* and *26* there were differences in the levels of satisfaction expressed by the home interviewees of different age/sex and different social class groups. They reflected differences in the criticisms made by these groups about different aspects of the consultation and the practice organization to which we have referred elsewhere in the book. Generally speaking, the young of both sexes, but more particularly the women, were the most likely to express less than total satisfaction, and more likely to express negative feelings. Manual workers were more likely to be very satisfied than the non-manual.

When we tried to see how far the presence of larger proportions of the most critical age/sex or social class groups accounted for the lower general level of expressed satisfaction in the group practices in 1975, we found that it did in part. There were more fifteen to thirty-four year-olds in the group practices (26 per cent at the

Table 25   *Percentage of home interviewees by age/sex category who were very satisfied, satisfied or not wholly satisfied with the general practitioner service in 1972 and in 1975*

	women							
level of satisfaction	16–34		35–64		65+		all	
	'72	'75	'72	'75	'72	'75	'72	'75
	%	%	%	%	%	%	%	%
very satisfied	55	41	71	64	81	64	69	59
satisfied	31	40	21	27	16	32	22	31
not wholly satisfied	14	19	8	9	3	4	9	10
N = 100%	(77)	(70)	(146)	(150)	(64)	(70)	(287)	(290)
	men							
very satisfied	61	47	68	56	75	79	68	57
satisfied	32	45	26	36	21	19	26	36
not wholly satisfied	7	8	6	8	4	2	6	7
N = 100%	(44)	(49)	(106)	(111)	(48)	(42)	(198)	(202)

Table 26   *Percentage of home interviewees by social class category who were very satisfied, satisfied, or not wholly satisfied with the general practitioner service in 1972 and in 1975*

satisfaction	non-manual		manual	
	1972	1975	1972	1975
	%	%	%	%
very satisfied	62	55	71	62
satisfied	28	35	22	31
not wholly satisfied	10	10	7	7
N = 100%	(162)	(172)	(305)	(208)

Avesbury and 37 per cent at the Barr) compared with the smaller practices (Cox 13 per cent, Erickson 21 per cent and Osmond 22 per cent). However, we also found that the most critical age group in the group practices were less likely to be very satisfied than their counterparts at the smaller practices. Similarly, the least critical groups in the smaller practices were more likely to be very satisfied than their counterparts in the larger practices. In *Table 27* we have used only one measure of satisfaction, the proportion of *very* satisfied, and shown only the percentage responses for the most and the least satisfied age groups, i.e. the under thirty-fives and the over sixty-fives, by practice in 1975. The numbers are small, especially in some practices, but they suggest a practice effect over and beyond the age effect.

Turning to social class, although the numbers were small, we found that the non-manual home interviewees in the group practices were less likely than their counterparts in the smaller

Table 27   *Percentage of under thirty-fives and over sixty-fives by practice who were very satisfied with the service in general in 1975*

practice	16–34		65 and over	
	%	(N = 100%)	%	(N = 100%)
Avesbury	28	(29)	62	(21)
Barr	41	(39)	65	(20)
Cox*	(5)*	(9)*	63	(24)
Erickson	53	(34)	81	(36)
Osmond*	(5)*	(8)*	73	(11)
All practices	44	(119)	70	(112)

* Numbers too small to percentage.

Table 28   *Percentage of non-manual home interviewees by practice and level of satisfaction in 1975*

level of satisfaction	Avesbury	Barr	Cox	Erickson	Osmond	All
	%	%	%	%	%	%
very satisfied	48	43	65	74	(6)*	55
satisfied	42	47	15	23	(1)*	35
not wholly satisfied	10	10	20	3	–	10
N = 100%	(50)	(60)	(20)	(35)	(7)*	(172)
non-manual as a % of home interviewees	50	40	23	24	21	34

* Numbers too small to percentage.

practices to be very satisfied (*Table 28*). As we have already shown (Chapter 2, p. 30), there were proportionately more of such patients in the group than in the smaller practices.

THE RESEARCH TEAM'S ASSESSMENT

It seemed to us possible to draw some interesting if limited conclusions from this review of some patient reactions to the practices in which their doctors worked.

First, for example, our analysis confirmed earlier ones by Cartwright (1967) and others that most patients appear to believe that the kind of practice organization in which their doctor works is a satisfactory one and that alternative methods which they have not experienced are unlikely to have advantages for them. We found little difficulty in finding evidence of this inherent conservatism. Thus most of the group practice home interviewees were not dissatisfied with the premises from which their practices moved to the Health Centre; but after the move they were even more satisfied with the new premises. Similarly, patients in the smaller practices did not want an appointments system to regulate their access to their doctors, while those in the group practices overwhelmingly favoured an appointments system. Whether or not a practice runs an appointments system may be a criterion used to select a practice in the first place; but it did not appear to figure as such in the responses of our home interviewees when asked why they had registered with their practice.

Whatever the system, however, the majority felt that the time they had to spend waiting before they saw the doctor was reasonable. Again, although there were differences in the arrangements for home visits, emergency calls, and repeat prescriptions at the smaller and larger practices, the majority were satisfied with the arrangements at their own practice.

At first sight, therefore, our results would lend support to the conclusion which Cartwright (1967) drew, namely that, in so far as primary medical care is concerned, pressure for change in practice organization is not likely to come from the patient body as such. It is likely to come only from the providers themselves. On the other hand, when changes do occur, they are likely to be acceptable to the majority who remain loyal to their doctors.

At the same time, however, our results suggested that, although the volume of specific criticisms of various facets of the practices and their organization diminished over time, so did the level of expressed satisfaction. In other words, there was some support for the doctors' own contention that patients as a whole were becoming more sceptical and less likely to accept without question the doctors' dicta. This was particularly true of the younger patients and those in middle-class occupations. We felt able to conclude, therefore, that, in so far as patients directly or indirectly persuade doctors to alter their clinical or organizational practices, practices with a greater proportion of young middle-class patients are the most likely to be influenced in this way.

Finally, we thought it significant that the overall level of expressed satisfaction with the service as a whole was more closely associated with levels of satisfaction with the doctor's empathic qualities and clinical skills than with facets of the practice's organization. This would suggest that it is what happens in the consulting room and not in the waiting room that has the greatest influence on patients' satisfaction or otherwise with the service.

PART IV

General Practice Strategies

17 Preparing the Ground for the 1980s

We began this book by suggesting that, in the 1960s, the future of British general practice was in jeopardy. The hospital, not only in Britain but throughout the industrial world, was the undisputed powerhouse where advances in the scientific base of medical knowledge were made and practices perfected. Those members of the medical profession associated with these advances, the hospital-based consultants in various specialties, had gained in prestige and standing, at the expense of the generalists. Excluded by the institutional arrangements of the National Health Service from the hospital, the latters' role appeared to be merely the subordinate one of sorting out the medically interesting wheat from the non-medically interesting chaff. The wheat was passed on to the hospital and the chaff was left to the general practitioner. To all intents and purposes, the hegemony of the specialist, in this country the hospital-based consultant, over the community-bound general practitioner, which had been growing for a century or more, appeared absolute and almost irreversible (Armstrong 1979).

Nevertheless, not all general practitioners, metaphorically relegated to the second division, had given up hope of reinstatement in the premier division alongside the consultants. Moreover, in the State, they had a powerful backer with a strong financial interest in securing their revival and in curbing the seemingly inexorable tendency for growth to occur in and around the hospital.

What we witnessed, particularly in the group practices we studied, can thus, in a sense, be seen as the strategy and tactics of some committed and ambitious general practitioners to ensure that they, and, by extension, the sector of the profession to which they belonged, obtained a better standing in the hierarchy of public and peer regard. Although their styles differed appreciably and their objectives were differently expressed, we could discern five kinds of steps taken by the Avesbury and Barr doctors to this end.

GENERAL PRACTICE ASSUMES THE OFFENSIVE

The first step was the creation of a multi-occupational work setting, in which the general practitioners were the centrepiece. Although still retaining the legal status of independent contractors, the increase in the size and complexity of their work units took them further away from the nineteenth-century image of the general practitioner as essentially a small, single-handed, business-oriented professional. It took them further along the road towards the kind of status which the hospital-based consultants enjoyed, that of being the key people, the king-pins, in a hierarchy of mutually dependent occupations, where they had the major voice in determining how the roles of others should interdigitate with their own. The expansion enabled the general practitioners, at least theoretically, to claw back from the hospital some part of the medical work which had drifted away from general practice in the previous decades. It enabled them, too, to become a significantly more important element in the panoply of community health and welfare services, some of which were now sited on general practitioners' premises. The expansion was not without its problems, of course, and these we deal with later.

The second step was to foster the development of closer contacts with hospital consultants, in particular through the invitation to some of them to perform on the general practitioner's own territory. This last was a way of signalling a significant change in the mutual relationships of the two kinds of medical men. It was possible to detect an element of condescension in the behaviour of some of the consultants, who may have interpreted the invitation as coming merely from those who were clients for their expertise and advice. Nevertheless, it was clear that the general practitioners themselves saw it as a method of bridging the gap which had yawned between them and the hospital and as doing it on their terms. They saw it as improving the image of the general practitioner held by the hospital consultants, because it gave the latter the opportunity to witness both the scope of their work and their expertise. It also helped to remind the consultants of their ultimate dependence on the goodwill of the general practitioner (Stevens 1966: 33).

The third step was to challenge, and challenge successfully, the exclusive right of the medical school staff and the associated hospital consultants to educate the profession's neophytes. It was true that the general climate of opinion had begun to change during the 1960s, when both the General Medical Council (1967) and the Royal Commission on Medical Education (1968) recommended that all students should be systematically introduced to general practice during their undergraduate education. The Royal Commission also recommended systematic postgraduate specialty training for those entering general practice. It needed, however, the efforts of general practitioners at local level to give substance to these recommendations; this, in turn, depended upon the development of facilities in the field itself. Only when these were forthcoming, as they were with the move to the Health Centre in 1973, were the group practice general practitioners able to make a major breakthrough on the educational front.

It is, of course, important not to exaggerate the scale of the victory gained by making the placements of medical students in general practice settings compulsory. The proportion of their time spent in such settings could still be regarded as so small as to make the exercise a token one, designed only to appease a growing lobby both inside and outside the health services. However, the impression we gained, admittedly on an unsystematic basis, was that their stint in general practice did at least confirm general practice as an attractive option for those who were already leaning towards it or, at any rate, had not closed their minds to it completely. It seemed, too, that even amongst those committed to other branches of medical practice, exposure to general practice, as practised in the Health Centre, made them less likely to see it as an uninteresting, unstimulating form of medical practice, fit only for those who could not face the competition and consequent anxieties generated by the pursuit of a career in hospital medicine.

The fourth step was to promote a view of what general medical practice was about which emphasized its difference from that of the hospital-based general physician, not its similarity. The distinction our study doctors drew between their own work and that of the hospital consultant owed much to the work of Michael Balint (1964). He had provided them with a holistic model of illness which refuted the mind–body dichotomy of much medical practice as it had developed in the nineteenth and twentieth centuries. The specialists, almost by definition, were still hoist on that petard. Balint's model suggested that alleviating the distress of those who sought medical advice involved understanding the complex interaction of mind and body. Illness was never solely a function of one or the other: it always involved both.

In asserting the equivalence, if not the superiority, of this explanatory and treatment model, the general practitioners had to deny the existence of trivia. Like present-day nutritionists, who have rediscovered the value of bran, once considered useless in the human diet, the general practitioners in our study rehabilitated trivia. Non-medical chaff was no longer unworthy of medical attention: it was a main, inescapable ingredient in every individual's illness and hence a fit subject for diagnosis and treatment.

The general practitioners' efforts to redress the balance of medical work in their favour was further assisted by the emphasis given in the 1970s to the concept of primary health care. It started initially as a reaction to the inappropriateness of much of the high-technology medicine foisted on developing, third world countries, when their overwhelming need was for the elemental provision of simple dispensaries and health advice centres and personnel; but it was not long before it was being argued that primary health care services were also underdeveloped in the richest industrialized societies, and that the concentration of resources in the tertiary section of health systems, besides being expensive, was signally failing to improve the health of their populations (Alma Ata Declaration 1978). While primary health care was intended by World Health Organisation spokesmen (Mahler 1975) to mean the greater use of minimally trained health personnel and a greater reliance on the unpaid work of kin and community, general practitioners in this country were eager to ally themselves and even to spearhead the movement, because it implied a lesser emphasis on the hospital and the specialist (Horder 1983).

The fifth step in the general practitioners' struggle to alter the intra-professional balance in their favour lay in gaining their patients' allegiance. The ascendancy of the medical specialist was due, in part at least, to the general support which they could command from the population at large. Those who were associated in the public mind with spectacular advances in life and death matters were becoming, with the assistance of the media, the folk heroes of the twentieth century. The general practitioners, with no spectacular rescues from the jaws of death to their credit, were unlikely to be put on the same pedestal or given the same degree of authority when they were consulted (Jefferys 1970).

In such circumstances, the only option open to general practitioners was to make a virtue of necessity. In other words, they had to win the trust and support of their patients, not by demanding an old-fashioned subservience which, at an earlier stage, they were usually able to secure, and which the older generation of patients might still be willing to accord them. Patients' allegiance now depended upon capitalizing on a growing societal trend to resist what appeared to be an unholy alliance of science, technology and bureaucratic growth which served to depersonalize the individual in need. They, the patients' personal doctors, had now to be seen as their protectors against these forces.

The emphasis which the doctors in our study placed on their desire to have a much more egalitarian relationship with their patients, one in which they listened, explored, and offered advice rather than conducted an inquisitorial investigation terminating in the obligatory 'doctor's orders', was consistent, of course, with their expressed belief that such a relationship was therapeutically the most appropriate. Yet it can also be interpreted as part of a strategy of distinguishing their role from that of the specialist, in such a way as not to invite invidious comparisons between the two.

INTER-OCCUPATIONAL RELATIONSHIPS IN THE GENERAL PRACTICE ARENA

So far in this chapter, we have considered the steps which our study practitioners took to re-position general practice in a more favourable way in relation to hospital-based specialist medicine. However, we think it would also be useful for our readers to think of the general practice units we studied as an arena in which relationships between occupational groups were being fashioned and refashioned. The occupations involved were, of course, those concerned with health and disease; but what was happening to their mutual relationships in the 1970s, although inevitably unique in some respects, may also be broadly illustrative of what was happening contemporaneously to the relationships of other occupational groups elsewhere in health service institutions and outside them. We need to look for explanations for what we found in our limited study, therefore, to society-wide trends in inter-occupational relationships.

As we suggested in Chapter 1, pp. 20–4, the period covered by our study, the 1970s, was one in which the unquestioned authority of certain occupational groups over others continued to be challenged (Haug 1976; Miliband 1978). In particular, the ability of what we have called the upper-stratum occupations (Chapter 9), not only to exercise autonomy in determining their own work, but also how the work of middle-stratum occupations should interdigitate with theirs, and how that of lower-stratum occupations should serve them, was no longer seen as unchallengeable.

Another, and in our view, crucial but complicating feature of the occupational changes which were occurring in the 1970s was the growth in the absolute and relative number of women, and especially of mature women, in the expanded middle-stratum occupational groups. In the 1950s and 1960s, it had been customary for married women after the birth of their first child to expect to undertake on an unpaid basis for the rest of their lives the work of child rearing, household management, and the care of dependent kin (Myrdal and Klein 1956). Changes in social values, however, had led by the 1970s to a more general acceptance that such work should not be solely performed in the domestic economy (Stacey 1981), as part of the mutual kinship system of rights and obligations, because it was exploitative of women, who were showing signs of unwillingness to perform on that basis. Nevertheless, the stereotypes of what kind of work was suitable for women persisted, and it was they, rather than men, who were available, and psychically prepared as well, to provide the expanded paid force of carers and educators which swelled the health and welfare public sector (Halmos 1970).

The growth in the size and organizational complexity of the model general practice unit, its slow conversion from a unicellular form of organization into the complex multi-occupational work team which began to characterize it in the 1970s, was essentially a process whereby the general practitioners, belonging to an upper-stratum occupation with a predominantly male image, were joined by members of middle-stratum occupational groups – nurses, health visitors, social workers, receptionists, secretaries – which had a predominantly female image (Huntington 1981). The imagery associated with the first was one of authority over patients and independence of judgement; the imagery associated with the others was essentially of caring and nurturing and of servicing the occupations in which males were dominant.

Furthermore, the union of occupations took place on territory belonging to or controlled by the general practitioners with their status of independent contractors. The members of the other groups, on the other hand, were employees either of the general practitioners or of a bureaucratic authority which had reached an agreement with the general practitioners to deploy staff in such a way as to further certain common objectives.

The units we studied were at different stages of this evolutionary process in general practice. When we began the study in the early 1970s, two of the three small practices were single-handed, with minimal receptionist support, and with some direct contact with health visitors who were partially attached to their practices. By the mid-1970s, largely as a result of urban renewal plans in which they were involuntarily caught up, the three had formed a group for the purpose of sharing common premises, while remaining independent as far as possible of one another. One of the practices had become a partnership; but, against this, another had elected to become single-handed on the retirement of a partner. Their common occupation of a group practice centre, however, had set them out on a path leading to greater involvement with attached Area Health Authority workers. The two group practices were both more complex work units when we first studied them. One, however, had gone considerably further than the other towards the multi-occupational enterprise which, by 1975, they had both become.

The adaptations required of individuals who are experiencing organizational change are very seldom entirely painless for all those involved. This is not to imply that there must always be losers, although few radical transformations of employment relationships have historically taken place without them.

Our study showed that the fashioning and refashioning of relationships between the occupational groups involved in the units were not accomplished without some misgivings and some feelings of loss on the part of some of the participants. Yet our overwhelming impression was that the absorption of the members of the middle-stratum groups into the general practice setting proceeded with remarkably little overt or covert conflict or anxiety.

REASONS FOR INTER-OCCUPATIONAL HARMONY IN ORGANIZATIONAL CHANGE

Assuming that our impressions were correct, to what can we attribute the generally peaceful transformation which we observed? We feel that there were five main reasons for the absence of marked inter-occupational tension in the units we observed; and the five reasons are related to each other.

The first reason was to be found in the size of the work unit. While we have emphasized the change in the size of the modal unit from the single-handed to the multi-person group in British general practice which took place in the 1960s and 1970s, the groups themselves still remained small when compared with the size of most working units in and outside health services. The comparatively small number of people involved in each occupational group encouraged wider unit loyalties and discouraged sectional cohesion at the expense of the unit as a whole. These tendencies were reinforced by an emphasis in the speech of all the participants on the symbiotic nature of their work and their relationships: and because this was clearly demonstrated in the day-to-day work in the unit it was acceptable to all the groups, including those in the middle and lower-strata occupations.

Second, it must be pointed out that the method of recruitment to the units, at every level, was also likely to reinforce inter-occupational as well as intra-occupational cohesion around the ideas and behaviour which characterized the groups (see Chapter 2). The partners, for example, selected newcomers to their ranks and their trainees and did so probably in their own image; they encouraged their receptionists and administrative staff to suggest like-minded individuals when they needed to fill a vacancy rather than rely on open recruitment; they had some say in the choice of those health authority workers who volunteered for attached posts with them. This last appears not to have been the case everywhere and may help to account, at least in part, for the conflicts which have been reported between general practitioners and other health workers in Health Centres elsewhere (Beales 1978).

The third reason for what we considered a high degree of inter-occupational harmony stemmed, in our view, from the attitudes to their own occupations of the incoming health workers. Many of them felt they had opportunities to do socially valuable work which made use, on a paid basis, of their nurturing capacities and desires. None of the realistic alternatives open to them, for instance, unpaid work in their own households, voluntary work in social welfare agencies, paid routine work in commerce and industry, most probably in large institutions, were likely to be seen as offering the same opportunities for self-fulfilment. In such circumstances, it was not surprising that most of them stressed the positive elements in their work.

Nor should it surprise us to find that not many of them were in the vanguard of the feminist movement, seeking, at a collective level, to enhance their occupational status, or to challenge the doctors to cede them greater autonomy in their work. In general, they did not interpret the doctors' behaviour to them as sexist or dominating. They recognized that their relationships with the doctors were not strictly egalitarian, but contained elements of authority and subordination. Nevertheless, unlike some other members of the same occupations who have felt that the male–female, husband–wife complementary image has been used to justify continued hegemony by male-dominated groups, they appeared to subscribe to an image of 'conjoint parenting', as one which symbolized their relationships and was seen by them as positive not negative.

The fourth clue to the apparent lack of much occupational-based tension in the groups was to be found, we thought, in the professed beliefs and the behaviour of the doctors in these groups.

Some of the sociological and iconoclastic literature on the professions in recent years has drawn attention to a discordance between professional protestations of disinterested altruism on the one hand, and what it is not difficult to display and interpret as a track record of professional self-aggrandizement on the other. (Zola 1972; Kennedy 1981). Part at least of this literature has drawn attention to the tactics, kid glove and naked fist, with which the medical profession has tried to strangle the professional ambitions of other occupational groups in the health and social welfare field if they appeared in any way to challenge the doctors' hegemony (Larkin 1983).

It was difficult for us to interpret the behaviour of the doctors we observed in this way, particularly in the light of the testimony about their activities which we obtained from the nurses, health visitors, geriatric visitors, and receptionists. Even the social workers, who were less likely to be euphoric than the other personnel about the general practitioners, were not prepared to interpret doctors' behaviour as in any way tainted by the desire to suppress the professional aspirations of others. On the contrary, the doctors' claims to us, that they were anxious to extend the competencies of those with whom they worked and to encourage them to work more autonomously, were largely confirmed by members of the other occupational groups whom we interviewed, and in particular by the surgery nurses.

How can the disparity between the analyses made by others of the collective stance of bodies claiming to represent doctors, or of the authoritarian behaviour of individual doctors with patients, and our own fine-grained observations be explained? It could be, and we cannot rule it out, that the doctors we studied succeeded in pulling the wool over only too willing or naïve eyes; that, given the nature of our assignment, we were predisposed to view their conduct of their relationships with other occupational groups in a favourable light (see Chapter 1, pp. 17–19). We must also remember that our interviews were held on the doctors' territory, and there may have been a reluctance on the part of nurses, social workers, and others to confide in us. There may well be some truth in these explanations; but we do not see our own findings as merely an artefact of interviewing methods and our personal biases. We favour another explanation.

We believe that the encouragement given by the doctors to the members of the occupational groups which joined them was genuine and that the tone was set, initially, by the Avesbury group, under the leadership of Dr Adams. His objective of a multi-occupational, non-hierarchical health care team serving a community was not shared in every particular by all his own colleagues, let alone by the Barr group doctors, whose approach was, organizationally at least, less radical than that of the Avesbury (see Chapter 2). Nevertheless, his enthusiasm for work-sharing was pervasive and, when the doctors were convinced that they had little to lose professionally in terms of status and authority and much to gain in terms of the warmth of regard they could obtain from co-workers, they were all willing to go some way along the same road with him. Given the composition of those selected to join the multi-occupational teams (mainly committed, caring women); and given the size of the units (still small compared to those elsewhere), such unconventional boldness posed no real threat to the averagely secure doctor. Indeed, by being a member of a work unit which, in some respects, resembled an ideal family rather more than it did a formal employing body, there was much to be gained in terms of personal satisfaction (Schumacher 1973).

A fifth, possible reason for the conflict-free relationships in the group practices was the belief, which was generally shared by all the participants, that they were part of an innovatory enterprise. Other observers (Brown 1973) have shown that, in the first stages of an innovation, especially when it is led by a charismatic figure, the sectional interests of the participants tend to be submerged in the enthusiastic ambience created by the leader and in the reflected sense of achievement which public or peer notice confer. The group practices, during the period of our study, were the frequent recipients of visits by distinguished persons and overseas visitors; it is likely that all those who worked in them were as stimulated to improve their performance as were the workers who were the subject of the Hawthorne experiments in the 1920s (Mayo 1933). The presence of the researchers may also have helped to persuade some that they were participating in an event of national significance.

WHERE DO WE GO FROM HERE?

It is customary in much health service research for the researchers to finish by making specific recommendations for policy which they see as arising from their findings and analyses. We do not propose to do it in this instance, although we have personal views on the direction we should like general practice to take in the future and the kind of inter-occupational relationships in primary health care teams we would like to see. Our reason is that we have felt our main responsibility as researchers to be to describe and analyze relationships and events in such a way that those who can make policy or apply it have more understanding of what may be involved in trying to change human behaviour or adapt social organizations in one way or another.

It can, of course, be argued that so many changes have occurred since we completed the fieldwork for this study that its results are likely to have only historical interest and cannot be used by those who are planning for the 1980s and 1990s. If all our research had to offer was an historical record, we would still see it as having some intrinsic merit. There is a need for detailed, documented studies of the ways in which individuals seek to control their work and their relationships in specific historical circumstances. If there were more such studies from the past, for example, we could make better analyses of contemporary human behaviour in varying work situations and the extent of its dependence on its social and political context, than we are now able to do. We believe, therefore, that future historians and analysts of general practice and medical care will welcome the documentary evidence we have provided of the day-to-day experiences and opinions of doctors, nurses, social workers, receptionists, and patients during the 1970s.

We believe, however, that our study is more than an interesting historical anecdote. The experiences and opinions we recorded, although not typical or in any sense average, were not very different from those of many other doctors, health workers, and patients scattered throughout the country, who were also responding to changes in the social climate and trying to make sense of their world and the best use of the opportunities it offered them.

Furthermore, the dilemmas and paradoxes of the 1970s remain with us in the 1980s. There are still conflicts of interest between those who work in the hospitals and those who work in the community. There is still competition for scarce resources. Many general practitioners still cling to single-handed practice and many feel that they have more to lose than gain from group practice or extended partnerships. Nurses and the members of other health occupations have still to negotiate their working relationships with general practitioners in such a way as to maximize their work satisfactions. Administrators still have to take decisions as to how big or small the general practice unit should ideally be and how much encouragement should be given to practitioners, or direction imposed on them, to achieve that ideal. Patients have still to weigh the importance to them of different kinds of emphasis in their general practitioner's approach to diagnosis and treatment. Professional social scientists and researchers still have to take decisions as to who and what it is possible or not possible to study. We hope that this study has some insights to offer all such people.

References

Abel-Smith, B. (1976) *Value for Money in the Health Services*. London: Heinemann.

Alma Ata Declaration (1978) *Primary Health Care: Report of the International Conference*. Geneva: World Health Organisation.

Armstrong, D. (1979) The Emancipation of Biographical Medicine. *Soc. Sc. and Med.* 13A: 1–8.

—— (1980) Health Care and the Structure of Medical Education. In H. Noack (ed.) *Medical Education and Primary Health Care*. London: Croom Helm.

Backett, M. (1976) We're All Ganging up on the Doctor. *The Observer Review* 19 September, 1976.

Balint, M. (1964) *The Doctor, His Patient and the Illness*. Revised 2nd edition. London: Pitman Medical.

—— (1973) Research in Psychotherapy. In E. Balint and J. S. Norell (eds) *Six Minutes for the Patient*. London: Tavistock Publications.

Balint, M., Hunt, J., Joyce, D., Marinker, M., and Woodcock, J. (1970) *Treatment or Diagnosis: A Study of Repeat Prescriptions in General Practice*. London: Tavistock Publications.

Baly, Monica E. (1973) *Nursing and Social Change*. London: William Heinemann Medical Books.

Barber, G. (1974) Pros of Single-handed Practice. *Update* 8, 109–14.

Barnett, B. (1971) Correspondence columns. *British Medical Journal* 1: 113.

Beales, J. G. (1978) *Sick Health Centres*. London: Pitman Medical.

Bedford College Social Research Unit (1979) *A Preliminary Analysis of the Visiting Patterns of Attached and Non-attached Health Visitors*. Unpublished report. Department of Health and Social Security.

Bell, K. M. (1965) The Development of Community Care. *Journal of the Royal Institute of Public Administration* 43: 419.

Berger, J. and Mohr, J. (1967) *A Fortunate Man*. London: Allen Lane, Penguin Press.

Bloom, S. W. (1965) *The Doctor and His Patient*. USA: Free Press.

Blythe, R. (1969) *Akenfield*. London: Allen Lane, Penguin Press.

Brandon, S. (1969) Medicine and Social Work. *Case Conference* 16 (7).

British Medical Association (1930) *Proposals for a General Medical Service for the Nation.*
—— (1938) *A General Medical Service for the Nation.*
—— (1950) *The Training of the General Practitioner.*
—— (1965) *A Charter for the Family Doctor Service.*
—— (1970) *Primary Medical Care.* Planning Unit Report No. 4.
British Medical Association/Department of Health and Social Security (1978) Joint letter to all general practitioners dated April, 1978.
British Medical Journal (1953a) The Organization of General Practices. Supplement, 2: 125.
—— (1953b) Report on Annual Representative Meeting at Cardiff Supplement, 2: 144.
—— (1954a) The GP and the Health Visitor. Supplement, 1: 125.
—— (1954b) Abuse of Barbiturates. Editorial, 2: 1534.
—— (1954c) Report on General Practice. Editorial, 2: 34–5.
—— (1960a) Retrospect to Pay Claim. Editorial, 1: 487.
—— (1960b) Report on BMA Annual Representative Meeting: Discussion of Health Centres, 2: 57.
—— (1963a) Annual Report of Council of BMA. Supplement, 1: 134.
—— (1963b) Report on Medical World Conference: Balint's Contribution, 2: 156.
—— (1963c) Present State of Medicine. Editorial, 2: 453–55.
—— (1963d) Report on Medicine in Parliament: Expenses Factor in Appointment System, 1: 959.
—— (1966) Attachment of Health Visitors. Motion Submitted to Council. Supplement, 2: 71.
—— (1967) Comment on Health Centres. Supplement, 2: 90.
—— (1969) The GMC's proposals. Editorial, 4: 60.
—— (1971) Report on Keith Joseph's Statement. Supplement, 4: 49.
—— (1972) Private lives. Editorial, 3: 189.
—— (1974) Vaccination Against Whooping Cough. Supplement, 2: 81.
Brooks, M. B. (1973) Management of the Team in General Practice. *Journal of the Royal College of General Practitioners* 23: 239–52.
Brotherston, J. H. F. (1967) The Changing Face of Medical Care and the Future Role of the Doctor. *Journal of the Royal College of General Practitioners* 13: 230–33.
—— (1971) Evolution of Medical Practice. In G. Mchachlan and T. Mckeown (eds) *Medical History and Medical Care.* London: Oxford University Press.
Brown, G. W. (1973) The Mental Hospital as an Institution. *Soc. Sci. and Med.* 7: 407–24.
Bulmer, M. (ed.) (1977) *Sociological Research Methods.* London: Macmillan.
Bunker, J. P. and Wennberg, J. E. (1973) Operation Rates, Mortality Statistics and the Quality of Life. *New England Journal of Medicine* 289: 1249.
Cardew, B. (1964) In James Farndale (ed.) *Trends in the National Health*

Service. Oxford: Pergamon Press.

Carpenter, M. (1977) The New Managerialism and Professionalism in Nursing in M. Stacey *et al.* (eds) *Health and the Division of Labour*. London: Croom Helm.

Cartwright, A. (1967) *Patients and Their Doctors*. London: Routledge and Kegan Paul.

Cartwright, A. and Anderson, R. (1981) *General Practice Revisited*. London: Tavistock Publications.

Cartwright A. and Marshall, R. (1965) General Practice in 1963. *Medical Care* 3: 69.

Clark, J. (1973) *A Family Visitor*. London: Royal College of Nursing.

Cohen, S. (1973) *Folk Devils and Moral Panics*. St Albans, Herts: Paladin.

Coles, L. (1950) The Teaching Hospital and the General Practitioner. *British Medical Journal* 1: 66.

College of General Practitioners (1964) Vocational Training for General Practice. *British Medical Journal.* Supplement, 2: 171.

―― (1965) *Special Vocational Training for General Practice*. Reports from General Practice I.

Collings, J. (1950) General Practice in England To-day. *Lancet* 1: 555–85.

Collins, J. (1965) *Social Casework in General Practice*. London: Pitman.

Committee of Enquiry on Children and Young Persons (1960) (Ingleby Report). Cmnd 1191. London: HMSO.

Committee of Enquiry into the Cost of the National Health Service (1956) (Guillebaud Report). London: HMSO.

Committee of Enquiry into the Relationship of the Pharmaceutical Industry with The NHS (1967) (Sainsbury Report). London: HMSO.

Committee on the Future of the Medical and Allied Services (Interim Report) (1920) (Dawson Report). London: HMSO.

Committee on Local Authority and Allied Personal Social Services (1968) (Seebohm Report). Cmnd 3703. London: HMSO.

Curwen, M. (1964) Lord Moran's Ladder. *Journal of the Royal College of General Practitioners* 7: 38–65.

Davies, K. (1969) Lysistrata and the Role of the Health Visitor. *Health Visitor*: 150.

Davis, F. (1960) Uncertainty in Medical Prognosis, Clinical and Functional. *American Journal of Sociology* LXVI: 41.

Davis, M. S. and Eichhorn, R. L. (1963) Compliance with Medical Regimens. *Journal of Health and Human Behaviour* 4: 240.

de Gruchy, S. (1970) Some Reflections on Relationships between Doctors and Social Workers. *Social Work Today* 1 (5).

Denzin, N. K. (1970) *The Research Act in Sociology*. London: Butterworth.

Department of Health and Social Security (1966) *Review Body on Doctors' and Dentists' Remuneration. Seventh Report*. Cmnd 2992. London: HMSO.

―― (1968) *Health Services and Public Health Act (Sections 10 and 11)*.

London: HMSO.

—— (1969a) *Annual Report.* Cmnd 4462. London HMSO.

—— (1969b) *The Functions of the District General Hospital* (Bonham Carter Report) (CHSC). London: HMSO.

—— (1971) *The Organization of Group Practice* (Harvard Davies Report.) London: HMSO.

—— (1972a) *Second Report of the Joint Working Party on the Organization of medical work in hospitals* (Cogwheel Report). London: HMSO.

—— (1972b) *Report of the Working Party on Medical Administration* (Hunter Committee). London: HMSO.

—— (1972c) *Management Arrangements for the Re-organized National Health Service.* London: HMSO.

—— (1974a) *Annual Report of the Department of Health and Social Security.* London: HMSO.

—— (1974b) *Statistics and Research Division.* London: HMSO.

—— (1976) *Fit for the Future: Report of the Committee on Child Health Services* (Court Report) vol. 1. London: HMSO.

Dopson, L. (1971) *The Changing Scene of General Practice.* London: Johnson.

Draper, P. (1967) Community Care Units as Alternatives to the District General Hospital. *Lancet* 2: 1406–409.

Dunnell, K. and Cartwright, A. (1972) *Medicine Takers, Prescribers and Hoarders.* London: Routledge and Kegan Paul.

Eimerl, T.S. (1956) Present State of Practice. Correspondence columns, *British Medical Journal.* Supplement, 1: 38.

Ennals, D. (1969) Hansard written answers. 31 January, 1969.

Finnerty, J. M. (1961) Leisure for GPs. Correspondence columns, *British Medical Journal.* Supplement, 1: 230.

Forman, J. A. S. (1974) Nurse Attachments to General Practice in South-west England. *Journal of the Royal College of General Practitioners* 24: 579–81.

Forman, J. A. S. and Fairbairn, E.M. (1968) *Social Casework in General Practice.* London: Oxford University Press.

Forsyth, G. (1966) *Doctors and State Medicine.* London: Pitman Medical.

Forsyth, G. and Logan, R. F. L. (1968) *Gateway or Dividing Line.* London: Oxford University Press.

Fox, R. (1957) Training for Uncertainty. In R. K. Merton, G. G. Reader, and P. L. Kendall (eds) *The Student Physician.* London: Oxford University Press.

Fox, T. F. (1956) The Greater Medical Profession. *Lancet* 2: 779–80.

—— (1960) The Personal Doctor and His Relation to the Hospital. *Lancet* 1: 743.

Freeman, J. and Byrne, P. S. (1976) The Assessment of Vocational Training for General Practice. *Report from General Practice No. 17.* Council of the Royal College of General Practitioners.

Freidson, E. (1961) *Patient Views of Medical Practice.* New York: Russell Sage.

—— (1970) *Profession of Medicine.* New York: Dodd, Mead.

—— (1975) *Doctoring Together*. New York: Elsevier.

Friedan, B. (1963) *The Feminine Mystique.*London: Victor Gollancz.

Fry, J. (1969) *Medicine in Three Societies*. Lancaster: MTP Press.

General Medical Council (1967) *Recommendations as to Basic Medical Education*. London: General Medical Council.

Glass, R. (1964) Introduction. In R. Glass (ed.) *London: Aspects of Change*. London: Cox and Wyman.

Gerth, H. H. and Mills, C. W. (1948) *From Max Weber*. International Library of Sociology and Social Reconstruction, London: Routledge and Kegan Paul.

Goldberg, E. M. and Neill, J. (1972) *Social Work in General Practice*. London: Allen and Unwin.

Goldthorpe, A. M. (1963) Militancy in the profession. *British Medical Journal*. Supplement, 2: 113.

Greer, G. (1971) *The Female Eunuch*. London: Paladin.

Hale, G. and Roberts, N. (1974) *A Doctor in Practice*. London: Routledge and Kegan Paul.

Hall, P., Land, H., Parker, R., and Webb, A. (1975) *Change, Choice and Conflict in Social Policy*. London: Heinemann.

Halmos, P. (1970) *The Personal Service Society*. London: Constable.

Hannett, C. and Williams, P. (1979) *Gentrification in London 1961–1971*. Centre for Urban and Regional Studies, University of Birmingham.

Harding, W. (1982) Personal communication.

Haug, M. (1976) Issues in General Practitioner Authority in the National Health Service. In M. Stacey (ed.) *The Sociology of the NHS. Sociological Review Monograph* 22.

Haug, M. R. and Sussman, M. B. (1971) Professionalization and Unionism. In E. Freidson (ed.) *The Professions and Their Prospects*. Beverly Hills/London: Sage Publications.

Health Visitor (1975) Report of Annual General Meeting. 48: 252–54.

Hewitt, R. M. (1963) Conditions of General Practice. Correspondence columns, *British Medical Journal*. Supplement, 1: 97.

Hockey, L. (1966) *Feeling the Pulse*. Queen's Institute of District Nursing.

—— (1968) *Care in the Balance*. Queen's Insitute of District Nursing.

Hodgkin, G. K. H. (1967) Saving the Doctor's Time with a Practice Nurse. In *The Team*. London: Royal College of General Practitioners.

Holme, A. and Maizels, J. (1978) *Social Work and Volunteers*. London: Allen and Unwin.

Home Office. *The Sexual Offences Act 1967*. London: Home Office.

Honigsbaum, F. (1979) *The Division in British Medicine*. London: Kogan Page.

Hopkins, P. (1974) The 'Cons' of Health Centre Practice. *Update* 8 (3): 348–54.

Horder J. P. (1977) Physicians and Family Doctors. *Journal of the Royal College of General Practitioners* 27: 391–96.

Horder, J. P. (1983) General Practice in 2000: Alma Ata Declaration. *British Medical Journal* 1: 191.

Horder, J. P. and Swift, G. (1979) The History of Vocational Training for

General Practice. *Journal of the Royal College of General Practitioners* 29: 24–32.

Hunnybun, N. K. (1954) Psychiatric Social Work. In C. Morris (ed.) *Social Casework in Great Britain*. London: Faber and Faber.

Hunter, E. (1959) The Relationship between the Public Health Nurse and the Social Worker. *Social Work* 16 (1): 2–9.

Huntington, J. (1981) *Social Work and General Medical Practice*. London: Allen and Unwin.

Huws Jones, R. (1971) *The Doctor and The Social Services*. Heath Clark Lectures, University of London, Athlone Press.

Illich, I. (1975) *Medical Nemesis*. London: Calder and Boyars.

Inter-departmental Committee on the Remuneration of General Practitioners (1946) (Spens Report). Cmnd 6810. London: HMSO.

Irvine, D. and Jefferys, M. (1971) General Practice Observed. *British Medical Journal* 4: 540.

Irvine, E. (1978) The Association of Psychiatric Social Workers. In E. Younghusband (ed.) *Social work in Britain 1950–1975* vol. 2. London: Allen and Unwin.

Jefferys, M. (1965) *An Anatomy of Social Welfare Services*. London: Michael Joseph.

—— (1970) The Doctors' Dilemma: A Sociological Viewpoint. *Social and Economic Administration* 4: 37–47.

Jewson, N. A. (1976) The Disappearance of the Sick Man from Medical Cosmology 1770–1870. *Sociology* 10: 225–43.

Johnson, M. L. (1975) Medical Sociology and Sociological Theory. *Social Science and Medicine* 9: 227–32.

Joint Working Party of the Royal College of Nursing and Royal College of General Practitioners (1974) *Nursing in General Practice in the Reorganized National Health Service*. London.

Journal of the Royal College of General Practitioners (1975) Nurses in General Practice. Editorial, 25: 157–58.

Kennedy, I. (1981) *The Unmasking of Medicine*. London: Allen and Unwin.

Klein, R. (1973) *Complaints against Doctors*. London: Charles Knight.

Lader, M. (1981) Benzodiazepine Dependence. In R. Murray *et al.* (eds) *The Misuse of Psychotropic Drugs*. Gaskell Special Publications no. 1. London.

The Lancet (1954) Shadow over Barbiturates. Editorial, 2: 75.

Larkin, G. V. (1983) *Occupational Monopoly and Modern Medicine*. London: Tavistock Publications.

Laurie, P. (1967) *Drugs*. London: Penguin Books.

Leiper, N. K. (1975) The Team: A Course for Practice Nurses. *Journal of the Royal College of General Practitioners* 25: 537–42.

Lewis, B. (1955) Burdens of the Doctor's Wife. Correspondence columns, *British Medical Journal*. Supplement, 2: 63.

Lindsey, A. (1962) *Socialized medicine in England and Wales: The National Health Service 1948–1961*. USA: University of North Carolina Press.

Lloyd, G. (1974) An Appointment System in a Teaching Practice. *Journal of the Royal College of General Practitioners* 24: 666–68.

McCleary, G. F. (1933) *The Early History of the Infant Welfare Movement*. London: H. K. Lewis.

McCullough, J. W. and Brown, M. J. (1969) Social Work in General Practice. *Medical Social Work* 22: 300–09.

McKeown, T. (1961) Limitations of Medical Care Attributable to Medical Education. *Lancet* 2: 1.

—— (1965) *Medicine in Modern Society*. London: Allen and Unwin.

McKinlay, J. B. (1977) The Business of Good Doctoring or Doctoring as Good Business: Reflections on Freidson's View of the Medical Game. *International Journal of Health Services* 7: 459–83.

McWhinney, I. R. (1964) *Observations in General Practice*. London: Pitman Medical.

—— (1966) General Practice as an Academic Discipline. *Lancet* 1: 419–24.

—— (1967) The Primary Physician in a Comprehensive Health Service. *Lancet* 1: 91–6.

Mahler, H. (1975) Health – Demystification of Medical Technology. *Lancet* 2: 829.

Mapes, R. (1980) Sociological Parameters of Increased Prescribing Rate. In R. Mapes *Prescribing Practice and Drug Usage*. London: Croom Helm.

Marinker, M. (1972) Prescriptions I. In P. Hopkins (ed.) *Patient-centred Medicine*. London: Regional Doctors Publications.

Martin, B. (1981) *A Sociology of Contemporary Cultural Change*. Oxford: Blackwell.

Mayo, E. (1933) *The Social Problems of an Industrial Civilization*. New York: Macmillan.

Mechanic, D. (1968) *Medical Sociology*. New York: Free Press.

Medical Officer (1966) Parliamentary Report. vol. 115: 80.

Medical Practitioners' Union (1963) Our Blueprint for the Future. London.

Medical Services Review Committee (1962) (Porritt Report). London: Social Assay.

Melville, A. and Mapes, R. (1980) Anatomy of a Disaster: The Case of Practolol. In R. Mapes (ed.) *Prescribing Practice and Drug Usage*. London: Croom Helm.

Miliband, R. (1978) A State of De-subordination. *British Journal of Sociology* 29 (4): 339–409.

Minister of Health Memorandum 101/MCW, 1925.

Ministry of Health (1954) *Report of the Committee on General Practice Within the NHS* (Cohen Report). London: HMSO.

—— (1956) *An Enquiry into Health Visiting* (Jameson Report). London: HMSO.

—— (1959) *Report of the Working Party on Social Workers in Local Authority and Health and Welfare Services* (Younghusband Report). London: HMSO.

—— (1963) *The Field of Work of the Family Doctor* (Gillie Report). London: HMSO.

—— (1964) Circular letter. HM (64) 69.

—— (1965) Circular no. 25.

Mitchell, J. (1971) *Woman's Estate*. Harmondsworth: Penguin Books.

Moran, C. (1960) *Minutes of Evidence to the Royal Commission on Doctors' and Dentists' Remuneration*. Cmnd. 3301. London: HMSO.

Myrdal, A. and Klein, V. (1956) *Women's Two Roles: Home and Work*. London: Routledge and Kegan Paul.

Nightingale, F. (1893) Sick-nursing and Health Nursing. In *Selected Writings of Florence Nightingale*. Compiled by L. Ridgely Segmer (1954). New York/London: Macmillan.

Noack, H. and Muller, H. R. M. (1980) Morbidity, Illness Behaviour and the Medical Model. In H. Noack (ed.) *Medical Education and Primary Health Care*. London: Croom Helm.

Norell, J. S. (1973) Introduction. In E. Balint and J. S. Norell (eds) *Six Minutes for the Patient*. London: Tavistock Publications.

Office of Health Economics (1975) *Medicines which Affect the Mind*. London.

Office of Population Censuses and Surveys (1970) *Classification of Occupations*. London: HMSO.

—— *Country of Birth Tables, Great Britain*. London: HMSO.

—— (1975) *Women at Work*. In *Population Trends 2*.

Parish, P. (1971) The Prescribing of Psychotropic Drugs. *Journal of the Royal College of General Practitioners*. Supplement, 4, 21: 61.

Parkin, F. (1979) *Marxism and Class Theory: A Bourgeois Critique*. London: Tavistock Publications.

Parsons, T. (1951) *The Social System*. London: Routledge and Kegan Paul.

Passmore, R. and Robson, J. S. (eds) (1974) *A Companion to Medical Studies*. vol. III. Oxford: Blackwell Scientific Publications.

Pearse, I. H. and Crocker, L. (1943) *The Peckham Experiment*. London: Allen and Unwin.

PEP (1937) *Report on the British Health Services*. London.

Powell, J. E. (1966) *Medicine and Politics*. London: Pitman Medical.

Rankin, A. M. (1968) Health Centres. Correspondence columns, *British Medical Journal* 1: 383.

Ratoff, L., Rose, A., and Smith, C. R. (1974) Social Workers and General Practitioners. *Social Work Today* 5 (16): 497.

Reedy, B. L. E., Philips, P. R., Newell, D. J. (1976) Nurses and Nursing in Primary Medical Care in England. *British Medical Journal* 2: 1304–306.

Review Body on Doctors' and Dentists' Remuneration (1966) *Seventh Report* Cmnd. 2992. London: HMSO.

Rex, J. and Tomlinson, S. (1979) *Colonial Immigrants in a British City*. London: Routledge and Kegan Paul.

Robertson, G. G. (1970) *Gorbals Doctor*. London: Jarrolds.

Rolfe, F. (1956) Burdens of the Doctor's Wife. Correspondence, *British*

Medical Journal. Supplement, 1: 3.

Rosenheim, M., McGregor, O. R., Harding, W., Jefferys, M., and Leck, I. (1968) Collaboration in Research and Teaching. *Lancet* 1: 912–13.

Royal College of General Practitioners, North London Faculty. (1967) *A Symposium on the Medical and Social Problems of an Immigrant Population in Britain.*

—— (1968) *The Practice Nurse. Report from General Practice* X: 47.

—— (1972) *The Future General Practitioner.*

Royal College of Nursing (1977) *Evidence to the Royal Commission on the NHS.*

Royal Commission on Doctors' and Dentists' Remuneration (1960). Cmnd. 939. London: HMSO.

Royal Commission on Medical Education (1968) (Todd Report). Cmnd. 3569. London: HMSO.

Rubsamen, D. S. (1979) Medical Malpractice. In G. L. Albrecht and P. C. Higgins (eds) *Health, Illness and Medicine.* Chicago: Rand McNally.

Runciman, W. G. (1966) *Relative Deprivation and Social Justice.* London: Routledge and Kegan Paul.

Scheff, T. (1966) Typification in the Diagnostic Practices Rehabilitation Agencies. In M. B. Sussman (ed.) *Sociology and Rehabilitation.* Washington, DC: American Sociological Association.

Schumacher, E. (1973) *Small Is Beautiful. A Study of Economics as if People Mattered.* London: Blond and Briggs.

Scott, R. (1963) *British Medical Journal.* Supplement, 1: 282.

Scott, W. R. (1965) Field Methods in the Study of Organizations. In J. G. March (ed.) *Handbook of Organizations.* Chicago: Rand McNally.

Shaw, G. B. (1906) *The Doctor's Dilemma.* Harmondsworth: Penguin Books. 1946 edition.

Sidel, V. W., Jefferys, M., and Mansfield, P. J. (1972) General Practice in the London Borough of Camden. *Journal of the Royal College of General Practitioners.* Supplement, 3: 22.

Simpson, R. (1979) Access to Primary Care. *Research Paper 6 of the Royal Commission on the National Health Service.* London: HMSO.

Snelling, J. C. (1954) Medical Social Work. In C. Morris (ed.) *Social Case Work in Great Britain.* London: Faber and Faber.

Socialist Medical Association (1933) *A Socialized Medical Service.*

Sowerby, P. R. (1974) Single-handed Practice. *Proceedings of the Royal Society of Medicine* 67: 623–26.

Sowerby, P. R. (1977) The Doctor, His Patient and the Illness: A Reappraisal. *Journal of the Royal College of General Practitioners* 27: 583–89.

Stacey, M. (1981) The Division of Labour Revisited or Overcoming the Two Adams. In P. Abrams *et al.* (eds) *Practice and Progress: British Sociology 1950–1980.* London: Allen and Unwin.

Standing Medical Advisory Committee (1981) *The Primary Health Care Team.* Report of the Joint Working Group (The Harding Report). London: HMSO.

Stevens, R. (1966) *Medical Practice in Modern England.* New Haven and

London: Yale University Press.

Stevenson, J. S. K. (1967) Appointment Systems in General Practice. How to Use Them. *British Medical Journal* 2: 827–29.

Subsachs, S. (1960) Square Deal for the Patient. *British Medical Journal* supplement 2: 65.

Swift, G. (1982) Recollections and Reflections: General Practice since 1946. *Journal of the Royal College of General Practitioners* 32: 471–79.

Swift, G. and MacDougall, I. A. (1964) The Family Doctor and the Family Nurse. *British Medical Journal* 1: 1697–699.

Teeling-Smith, G. (1980) *A Question of Balance: The Benefits and Risks of Pharmaceutical Innovation.* London: Office of Health Economics.

Thomas, K. B. (1974) Temporary Dependent Patients in General Practice. *British Medical Journal* 1: 625–26.

Titmuss, R. M. (1958) *Essays on the Welfare State.* London: Allen and Unwin.

Trounce, J. R. (1970) Pharmacology for Nurses. London: J. and A. Churchill.

Waitzkin, H. (1979) Medicine, Superstructure and Micropolitics. *Soc. Sc. and Med.* 13A: 601–09.

Warin, J. F. (1968) General Practitioners and Nursing Staff: A Complete Attachment Scheme in Retrospect and Prospect. *British Medical Journal* 2: 41–5.

Westergaard, J. and Resler, H. (1975) *Class in a Capitalist Society.* London: Heinemann.

Weston Smith, J. and Donovan, J. B. (1970) The Practice Nurse – a New Look. *British Medical Journal* 4: 673–74.

Weston Smith, J. and Mottram, E. M. (1967) Extended Use of the Nursing Services in General Practice. *British Medical Journal* 4: 672–74.

Williams, D. L. (1967) Correspondence. *British Medical Journal* 4: 803.

Zola, I. K. (1972) Medicine as an Institution of Social Control. *Sociological Review* 20: 487–504.

Name Index

Fictionalized names of medical personnel can be found in the subject index

Subject Index

This index also contains the fictionalized names of the practices and personnel studied.

The following abbreviations are used:

Ave = Avesbury practice
Barr = Barr practice
C.C. = Charlton-Cox practice

Erik = Erickson practice
Os = Osmond practice